D1562778

Unless Recalled

*Functions of the Right
Cerebral Hemisphere*

Functions of the Right Cerebral Hemisphere

Edited by

Andrew W. Young
Department of Psychology
University of Lancaster
Lancaster, UK

1983

 ACADEMIC PRESS, INC.

Harcourt Brace Jovanovich, Publishers
London   Orlando   San Diego
New York   Austin   Toronto   Montreal
Sydney   Tokyo

RECEIVED

OCT 2 5 1985

MSU - LIBRARY

QP
381
.F85
1983

ACADEMIC PRESS INC. (LONDON) LTD
24-28 Oval Road,
London NW1

U.S. Edition published by
ACADEMIC PRESS, INC.
Orlando, Florida 32887

Copyright © 1983
by ACADEMIC PRESS INC. (LONDON) LTD

All Rights Reserved

No part of this book may be reproduced in any form by photostat,
microfilm, or any other means without written permission from the publishers

British Library Cataloguing in Publication Data

Functions of the right cerebral hemisphere.
  1. Cerebral hemispheres   2. Psychology,
  Physiological
  I. Young, Andrew W.
  612'.825   QP381

  ISBN 0-12-773250-0

  LCCN 83-70440

PRINTED IN THE UNITED STATES OF AMERICA

10370873
85 86 87 88   9 8 7 6 5 4 3 2

1.14.86 AC

CONTRIBUTORS

J. GRAHAM BEAUMONT, *Department of Psychology, Leicester University, Leicester LE1 7RH, UK*

MAX COLTHEART, *Department of Psychology, Birkbeck College, London University, Malet Street, London WC1E 7HX, UK*

HADYN D. ELLIS, *Department of Psychology, Aberdeen University, Old Aberdeen AB9 2UB, UK*

HAROLD W. GORDON, *Western Phychiatric Institute, University of Pittsburgh, 3811 O'Hara Street, Pittsburgh PA 15213, USA*

JOSEPH E. LE DOUX, *Department of Neurology, Cornell Medical Center, 525 East 68th Street, New York 10021, USA*

GRAHAM RATCLIFF, *Western Psychiatric Institute, University of Pittsburgh, 3811 O'Hara Street, Pittsburgh PA 15213, USA*

ALAN SEARLEMAN, *Department of Psychology, St. Lawrence University, Canton, New York 13617, USA*

ANDREW W. YOUNG, *Department of Psychology, Lancaster University, Lancaster LA1 4YF, UK*

PREFACE

NEAR THE beginning of Ian Fleming's book, *Dr No*, we are informed that James Bond need not be concerned about the injuries sustained on his last mission because an average person can manage without his gall-bladder, spleen, tonsils, appendix, one kidney, one lung, two quarts of blood, two-fifths of his liver, most of his stomach, four feet of intestines, and half his brain.

The last item on this list of expendables derives from a long tradition of neuropsychological thinking. As is now well known, interest in cerebral asymmetries was originally stimulated by the discovery made during the nineteenth century, that for most people the left cerebral hemisphere plays an important role in the production and perception of speech. Because of the 'crossed' arrangement of much of the nervous system the left hemisphere is also important in initiating and controlling movements of the right hand. The fact that for most people the left hemisphere is thus important both for language and for movements of the preferred hand was then interpreted as indicating that the left hemisphere is the dominant hemisphere. The right hemisphere was regarded as non-dominant, or minor.

Although this conception of the nature of cerebral asymmetry, and of the role of the right cerebral hemisphere in particular, was always resisted in some quarters, it became sufficiently widespread to influence popular thinking. It is, however, a curiously inconsistent position that maintains that the cerebral cortex has evolved to make complex mental abilities possible but that half of it doesn't really have a very important role to play. For this reason alone, it might have been thought that the minor hemisphere concept was wrong. More convincing reasons have indeed emerged during the last 40 years, with a continuous accumulation of examples of tasks on which the right hemisphere is in fact superior in performance to the left.

The purpose of this book is to take stock of our current knowledge of right hemisphere function. To this end, the first three chapters look at the right hemisphere's abilities in areas where some degree of right hemisphere superiority seems to arise; visuospatial abilities (Chapter 1, by Graham Ratcliff and myself), face perception (Chapter 2, by Hadyn Ellis), and musical skills (Chapter 3, by Harold Gordon). All three reviews point out that although substantial right hemisphere superiorities can be found, they are not absolute superiorities, and the left hemisphere's contribution should not be disregarded. Moreover, all three agree that it is now essential to direct attention toward efforts to specify more precisely for what aspects or components of visuospatial abilities, face recognition and musical skills the right hemisphere is superior.

In Chapter 4, Alan Searleman examines the language abilities of the right hemisphere. Although these are clearly somewhat limited in comparison with those of the left hemisphere, it is none the less important to know how extensive they are, and what the nature of the difference between left and right hemisphere language abilities might be.

The study of cerebral asymmetries is rendered difficult not only by the complexity of the phenomena investigated, but also by the fact that there is at present no perfect research method. A variety of methods have been devised, but they all have their own characteristic advantages and limitations. These are carefully considered by Graham Beaumont in Chapter 5. It is clear from his review that although all of the methods have their limitations, these are quite different from one method to another, so that it is possible to have considerable confidence in results that are corroborated by a number of methods. This point is reiterated in several of the other chapters, especially in terms of the importance of securing complementary evidence deriving from investigations with normal and clinical subject populations.

Chapters 1 to 4, then, review our knowledge of right hemisphere function in adults, and Chapter 5 considers the research methods that have been used. Chapters 6 and 7 look at right hemisphere function from rather different perspectives. Chapter 6 considers the way in which the right hemisphere abilities found in adults are established during development from infancy to adulthood. In Chapter 7, Max Coltheart considers the contribution of the right hemisphere to the patterns of abilities and disabilities seen in disorders of reading. This is an interesting exercise because, in the other chapters, clinical subject populations have been studied for the light they can shed on normal function. In this case, however, the conclusions that have been drawn concerning normal function are then used in trying to understand disordered function itself.

A point made in different ways by all the contributors to this book is that it is important not to lose sight of the fact that the right hemisphere functions as part of an integrated system together with the rest of the brain. It is *not* isolated, and thinking about it as if it were can distort our understanding. This point is so important that it is considered and developed in the final chapter (Chapter 8) by

Joseph Le Doux. He also spells out the dangers implicit in too readily using findings of cerebral asymmetries as a basis for postulating more general hemisphere asymmetries.

It must be admitted that what is not included in a book of this type can often be as revealing as what went in. There are two areas, in particular, which were considered but omitted. These concern individual differences in right hemisphere function and the importance of the right hemisphere to emotions. In both cases interesting work has been done, but I did not think that it was yet sufficiently extensive for detailed review. This is an editorial decision which still seems to me correct at the time of writing, and for which I, of course, take full responsibility.

Edited works always run the risk of being little more than a collection of different views put forward by different people. We hope that in this book this danger has been avoided. Although the topics dealt with in each chapter are, of course, quite diverse there is a considerable degree of agreement in the themes that are emphasised. As already mentioned, these include the use of normal and clinical studies to complement and enrich each other, the need to increase our knowledge of the precise nature of the right hemisphere's contribution to a number of abilities, and the importance of understanding the right hemisphere's role as part of an integrated system.

ANDREW YOUNG
Lancaster, August 1983

CONTENTS

6. **The Development of Right Hemisphere Abilities**
   Andrew W. Young

7. **The Right Hemisphere and Disorders of Reading**
   Max Coltheart

CONTENTS

1

VISUOSPATIAL ABILITIES OF THE RIGHT HEMISPHERE

Andrew W. Young and Graham Ratcliff

Introduction

IN THIS chapter we will examine the right cerebral hemisphere's contribution to abilities that are often referred to as 'visuospatial'. This rather loose term is used to group together cognitive and perceptual processes involved in perceiving and understanding the shapes and locations of objects. We will consider perception involving the modalities of vision and touch, but will avoid discussion of the potentially special case of face recognition, which is considered in Chapter 2 of this book.

There is a considerable body of evidence indicating that the right hemisphere makes a substantial contribution to the processing of visuospatial information (Joynt and Goldstein, 1975). Most of the available studies have, however, been content to simply demonstrate the importance of the right hemisphere without analysing more precisely the nature of its contribution. Whilst this has been a reasonable means of establishing the right hemisphere's importance to visuospatial abilities, this is no longer disputed, and recent reviews have begun to explore the nature of the contribution the right hemisphere makes to visuospatial abilities and the reasons for its apparent superiority over the left hemisphere on certain visuospatial tasks. Corkin (1978) looks at the contribution of the right hemisphere to tactile perception, using data deriving from normal and clinical subject populations. Davidoff (1982) reviews studies of the processing of nonverbal visual stimuli laterally presented to normal adults.

FUNCTIONS OF THE RIGHT CEREBRAL HEMISPHERE
0-12-773250-0 *Copyright © 1983 by Academic Press, London.
All rights of reproduction in any form reserved.*

Moscovitch (1979) provides an overview of studies of cerebral hemisphere differences in both normal and clinical subjects involving a wide range of tasks and stimuli, and Ratcliff (1982) examines the various disturbances of spatial orientation associated with different cerebral lesions.

Although clearly diverse with respect to the actual visuospatial abilities discussed and with respect to the sources of evidence considered, these recent reviews are in agreement that the right hemisphere does not inevitably show superiority over the left hemisphere on any task with a visuospatial component. Instead, it is held that the right hemisphere's contribution is more important in the case of relatively complex and 'high-level' visuospatial abilities, with relatively simple or 'low-level' abilities being represented more or less equally effectively in both cerebral hemispheres. The way in which this distinction is made does, however, differ; Corkin (1978) contrasts elementary with higher-order functions, Davidoff (1982) uses the idea of non-categorical and categorical functions, Moscovitch (1979) refers to early and late stages of information processing, and Ratcliff (1982) distinguishes low-level sensory analysis from high-level perceptual integration.

The present review is intended to integrate findings from studies of the right hemisphere's visuospatial abilities involving both normal and clinical subject populations. We will not, however, attempt a comprehensive review of such studies, because of their large number. Instead, we will be more concerned to continue the trend noticeable in the other recent reviews cited, of trying to specify more precisely the nature of the right hemisphere's superiority on visuospatial tasks. For this reason we will give most attention to studies that can further this aim of clarifying the nature of hemisphere differences in visuospatial tasks, and will give less attention to studies that simply demonstrate that such differences exist. In order to do this we will try to develop a theoretical framework that can both encompass existing findings and suggest further topics for investigation. We will not consider questions of individual differences in cerebral organisation, such as those known to be associated with handedness, and findings from the studies of normal subjects to be discussed involve right handed people unless otherwise stated.

'Levels' of Representation

As already mentioned, reviews by Corkin (1978), Davidoff (1982), Moscovitch (1979) and Ratcliff (1982) have all argued that the right hemisphere's contribution to visuospatial information processing is more important to relatively complex than to elementary visuospatial abilities. None the less, these authors all differ in the way in which they try to make this distinction. The differences are largely due to the difficulty of achieving satisfactory definitions of the different types of visuospatial ability. This in turn reflects the absence of an adequate psychological theory of visuospatial information processing, from which the necessary distinctions would follow.

In the absence of an adequate psychological theory, we wish to suggest that Marr's (1980) work on the computational theory of human vision may be of some use. Marr takes as his starting point the assumption that vision involves the construction of efficient symbolic descriptions (or representations) from images of the world. His basic questions are thus those of what types of representation are necessary and what computational problems their construction involves. He suggests an analysis which proceeds through a sequence of three representations.

1. The primal sketch. This is a representation of intensity changes across the field of vision, and the two-dimensional geometry of the image. Such features as edges will, of course, usually produce quite abrupt intensity changes, whereas shadows and the like tend to be more gradual.

2. The 2½-D sketch. A representation of the spatial location of visible surfaces from the viewer's position. Marr's idea is that conventional sources of information concerning depth and location (stereopsis, texture gradients, shading and so on) are computed as part of the primal sketch and then assembled into the 2½-D sketch. The disadvantage of this 2½-D representation is that, being centred on the viewer's position, it lacks generality since it varies not only with the structure of observed shapes but also with the observer's viewpoint.

3. The 3-D model representation. This is a representation of the objects and surfaces viewed which is independent of the viewer's position, and specifies the real shape of these objects and surfaces and how they are positioned with respect to each other. Marr describes it as being object centred.

The interest of Marr's work for present purposes lies in the fact that he does try to specify precisely what kinds of visual representation must be created. He sees the key to specifying how these representations may be constructed as lying in the discovery of valid constraints on the physical properties of the world. In other words, a single image will not usually itself provide enough information to allow the construction of a 3-D model representation, but this can be achieved if certain assumptions are made about the nature of objects and surfaces. These assumptions will have to be made on the basis of known constraints on the types of objects and surfaces that exist, or that are usually encountered.

Whether the particular algorithms Marr suggests for the purposes of constructing these representations are valid, and whether they relate to the methods used by the human brain, are not questions of direct importance to the present discussion. We are simply interested in his specification of the different kinds of representation that are necessary. However, there are problems in making use of Marr's work.

The principal difficulty is that most of the studies we will discuss have not achieved the same precision as Marr in specifying what they are investigating. A second difficulty is that Marr concentrates on the analysis of a single image, and gives little indication as to how an integrated representation is constructed and updated from a series of images from different positions. This is unfortunate since movement is so typical of everyday life that the integration of information from images seen from different positions must be frequently necessary. However, the difficulty created by the lack of satisfactory analysis as to how this is achieved is not as pressing as it at first appears, since many of the studies we will consider have presented stimuli in the form of pictures or photographs, which in effect provide images from only a single position. A third difficulty in utilising Marr's work is that since he is concerned with the creation of representations he does not specify what operations may be carried out on 3-D model representations, i.e. the uses to which they can be put. Many of the studies we will consider here involve both factors, so that it is often difficult to specify whether obtained right hemisphere superiorities relate to the construction of representations or to operations (such as matching or enumeration) on those representations. Finally, there is also the obvious difficulty that Marr's work concerns itself only with the construction of visual representations, whereas we are interested here in both visual and tactile representations. We will simply assume that his conception of the different levels of representation needed for effective vision can be extended to the sense of touch, though we do not wish to imply strict isomorphism of visual and tactile processes.

The attractions of trying to apply Marr's ideas to the question of the right hemisphere's contribution to visuospatial information processing outweigh these difficulties, because they are more precisely specified than alternative psychological theories, but it will obviously prove to be the case that a neat and direct application is not always possible. Some of the ingredients of Marr's primal sketch have been investigated, and these will be reviewed in a section of the chapter concerned with analysis of basic perceptual properties. However, most investigations of the higher level abilities have neither distinguished 2½-D sketch from 3-D model representations, nor distinguished the creation of such representations from operations carried out on those representations. For this reason we will consider together those studies which have involved creating and operating on representations.

Issues of Method

As one of our principal concerns is to integrate findings from studies of normal and clinical subject populations it is necessary to explain the advantages, limitations and assumptions involved in the methods employed. These comments will be brief because a full review of this topic is provided in Chapter 5 of this book.

The studies we will consider fall into four main types, involving the presentation of lateralised visual stimuli to normal subjects, the presentation of lateralised tactile stimuli to normal subjects, studies of patients with unilateral cerebral injuries, and studies of commissurotomy (split-brain) patients.

The methods involved in studies using the lateralised presentation of visual stimuli to normal subjects have been reviewed by Young (1982). Nerve fibres from the retina of each eye divide in such a way that information falling to the left of the point at which a person is looking (in the left visual hemifield, or LVF) is initially projected to the right cerebral hemisphere, whilst information falling in the right visual hemifield (RVF) is initially projected to the left cerebral hemisphere. Thus, provided we know where a person is looking, it is possible to present stimuli to the left or to the right cerebral hemisphere. It is important to note that such stimulus presentations must be brief, in order to prevent any eye movements that would bring them into central vision, and this requirement seriously limits the range of stimuli and tasks that may be employed. In addition, the method only determines the initial projection of stimuli to one or the other of the cerebral hemispheres, and little is understood concerning the ways in which information is then integrated and coordinated by means of the cerebral commissures. Despite these limitations, however, the method has the advantage that it can be used to study asymmetries of visual information processing in the normal, intact brain.

The arrangement of nerves mediating touch is rather different to the case of vision. Information about stimuli felt by the left hand is projected to the right cerebral hemisphere by contralateral nerve fibres, and also to the left cerebral hemisphere by ipsilateral nerve fibres. Information about stimuli felt by the right hand is projected to the left cerebral hemisphere by contralateral nerve fibres, and also to the right cerebral hemisphere by ipsilateral nerve fibres. These ipsilateral and contralateral nerve projections are, however, organised into discrete systems that probably serve different purposes (Wall, 1975). It is thought that in the case of 'active' touch and proprioception (Gibson, 1962) the contralateral pathways predominate, so that information about left hand stimuli is projected to the right hemisphere and information about right hand stimuli to the left hemisphere. As in the case of vision it is not known how information is then integrated by means of the cerebral commissures, but again the method has the advantage of allowing the study of asymmetry of function in the normal, intact brain.

Patients with cerebral lesions differ in several respects from the typical undergraduate sample of the experimental psychologist. Apart from the obvious fact that they do not have normal, intact brains they are usually two, three or even four decades older with much greater between-subject differences in age and level of education. They are also often ill and taking medication, more liable to fatigue, and they may be depressed, worried or resentful of what has happened to them. In addition, the lesions themselves are rarely equivalent between subjects and the effects of a cerebral lesion vary with the age of the patient, the aetiology, size and site of the lesion (which itself may be difficult to determine) and the length of time that has elapsed since it occurred. All of these factors increase the within-group variance and militate against the use of long or difficult experimental tasks, making it difficult to transfer the techniques of the experimental psychology laboratory to the clinic or to search for subtle differences between patient groups.

It is also more difficult than is sometimes realised to ensure equivalence between groups of patients with right and left hemisphere lesions, even on a group basis and even when aetiology of lesion and length of time since onset are controlled. Patients who exhibit severe visuospatial disorders typically have lesions involving the posterior half of the right hemisphere and frequently, though not invariably, these cause left homonymous hemianopia and left hemiplegia (blindness in the left half field and paralysis on the left side of the body). However, patients with left posterior lesions causing these symptoms on the right side of the body are frequently severely aphasic and extremely difficult or impossible to test. There is thus a tendency to exclude them and, consequently, to compare groups of patients who differ systematically with respect to the size or site of their lesions. The reader is cautioned to check the incidence of visual field defect and hemiplegia in left and right hemisphere lesion groups as a rough test for this artifact before accepting performance differences between groups as evidence of hemispheric asymmetry of function.

Finally, there is the problem that in studying patients with cerebral lesions one is studying dysfunction and inferring function rather than studying function directly. This problem has both logical and practical aspects. The anology of a radio which begins to hum when a valve dysfunctions and the erroneous conclusion that the purpose of the valve is to supress hums is often quoted to illustrate the logical problem. In neuropsychology there are several examples of syndromes (e.g. conduction aphasia, dyslexia without dysgraphia) which, it has been argued, occur because of a disconnection between parts of the brain (Geschwind, 1965) rather than because of damage to structures constituting 'centres' responsible for a given function, although the disconnection explanation is not universally accepted (Warrington and Shallice, 1979). It must always be born in mind that the brain is a multiply interconnected, poorly understood information processing system and that it is extremely unlikely that a lesion will ever destroy a single processor (or the neural substrate for a single box in a cognitive model) without impingeing on other functionally distinct systems or disrupting the connections between them.

The further practical problem for those who are interested in using clinical evidence to develop theories of cognitive function is that this has *not* been the purpose of many of the studies of patients with cerebral lesions. It is quite legitimate for clinical neuropsychologists to be interested in dysfunction *per se* and to design their experiments with a view to achieving a better understanding of the disorders suffered by their patients and better ways of detecting them — even a better description of their deficits — and to pay less attention to questions which are of more interest to experimental psychologists. It may, of course, be the case that these clinical aims would be more readily achieved if more attention were paid to the progress that has recently been made in cognitive psychology, but the fact remains that clinical and experimental data do not always bear on the same issues.

In the light of all these problems it is fortunate from the scientific point of view that clinical studies have compensating advantages. Cerebral lesions can produce profound disorders of visuospatial function that swamp between-subjects variance and dwarf the visual field effects seen in normal subjects. Typical hemispheric differences are still seen in populations in which the sampling biases mentioned above are minimal, like patients with chronic penetrating missile wounds (Newcombe, 1969) and patients who have undergone temporal lobectomy for relief of epilepsy (Milner, 1971). Recently we have also seen the revival of the single case study in a new and more rigorous form which makes it a powerful investigative tool (Shallice, 1979), although the new generation of case studies has not yet made much impact on our understanding of visuospatial abilities, probably in part because of the relative dearth of testable theories of spatial cognition.

Split-brain patients have the obvious advantage over normal subjects as subjects for research in laterality that the opportunity for communication of information between the hemispheres is likely to be greatly reduced in the former group. One is therefore much safer in assuming that one is testing the function of the hemisphere to which the lateralised stimulus has been presented or from which a response is required, although in the more recent split-brain patients in whom the anterior commissure has been spared (Wilson *et al.*, 1977) this assumption is less secure (Risse *et al.*, 1978). The development of a contact lens system which allows lateralised visual stimuli to be presented for an indefinite period of time (Zaidel, 1975) has allowed quite elaborate tests to be conducted on the split-brain patients and, together with hemispherectomy patients, they are unique in that they allow one to explore the positive capacity of a (relatively) isolated hemisphere. Much of the information about the language competence of the right hemisphere (Zaidel, 1976, 1977, 1978), for example, could not have been derived from any other source.

However, there is the compensating disadvantage that split-brain patients are few in number and they are unlikely to have had normal brains prior to surgery

(Bogen and Vogel, 1975). Thus, the isolated hemisphere under study is likely to be damaged, or to have been subject to abnormal functional development because of damage to the other hemisphere, or both. Nor can we be sure of the effects of disconnection itself on cognitive function. It seems, for example, that cerebral commissurotomy is followed by general impairment of memory (Zaidel and Sperry, 1974).

It is clear that the methods of investigation used with normal and clinical subject populations each have their own distinct advantages and limitations. Thus, despite the criticisms that can be made of each individual method it is, as Cohen (1977) explains, unlikely that findings that are independently confirmed by such disparate methods can arise on any artifactual basis. It is for this reason that we see the integration of findings deriving from studies of normal and clinical subject populations as being of such importance.

Analysis of Basic Perceptual Properties

Under this heading we will consider cerebral hemisphere differences in processing the kinds of information needed for what Marr (1980) calls the 'primal sketch'. Although no one disputes that such abilities are bilaterally represented, it is sometimes suggested that the right hemisphere is none the less more efficient. Vision and touch will be considered separately with vision being subdivided under the headings detection, intensity differences, location, orientation, stereoacuity, and colour, and touch under the headings sensitivity, location, and orientation.

Vision

A. Detection

The simplest of all visual tasks would seem to be to report on the presence or absence of a stimulus. In some studies of normal subjects visual hemifield differences in dot detection have not been found (e.g. Filbey and Gazzaniga, 1969; Bryden, 1976), whilst others have reported LVF (and hence presumably right hemisphere) superiorities (Jeeves and Dixon, 1970; Davidoff, 1977; Berlucchi et al., 1977). It should be pointed out that these LVF superiorities did not hold for all of the conditions or subject groups of the studies concerned. However, RVF superiorities have not been reported, so that it is unlikely that such LVF superiorities have simply arisen by a combination of chance and what is believed to be the widespread practice of not reporting negative results. Rather, it would seem to be the case, as Davidoff (1982) argues, that there is a right hemisphere superiority for dot detection, but one that is so small that it can itself only be detected under ideal conditions. Such ideal conditions would include not relying on any timing of vocal responses, which are presumably initiated by the left hemisphere, the minimisation of stimulus-response compatibility effects, in which the left hand responds most quickly to LVF stimuli and the right hand to RVF stimuli, and the use of sensitive measures and relatively large numbers of trials.

The clinical literature contributes little useful evidence on this point. Patients with right hemisphere lesions may be less able to detect stimuli in the sense of failing to notice those on the side contralateral to the lesion in overt visual or tactile search tasks than patients with left hemisphere damage (De Renzi et al., 1970) and they more frequently omit contralateral elements in drawing tasks (Oxbury et al., 1974; Heilman, 1979), but these are hardly detection tasks in the sense of the psychophysicist. It has also been reported in a number of studies that patients with right hemisphere lesions show a greater increase in latency of response to a simple visual stimulus than patients with left hemisphere damage (Arrigoni and De Renzi, 1964; De Renzi and Spinnler, 1966a,b) and in at least one study (Benson and Barton, 1970) this difference does not appear to have been attributable to differences in lesion size between the groups, but the location of the lesion within the hemisphere also affects reaction time (Benton and Joynt, 1959) and an asymmetric distribution of lesions might conceivably account for the finding. In any case, similar results have been reported for auditory reaction time (Howes and Boller, 1975) and the possibility that all these findings are attributable to alterations in response speed or some kind of arousal mediated by the right parietal cortex (Van den Abell and Heilman, unpub.) has not been definitely excluded.

B. Intensity differences

There are few modern studies of this topic, and the historic studies reviewed by Davidoff (1982) did not use many subjects. Davidoff (1975) found that LVF stimuli were perceived as rather lighter than stimuli presented in the RVF, whilst Basso et al. (1977) found that the effect of different LVF and RVF background contrasts on a grey rectangle extending through both visual hemifields reflected an averaging of LVF and RVF stimulation. The latter result was taken to reflect the high degree of interhemispheric coordination existing at this level.

C. Location

The accuracy with which people can specify the location of stimuli presented in the LVF or RVF has been investigated in a number of studies. The usual method has been to present a dot stimulus, whose position the subject must then locate on a matrix of all the possible positions used in the experiment. Although simple to set up, there are a number of difficulties in interpreting results obtained with this technique. It is not clear whether it is the subjects' perception of the dot's location that is being studied, or their memory of its location across the time interval needed to make the report. Moreover, subjects will have at their disposal a range of different strategies for performing the task, the most obvious of which involve some form of verbal coding (e.g. 'top left'). The use of these strategies may itself be influenced by a range of subject and procedural variables, such as the presence or absence of a clearly marked frame of reference (Bryden, 1976), and it is always risky to lump together results obtained from people who are effectively doing different things. Moreover, if the task is made too difficult, LVF superiorities for dot detection (as opposed to location) may begin to emerge, as Bryden's (1976) study demonstrates.

Despite these difficulties of design and interpretation location tasks are of undoubted interest since they involve what can be construed as the simplest possible spatial component. It is not, however, perhaps surprising that results have been inconsistent. The literature contains reports of LVF superiorities (Kimura, 1969; Levy and Reid, 1976; Robertshaw and Sheldon, 1976), no visual hemifield differences (Bryden, 1976; Birkett, 1977) and RVF superiorities (Pohl *et al.*, 1972; Bryden, 1973). These inconsistencies may be seen as reflecting the need to control still more carefully the procedural factors already explained or as indicating that there is in fact no measurable hemisphere difference in location ability.

The clinical literature distinguishes between 'absolute' localisation, i.e. localisation of a single stimulus with respect to the observer, and 'relative' localisation, appreciation of the spatial relationship obtaining between two or more external stimuli (Benton, 1979). The former ability is usually tested by asking the subject to reach for or point to a single visual stimulus and is affected by posterior cerebral lesions. When the lesion is bilateral the disorder can affect the ability to locate stimuli in all parts of the field including the fixation point (Holmes, 1918, 1919; Holmes and Horrax, 1919), but when the lesion is unilateral the disorder is largely restricted to the contralateral half-field and independent of the arm which is used in reaching (Cole *et al.*, 1962; Ratcliff and Davies-Jones, 1972), although cases have been described in which only a specific arm/field combination appears to be affected (Bálint, 1909; Rondot *et al.*, 1977). Preservation of the ability to point relatively accurately to targets in the ipsilateral half-field and to tactile stimuli on the surface of the body is usually taken as evidence that the disorder is not a trivial consequence of inability to put the arm in the desired position but a true failure to locate the target or, at least, a failure to provide accurate target information to the motor system (Ratcliff, 1982).

Defective localisation, assessed in this way, is just as common after left hemisphere damage as it is in patients with right hemisphere lesions and at least as severe (Ratcliff and Davies-Jones, 1972). These clinical data lend some support to the suggestion, derived from studies of normal subjects, that the hemispheres do not differ in location ability, but the tasks used are so different that it is by no means certain that the same ability is being measured in the two settings. In addition to the differet response modes, the clinical studies use stimuli in the peripheral visual field rather than the central 8–10° field of a tachistoscope, and the errors are an order of magnitude larger and less precisely measured— Ratcliff and Davies-Jones (1972) recorded a mean error of nearly 20° in the contralateral half-field of one of their patients and could not have detected errors of less than 1°.

Hemispheric differences begin to appear when patients with cerebral lesions are asked to perform tasks which approximate more closely the experimental paradigm used with normal subjects. Hannay et al. (1976) found that patients with right hemisphere lesions were significantly worse than those with left hemisphere damage at locating one or two dots flashed on a screen by reference to a card presented two seconds later on which all possible dot positions were indicated by numbers. Warrington and Rabin (1970) used a series of matching tasks in which patients were required to make same-different judgements with respect to pairs of stimuli including single dots occupying potentially different positions in a square framework, lines of potentially different slopes, and contours with gaps of potentially different size. The results of all three tasks were combined in the statistical analysis and patients with right hemisphere lesions were found to be significantly worse than the control and left hemisphere groups, which did not differ. Inspection of the data suggests that each of the three matching tasks contributed roughly equally to the overall score. Similar results have been obtained for tachistoscopic number estimation in patients with right hemisphere lesions (Kimura, 1963; Warrington and James, 1967a) and interpreted as an impairment of the ability to specify the position of the dots to be counted.

D. Orientation

A number of studies have sought to demonstrate cerebral hemisphere differences in the perception of line orientation. In several cases LVF superiorities have been found for normal subjects (Fontenot and Benton, 1972; Kimura and Durnford, 1974; Phippard, 1977; Sasanuma and Kobayashi, 1978). The critical conditions for obtaining a LVF superiority would seem to be the use of a fairly difficult task (often involving a relatively brief stimulus exposure) and a comparatively large number of possible stimulus orientations that are not readily verbally coded (Umilta et al., 1974). With a sensitive measure and a sufficiently difficult orientation task (reading the time from a clock face) a LVF superiority has been found to be demonstrable even with verbal coding and a vocal response by Berlucchi et al. (1979).

Perception of orientation has traditionally been investigated in brain damaged patients by asking them to set a rod or draw a line to indicate the horizontal and vertical planes. The inability to do so, known in the older literature as 'deformation of the optic coordinates' appears to have been more frequent after right hemisphere damage (Lenz, 1944; Bender and Jung, 1948; McFie *et al.*, 1950; McFie and Zangwill, 1960) and significant impairment of patients with right hemisphere lesions has been reported in tasks in which the patient must set a rod to vertical under conditions of body tilt (Teuber and Mishkin, 1954) or set a rod to match the position of a standard (De Renzi *et al.*, 1971). Pairs of lines of potentially different slope were one of the types of stimuli included in Warrington and Rabin's (1970) perceptual matching study in which they demonstrated selective impairment after right hemisphere damage, and the same result has been obtained with a similar task by Bisiach *et al.* (1976) and in two different multiple choice versions (Benton *et al.*, 1975; Benton *et al.*, 1978a).

E. Stereoacuity

Although Durnford and Kimura (1971) report a LVF advantage for stereoacuity, depth perception (defined in a variety of ways and assessed by various means) has been reported to be impaired by damage to either hemisphere (Hécaen and Angelergues, 1963; Rothstein and Sacks, 1972; Lehman and Walchli, 1975; Danta *et al.*, 1978). The incidence of impairment varies considerably between studies, even when the same test has been used (Hamsher, 1978a,b; Ross, in press), and gross impairments of depth perception, sufficient to make the world appear flat to the patient (see for example, Holmes and Horrax, 1919), probably only occur after bilateral lesion. Some clinical studies have found more frequent impairment of depth perception after right hemisphere damage under some conditions (Birch *et al.*, 1961; Danta *et al.*, 1978; Ross, in press), whereas no substantial study has found the reverse pattern, but one has to be much more cautious about interpreting this asymmetry in reports as an indication of an asymmetry in the cerebral basis for depth perception than would be the case with reports in the experimental literature because of the sampling biases discussed earlier. Indeed, some authors specifically note the possibility of such an artifact in their studies (Birch *et al.*, 1961; Danta *et al.*, 1978) and one wonders whether the disorders of depth perception described in the clinical literature are true disturbances of stereoacuity or manifestations of a more complex, higher level perceptual disorder.

F. Colour

Although the processing of colour information is not really of interest to Marr (1980), it would clearly seem to belong to the primal sketch level of his scheme. Colour naming and discrimination tasks have been found to give LVF superiorities provided they are made sufficiently difficult (Davidoff, 1976; Pennal, 1977; Hannay, 1979; Grant, 1980, 1981) whereas relatively easy versions of such tasks have yielded no visual hemifield differences or RVF superiorities (Dimond and Beaumont, 1972a; Dyer, 1973; Malone and Hannay, 1978; McKeever and Jackson, 1979). Although De Renzi and Spinnler (1967) reported greater impairment on a colour sorting task after right hemisphere damage, this was a task which patients with right hemisphere lesions might be expected to fail because of its spatial component, and the necessary control condition using grey stimuli was not included.

Touch

In considering the evidence from studies of touch we will assume that the levels of representation involved in tactile information processing correspond to those described by Marr (1980) for visual information processing. In so doing we do not seek to imply that homologous computational processes are involved, but simply that the distinction of levels of representation is again useful.

In this section we consider tactile information processing at a level equivalent to that of the primal sketch.

A. Sensitivity

The evidence on left and right side sensitivity to pressure and vibration has been thoroughly reviewed by Corkin (1978). Such tasks may be seen as tactile analogues of the visual detection tasks. Whilst sensitivity differences between the hands or sides of the body, have been reported for normal subjects (e.g. Semmes et al.. 1960), they have not been found in most of the existing studies (Goff et al., 1965; Fennel et al., 1967; Carmon et al., 1969; Perret and Regli, 1970). It is thus evident that there is probably no asymmetry in left and right side sensitivities to pressure and vibration, and that if any degree of asymmetry does exist it is extremely weak and difficult to demonstrate.

B. Location

No laterality effects were found in studies by Semmes et al. (1960) and Weinstein (1968).

C. Orientation

The report of the orientation of a tactually perceived line has become a popular task for use with normal subjects and, as with its visual equivalent, convincing and reliable right hemisphere superiorities have been demonstrated (Benton et al., 1973, 1978b; Varney and Benton, 1975). Comparable deficits have been shown after right hemisphere damage on similar tasks (Carmon and Benton, 1969; Fontenot and Benton, 1971), and on a tactile version of De Renzi et al's (1971) rod setting task.

By using simultaneous stimulation of both the left and right hands

Oscar-Berman *et al.* (1978) were able to demonstrate that there is no apparent perceptual asymmetry for readily discriminable orientations, as shown by the absence of a hand difference on subjects' first reports. With second reports, however, for which a greater memory component is involved, Oscar-Berman *et al.* (1978) found a left hand (and hence apparently right hemisphere) superiority. The conclusion that right hemisphere superiorities for reports of stimulus orientations can be demonstrated in normal subjects for tasks involving relatively difficult discriminations or a relatively substantial memory component is consistent with the conclusions drawn on the basis of findings from analogous visual tasks.

Creating and Operating on Representations

Although many of the studies of 'low-level' visual and tactile information processing considered in the preceding sections have taken considerable care to try accurately to identify the processes responsible for any laterality effects found, this is in general less true of investigations of relatively 'high-level' information processing, where the difficulties of any such enterprise are considerably increased. Many tasks involve both the creation of 2½-D sketch or 3-D model representations (which in the special case of two-dimensional stimuli that lack implied or pictorial depth do not differ in any important way) and operations carried out on those representations, with the various contributions of each being very difficult to identify with any degree of precision. For this reason we are considering together the whole range of studies involving creating and operating on representations, but giving more detailed treatment of those studies that have tried to specify what processes contribute to obtained laterality effects. In the case of such 'high-level' processes it is more convenient to reverse the organisation we imposed on our discussion of basic perceptual properties, considering the modalities of vision and touch under common headings but largely separating studies of normal subjects from those which consider the patients with cerebral lesions, because of the very different types of task used with the two populations.

Studies of Normal Subjects

A. Form recognition

In considering studies of form recognition it is necessary to draw attention to two dimensions on which stimuli may differ. Firstly, the extent to which such forms as letters, numbers, signs, object outlines and simple geometric shapes are readily named must be considered, and these must be distinguished from forms that are not readily named. Secondly, it is necessary to consider the 'perceptual complexity' of the forms themselves. The evidence that both factors are important in understanding cerebral asymmetries in form recognition is strong.

The overwhelming majority of studies involving recognition of readily named stimuli (usually described as verbal stimuli) visually presented to normal subjects have led to the expected RVF superiorities (see Beaumont, 1982, for a full review). What are more worthy of note in discussing the question of the right hemisphere's contribution to visuospatial information processing are the cases where RVF recognition superiorities are not found with visually presented verbal stimuli, of which a simple list can readily be constructed.

The most well known example comes from the study of Bryden and Allard (1976), in which letters were only associated with RVF recognition superiorities when presented in print-like form, with script-like letters tending to give LVF superiorities. LVF superiorities have also been found when both deaf and hearing subjects were asked to identify pictures of hand positions used in sign language (e.g. McKeever et al., 1976; Poizner and Lane, 1979). The recognition of simple geometric stimuli often produces no visual hemifield differences (White, 1972). Findings of LVF superiority or no visual hemifield difference have also been made when pictures of common objects were used as stimuli (Paivio and Ernest, 1971; Klatzky, 1972; Schmuller and Goodman, 1980; Young et al., 1980; Young and Bion, 1981), though small RVF advantages have also been found for picture recognition (Wyke and Ettlinger, 1961; Bryden and Rainey, 1963) and for the brief memory storage of laterally presented pictures (Young et al., 1980; Young and Bion, 1981). Words written in the Japanese Kanji script, which is ideographic, have also been found to give LVF superiorities or no visual hemifield differences when presented to Japanese subjects (Hatta, 1977a,b; Sasanuma et al., 1977; Elman et al., 1981a,b).

The effect of stimulus complexity is readily seen in this list of verbal forms that have not produced consistent RVF recognition superiorities, with a clear tendency for the more complex stimuli to yield LVF superiorities. The main exception to this rule would be simple geometric stimuli, which do not give consistent RVF superiorities despite being less complex than letters or numbers.

In order directly to investigate the role of stimulus complexity, studies have used shapes that have no commonly accepted names. These have included random shapes generated using Vanderplas and Garvin's (1959) method, for which a simple measure of complexity can be given in terms of the number of points used in generating each shape. Geometric figures with differing numbers of sides have also been used. Such methods minimise the possibility of subjects relying on verbal coding of stimuli, though they cannot eliminate this possibility entirely since some degree of verbal coding can always be achieved, especially for relatively simple stimuli.

Fontenot (1974) was perhaps the first to show both a LVF superiority for recognition of complex (12 point) shapes and no visual hemifield difference in the recognition of simple shapes. The general conclusion that LVF superiorities can be found for the recognition of complex shapes, with no visual hemifield differences or small RVF superiorities for the recognition of simple shapes is borne out by the findings of several other studies, including those of Dimond and Beaumont (1972b), Beaumont and Dimond (1975), Hellige and Cox (1976), Axelrod *et al.* (1978), Endo *et al.* (1978), Polich (1978), Umilta *et al.* (1978), and Hatta and Dimond (1980). There is, however, a hint of a U-shaped function, with recognition of *very* complex figures again producing no visual hemifield differences in some studies (Oscar-Berman *et al.*, 1973; Hellige, 1978). Paradoxically, the results of studies using similar stimuli exposed in free vision to patients with cerebral lesions seem to implicate the left hemisphere in shape discrimination (Bisiach and Faglioni, 1974; Bisiach *et al.*, 1979) or reveal no hemispheric difference (Newcombe and Ratcliff, 1979).

As well as visual hemifield differences, differences in form recognition between the left and right hands have been investigated in normal subjects. These studies are much less numerous than the visual hemifield studies, and the relevant factors have consequently been less systematically examined. Left hand superiorities for the recognition of unfamiliar shapes have been demonstrated by Witelson (1974), Gardner *et al.* (1977), Dodds (1978), Webster and Thurber (1978), Cioffi and Kandel (1979), and Flanery and Balling (1979). It does, however, seem 'easier' to obtain a left hand than a LVF superiority, since some of these studies used relatively simple stimuli. Moreover, no overall hand differences in the perception of letters were found by Witelson (1974) and for pairs of letters by Cioffi and Kandel (1979). These are stimuli which might be expected to produce RVF superiorities when presented visually, again confirming the bias toward findings of right hemisphere advantages in tactile tasks. Cioffi and Kandel (1979) were, however, able to report a right hand superiority for the perception of two-letter words.

These visual and tactile form recognition tasks used with normal subjects all involve the recognition of forms varying on only two spatial dimensions. Thus the key level of representation in each case is that of the 2½-D sketch, which in the special case of effectively flat stimuli will not differ in any important way from the 3-D model representation. In addition, all of the tasks involve the execution of operations on these representations, in order to effect recognition. The precise nature of these operations will, however, have varied considerably from study to study because of differences in such factors as numbers of target and non-target stimuli, the familiarity of stimuli to subjects, the degree to which targets and non-targets differ, whether any necessary comparisons are to be made to previously or to subsequently presented stimuli, stimulus presentation times, and interstimulus intervals. Given the wide range of possible operations involved it would seem unlikely that the LVF and left hand superiorities found in the studies cited arose exclusively from this source, and a right hemisphere superiority in constructing the 2½-D sketch representations would seem to be implicated. The findings of the visual hemifield studies emphasise, however, that the left hemisphere is also quite capable of forming 2½-D sketches, and that the right hemisphere's superiority can only be readily detected for stimuli of an optimum degree of complexity.

B. Recognition and enumeration of stimulus configurations

As well as examining recognition of discrete forms, it is possible to investigate left and right hemisphere abilities to process information given by configurations made up of a number of discrete stimuli. In particular, the recognition and enumeration of stimulus configurations have been studied.

Gross (1972) demonstrated a LVF superiority in normal subjects' recognition of irregular patterns of filled and unfilled squares contained in a regular matrix, and Umilta et al. (1979) showed right hemisphere superiorities in ability to report the presence of a solid dot in an array of otherwise empty dots. LVF superiorities for the enumeration of visually presented collections of dots have been found by Kimura (1966), McGlone and Davidson (1973) and Young and Bion (1979). As already mentioned, Kimura (1963) and Warrington and James (1967a) noted that patients with right cerebral injuries performed worse than patients with left cerebral injuries in a similar task of estimating the number of dots in a briefly presented configuration. There is thus evidence from a number of converging sources pointing to a right hemisphere superiority in some aspect of the processing of visually presented stimulus configurations.

The evidence with respect to tactile configurations is also consistent and convincing. Most of the existing studies have involved the presentation of patterns of raised dots of the type used in Braille. Left hand superiorities in reading Braille and in learning to identify the raised dot patterns have been found in both blind and sighted people (Hermelin and O'Connor, 1971; Rudel et al., 1974, 1977; Harriman and Castell, 1979). Young and Ellis (1979) found a left hand superiority for enumerating the number of dots in configurations of this type, and also demonstrated that this was not due to a right hemisphere superiority for enumeration per se, by finding no difference between left and right hand performance at enumerating collections of dots arranged in straight lines. It would thus seem that it is the spatial complexity of the raised dot patterns used in such studies that is the crucial factor implicated in the obtained left hand superiorities.

Taken together, the studies of left and right hemisphere abilities to recognise and enumerate stimulus configurations are consistent with the conclusion reached for form recognition, that the right hemisphere shows a superiority in constructing 2½-D sketch representations. That this superiority has been so consistently demonstrated for configurational stimuli is probably attributable to the spatial complexity of the configurations that have typically been chosen.

Studies of Patients with Cerebral Lesions

Clinical studies of visuospatial ability have overwhelmingly concentrated on complex tasks which, in our terms, presumably involve creating and operating upon representations of the external world. While our review of the literature on basic perceptual asymmetries has not been exhaustive it includes reference to most of the relevant clinical data of which we are aware, but it would be quite impossible to be as comprehensive with respect to more complex disorders. In addition to the reviews mentioned earlier the reader is referred to De Renzi (1982), who provides by far the most complete account of disorders of spatial orientation currently available.

There is the additional problem that the clinical data are difficult to integrate with the findings from studies of normal subjects and not easily interpreted in terms of the level of representation or cognitive processes thought to be deficient. Many studies deal with phenomena which either do not occur in normal subjects or are difficult to investigate in the lateralised presentation paradigm, and few authors have designed their experiments in such a way as to allow one to specify the functional locus of the impairments they detect or included controls to establish the integrity of basic perceptual processes in their subjects. Constructional apraxia and topographical disorientation, for example, are almost certainly multifactorial deficits and do not lend themselves to study in normal subjects, while unilateral neglect probably does not exist in any comparable form in any other situation. Nevertheless, these and other similar topics loom so large in the clinical literature that a brief discussion of their implications seems to be in order before we proceed to other phenomena.

A. Perception, exploration, memory, learning and reproduction of spatial configurations

These different aspects of spatial information processing are so thoroughly confounded in most of the clinical literature that we will not always distinguish them here, but they are all likely to involve the creation of higher level representations or the performance of some operation upon such a representation. To the extent that this is true, selective deficits in these areas after right hemisphere damage contribute evidence suggestive of a right hemisphere predominance for these functions.

Perhaps the most easily isolated disorder is neglect of the contralateral half of space after a unilateral cerebral lesion, which seems to be more frequent after right hemisphere damage even after sampling biases have been taken into account (see Heilman, 1979; De Renzi, 1982, for reviews). The presence of visual field defect, oculomotor disorders, and defective arousal have all been suggested as possible causes of the disorder, and all are probably implicated in some cases, but none of them account for all the data and an intriguing recent report from Bisiach and Luzzatti (1978) suggests that a more central representation of the external world may be involved. They found that two patients with right hemisphere lesions and the typical symptoms of left-sided neglect also failed to describe the left side of a familiar scene which they were asked to imagine. The results of more formal visual and tactile search tasks also suggest that the right hemisphere has a special role in the exploration of space (De Renzi *et al.*, 1970) although precisely what that role is remains to be determined.

Although neglect of the left is readily apparent in drawings made by patients with right hemisphere lesions, it cannot explain all of the difficulty they have with such tasks. Errors are also made on the right side of the drawing (Ratcliff, 1982) and attempts to draw plans or maps may include all relevant details but be so spatially disorganised as to give no information about the spatial relationships obtaining between them (McFie *et al.*, 1950). The inability accurately to reproduce drawings or patterns made up of blocks or sticks is also seen after left hemisphere damage, but in seven studies reviewed by De Renzi (1982) the incidence of impairment after left hemisphere damage never exceeded that observed in the right hemisphere group and in three of them it was less than half as frequent.

Visual and tactile stylus maze-learning (Corkin, 1965; Milner, 1965; Newcombe, 1969) and other tasks involving spatial memory are selectively affected by right hemisphere damage (e.g. Milner, 1971; De Renzi *et al.*, 1977a) and because of the nature of the patient groups in most of these studies one can be confident that this is not a consequence of sampling bias. The possibility that it is attributable to a disorder of elementary perception has not been formally excluded, but this seems unlikely. It will be recalled, for example, that Ratcliff and Davies-Jones (1972) found that patients with left hemisphere lesions were just as impaired as their right sided counterparts at visual localisation of a single stimulus but the left hemisphere group reported by Ratcliff and Newcombe (1973), which was largely comprised of the same patients, was unimpaired at maze learning.

The situation with respect to topographical disorientation, topographical memory loss and defective route finding in locomotor space is less clear. A case has been made for a right hemisphere substrate for topographical memory (De Renzi *et al.*, 1977b), and right hemisphere or bilateral damage is the rule in case reports of topographical disorientation (De Renzi, 1982), but two out of four studies using an experimental locomotor route-finding task have failed to provide any evidence for hemispheric differences (Semmes *et al.*, 1955; Ratcliff and Newcombe, 1973) while the remaining two gave contradictory indications (Semmes *et al.*, 1963; Hécaen *et al.*, 1972).

In summary, it seems that right hemisphere damage is more likely to affect performance on a variety of complex spatial tasks than is comparable left hemisphere damage although, because of the complexity of the tasks involved, it is not entirely clear for which aspects of spatial information processing the right hemisphere predominates. Some support for this general conclusion comes from studies and case reports of split-brain patients which suggest superior performance of the isolated right hemisphere on tasks with similar implications (Levy-Agresti and Sperry, 1968; Nebes, 1973; Sperry, 1974; Bogen and Vogel, 1975).

B. Object recognition

Failure to recognise real, three-dimensional objects (as opposed to failure to name them) is rare (see Rubens, 1979; Ratcliff and Newcombe, 1982, for recent reviews). When it does occur it is either the result of a lesion which can reasonably be supposed to have disconnected the visual and language areas of the brain, or it is associated with large bilateral lesions or diffuse cerebral disease. However, a number of studies have shown that patients with right hemisphere lesions are disproportionately impaired when the task is made sufficiently difficult by using degraded stimuli, such as overlapping line drawings and the Street Completion Figures (De Renzi and Spinnler, 1966b), the Mooney Faces (Newcombe and Russell, 1969), the Gollin Figures (Warrington and James, 1967b) and photographs of objects taken from unusual angles (Warrington and Taylor, 1973, 1978). Again, basic perceptual disorders have not definitely been excluded as a cause of impairment on these tasks, but they seem unlikely to be the whole explanation. Warrington and Rabin (1970) found no correlation between performance on the Gollin Figures Test and their perceptual matching tasks discussed earlier (although it must be confessed that they also failed to replicate the finding of a right hemisphere deficit on the former task) and there was no right hemisphere deficit in Warrington and Taylor's (1973) study when photographs taken from more conventional angles but of roughly equal complexity were used.

Two of these studies deserve additional comment. Newcombe and Russell (1969) provide evidence showing that the ability to recognise degraded stimuli and the ability to learn a stylus maze are independent of each other although both depend on the integrity of the right hemisphere. They found that patients with right parietal lesions were unimpaired on the recognition task although they were significantly impaired on the stylus maze, while patients with more inferior lesions in the region of the temporo-parieto-occipital junction exhibited the reverse pattern.

Warrington and Taylor's (1978) matching version of the Unusual Views Test is of particular interest because rotation of a stimulus to an angle which makes its principal axis difficult to determine could be expected to make it difficult to construct a 3-D model representation which would match that derived from the conventional view (Marr and Nishihara, 1978a,b). Conversely, the ability to derive adequate 3-D model representations should facilitate matching of two different views of the same object although the primal sketches would be quite different.

The matching version of the Unusual Views Test has the advantage that it only requires the subject to decide whether two different photographs are representations of the same object and not to state what the object is. It can thus be used with the rare agnosic patients who cannot identify even real objects from familiar view points. One such patient, whose matching of physically identical stimuli was virtually error free and who made excellent copies of drawings of objects that he could not identify, was near chance on the Unusual Views Test (Ratcliff and Newcombe, 1982) and on the basis of this result and other data the authors concluded that his deficit was at the stage of the 3-D model representation. This suggests that the Unusual Views Test is testing an ability which is necessary for the recognition of real objects and, to the extent that it is differentially sensitive to right hemisphere damage, that this ability is predominantly subserved by the right hemisphere. It cannot be the exclusive responsibility of right hemisphere processors, however, because unilateral right hemisphere lesions do not cause gross disturbances of the ability to recognise objects except under conditions of stimulus degredation.

Some agnosic patients (who, incidentally, can match usual and unusual views of objects normally even though they do not recognise the objects) seem to fail in object recognition tasks because the stimulus does not evoke the appropriate central representation in semantic memory (Warrington, 1975). There is now converging evidence from several sources in the neurological literature which appears to indicate that semantic memory may be divided into several partially separable components (Shallice, 1981) and there is just a suggestion that one of the divisions may reflect differential coding of information by the hemispheres (Wilkins and Moscovitch, 1978), the right hemisphere storing (or having privileged access to) information about size (and possibly physical attributes in general) and the left hemisphere being more concerned with information about function and semantic category.

C. Other clinical evidence

Global stereopsis, the ability to perceive a form standing out (or back) in a random element stereogram (Julesz, 1971) has been found to be more impaired by right than left hemisphere lesions (Carmon and Bechtoldt, 1969; Benton and Hécaen, 1970; Hamsher, 1978a). In one of these studies impaired stereoacuity was excluded as a possible cause of failure (Hamsher, 1978a) and patients with right hemisphere lesions who could not achieve stereopsis were also unable to perceive 'anomalous' or 'illusory' contours (Hamsher, 1978b). This would seem to suggest that impaired global stereopsis in this group is related to difficulty in extracting a coherent shape standing out in depth, but a right hemisphere deficit for global stereopsis independent of stereoacuity has not been confirmed (Ross, in press; Lawler, 1982).

The right hemisphere of split-brain patients is superior to the left at selecting from several alternatives a circle with the same radius as a previously palpated arc (Nebes, 1971), at recognising shapes when they have been exploded (Nebes, 1972), and at detecting the structure in regular patterns (Nebes, 1973). Performance on all of these tasks would presumably be facilitated by the ability to generate representations of the stimuli or, in more traditional terminology, to form gestalten. However, another task which has been widely used in patients with cerebral lesions and which would also seem to involve gestalt formation, the Gottschaldt Hidden Figures Test, has never produced convincing evidence for hemispheric asymmetry and seems to be sensitive to the size rather than site of the lesion (Corkin, 1979).

Finally, we note two experiments which speak to the issue of 'spatial thought', a form of mental activity which has frequently been postulated in the clinical literature on spatial disorders (e.g. Critchley, 1953; Ettlinger *et al.*, 1957; Butters *et al.*, 1970; Benton *et al.*, 1974). Franco and Sperry (1977) required split-brain patients to decide whether geometrical shapes did or did not belong to a set which was defined, in different phases of the experiment, in terms of Euclidean, affine, projective or topological geometry. As the number of properties defining the set declined in the progression from Euclidean to topological space so did the performance of the right-hand and left-hemisphere combination, whereas the left-hand and right-hemisphere combination performed equally well under all conditions. This result was interpreted in terms of differential strategies; feature analysis supposedly being employed by the left hemisphere and being progressively less adequate as the number of defining features declined whereas the more global analysis supposedly characteristic of right-hemisphere processing remained efficient. However, these findings could also reflect superior ability on the part of the right hemisphere to represent shapes in more abstract, sophisticated or flexible ways. Indeed these two interpretations may be different ways of saying the same thing.

There is also evidence pointing to a right hemisphere superiority for performing mental operations on representations. Ratcliff (1979) exposed schematic drawings of a human figure, either upright or inverted, to patients with unilateral cerebral lesions. One of each manikin's hands was marked with a black disc and the subject's task was to say 'right' or 'left' depending on which hand was marked. There is independent evidence indicating that subjects mentally re-orient inverted stimuli in this task before making the right/left judgement (Benson and Gedye, 1963) and analysis of variance revealed a significant group × orientation interaction, the right hemisphere group being selectively impaired in the inverted condition, presumably because of difficulty in mentally re-orienting the stimuli.

Although some of these miscellaneous experiments may individually be susceptible to alternative explanation, the unifying theme which runs through them is the suggestion that the right hemisphere has a special role in creating and operating upon higher-level or more abstract mental representations of external stimuli. Collectively they constitute persuasive, if circumstantial, evidence for this hypothesis.

Summary and Conclusions

A number of points emerge from this review of right hemisphere superiorities for visuospatial information processing. It is perhaps worthwhile to restate the main ones.

Firstly it is clear that, taken together, studies of normal and clinical subject populations provide completely convincing evidence of right hemisphere superiorities for at least some aspects of visuospatial information processing. Although none of the available research methods are free from intrinsic limitations and problems of interpretation, such difficulties tend to be specific to particular methods, and the extent to which studies using entirely different techniques confirm and substantiate each other can leave no doubt that the case for right hemisphere superiorities is not grounded in artifact.

A second point concerns the need for a theory of visuospatial information processing that will inform the attempts that must now be made to specify more precisely the nature of these right hemisphere superiorities. We have suggested that Marr's (1980) views on the levels involved in the creation of visual representations may be of some use in this respect. From applying our interpretation of Marr's work to the studies that have been carried out, it has been argued that right hemisphere superiorities can be demonstrated at all of the levels of representation Marr described, but that those involved in the relatively low levels of representation are small and can only be detected under sensitive conditions.

As well as the need for an explicit theory of visuospatial information processing, some changes in research strategy are also necessary, and are beginning to be used. The dominant tactic in research to date has been to collect more and more examples of tasks that give or do not give right hemisphere superiorities. This tactic has been of great value in substantiating the conclusion that right hemisphere superiorities for visuospatial information processing exist. However, it is less helpful in clarifying the nature of the right hemisphere superiorities that have been found, because the numerous procedural differences between different studies often make comparisons across studies either tentative or impossible. One solution to this difficulty might lie in the appearance of a set of 'standard' experimental conditions for each type of study, but for obvious reasons this is most unlikely to ever come about. A more realistic approach is for investigators to demonstrate, within a single study, tasks or stimuli varying on only one factor which leads to the presence or absence of right hemisphere superiorities. The demonstration of such hemisphere × task, or hemisphere × stimulus, interactions allows relatively strong inferences to be drawn concerning the nature of the right hemisphere's contribution. Although this technique has at present only been used in a few studies (e.g. Bryden and Allard, 1976; Umilta *et al.*, 1978; Young and Ellis, 1979) it would seem to offer much promise for future research.

References

ARRIGONI, G. and DE RENZI, E. (1964). Constructional apraxia and hemispheric locus of lesion. *Cortex* **1**, 180-197.
AXELROD, S., LEIBER, L. and NOONAN, M. (1978). Classification of random forms and distortions presented to the left or right visual field. *Perceptual and Motor Skills* **27**, 615-621.
BÁLINT, R. (1909). Die Seelenlähmung des Schauens, optische Ataxie, Räumliche Störung der Aufmerksamkeit. *Monatsschrift für Psychiatrie und Neurologie* **25**, 51-81.
BASSO, A., BISIACH, E. and CAPITANI, E. (1977). Decision in ambiguity: hemispheric dominance or interaction. *Cortex* **13**, 96-99.
BEAUMONT, J. G. (1982). Studies with verbal stimuli. In *Divided Visual Field Studies of Cerebral Organisation* (J. G. Beaumont, ed.), pp.57-86. Academic Press, London and New York.
BEAUMONT, J. G. and DIMOND, S. J. (1975). Interhemispheric transfer of figural information in right- and non-right-handed subjects. *Acta Psychologica* **39**, 97-104.
BENDER, M. and JUNG, R. (1948). Abweichungen der subjectiven optischen Verticalen und Horizantalen bei Gesunden und Himverletzen. *Archive für Psychiatrie* **181**, 193-212.
BENSON, A. J. and GEDYE, J. L. (1963). Logical processes in the resolution of orientation conflict. *RAF Institute of Aviation Medicine Report No.* **259**. Ministry of Defence (Air), London.
BENSON, D. F. and BARTON, M. I. (1970). Disturbances in constructional ability. *Cortex* **6**, 19-46.
BENTON, A. L. (1979). Disorders of spatial orientation. In *Handbook of Clinical Neurology* (P. J. Vinken and G. W. Bruyn, eds). North Holland, Amsterdam.
BENTON, A. L. and HÉCAEN, H. (1970). Stereoscopic vision in patients with unilateral cerebral damage. *Neurology* **20**, 1084-1088.
BENTON, A. L. and JOYNT, R. J. (1959). Reaction time in unilateral cerebral disease. *Confinia Neurologica (Basel)* **19**, 247-256.
BENTON, A. L., LEVIN, H. S. and VARNEY, N. R. (1973). Tactile perception of direction in normal subjects. *Neurology* **23**, 1248-1250.
BENTON, A. L., LEVIN, H. S. and VAN ALLEN, M. W. (1974). Geographic orientation in patients with unilateral cerebral disease. *Neuropsychologia* **12**, 183-191.
BENTON, A. L., HANNAY, J. and VARNEY, N. R. (1975). Visual perception of line direction in patients with unilateral brain disease. *Neurology* **25**, 907-910.

BENTON, A. L., VARNEY, N. R. and HAMSHER, K. de S. (1978a). Visuospatial judgement: a clinical test. *Archives of Neurology* **35**, 364-367.

BENTON, A. L., VARNEY, N. R. and HAMSHER, K. de S. (1978b). Lateral differences in tactile directional perception. *Neuropsychologia* **16**, 109-114.

BERLUCCHI, G., CREA, F., DI STEFANO, M. and TASSINARI, G. (1977). Influence of spatial stimulus-response compatability on reaction time of ipsilateral and contralateral hand to lateralised light stimuli. *Journal of Experimental Psychology: Human Perception and Performance* **3**, 505-517.

BERLUCCHI, G., BRIZZOLARA, D., MARZI, C. A., RIZZOLATTI, G. and UMILTA, C. (1979). The role of stimulus discriminability and verbal codability in hemispheric specialization for visuospatial tasks. *Neuropsychologia* **17**, 195-202.

BIRCH, H. G., PROCTOR, F. and BORTNER, M. (1961). Perception in hemiplegia: III The judgement of relative distance in the visual field. *Archives of Physical Medicine and Rehabilitation* **42**, 639-644.

BIRKETT, P. (1977). Measures of laterality and theories of hemispheric processes. *Neuropsychologia* **15**, 693-696.

BISIACH, E. and FAGLIONI, P. (1974). Recognition of random shapes by patients with unilateral lesions as a function of complexity, association value and delay: an analysis of sensitivity and response criterion. *Cortex* **10**, 101-110.

BISIACH, E. and LUZZATTI, C. (1978). Unilateral neglect of representational space. *Cortex* **14**, 129-133.

BISIACH, E., NICHELLI, P. and SPINNLER, H. (1976). Hemispheric functional asymmetry in visual discrimination between univariate stimuli: an analysis of sensitivity and response criterion. *Neuropsychologia* **14**, 335-342.

BISIACH, E., NICHELLI, P. and SALA, C. (1979). Recognition of random shapes in unilateral brain damaged patients: a reappraisal. *Cortex* **15**, 491-499.

BOGEN, J. E. and VOGEL, P. J. (1975). Neurologic status in the long term following complete cerebral commissurotomy. In *Les Syndromes de Disconnexion Calleuse Chez l'Homme* (Colloque International de Lyon, 1974) F. Michel and B. Schott, eds. Hôpital neurologique de Lyon, Lyon.

BRYDEN, M. P. (1973). Perceptual asymmetry in vision: relation to handedness, eyedness and speech lateralization. *Cortex* **9**, 418-435.

BRYDEN, M. P. (1976). Response bias and hemispheric differences in dot localization. *Perception and Psychophysics* **19**, 23-28.

BRYDEN, M. P. and ALLARD, F. (1976). Visual hemifield differences depend on typeface. *Brain and Language* **3**, 191-200.

BRYDEN, M. P. and RAINEY, C. A. (1963). Left-right differences in tachistoscopic recognition. *Journal of Experimental Psychology* **66**, 568-571.

BUTTERS, N., BARTON, M. and BRODY, B. A. (1970). Role of the right parietal lobe in the mediation of cross-modal associations and reversible operations in space. *Cortex* **6**, 174-190.

CARMON, A. and BECHTOLDT, H. P. (1969). Dominance of the right cerebral hemisphere for stereopsis. *Neuropsychologia* **7**, 29-40.

CARMON, A. and BENTON, A. L. (1969). Tactile perception of direction and number in patients with unilateral cerebral disease. *Neurology* **19**, 525-532.

CARMON, A., BILSTROM, D. E. and BENTON, A. L. (1969). Thresholds for pressure and sharpness in the right and left hands. *Cortex* **5**, 27-35.

CIOFFI, J. and KANDEL, G. L. (1979). Laterality of stereognostic accuracy of children for words, shapes, and bigrams: a sex difference for bigrams. *Science* **204**, 1432-1434.

COHEN, G. (1977). *The Psychology of Cognition.* Academic Press, London and New York.

COLE, M., SCHUTTA, H. S. and WARRINGTON, E. K. (1962). Visual disorientation in homonymous half-fields. *Neurology* **12**, 257-263.

CORKIN, S. (1965). Tactually guided maze learning in man: effects of unilateral cortical excisions and bilateral hippocampal lesions. *Neuropsychologia* **3**, 339-351.

CORKIN, S. (1978). The role of different cerebral structures in somesthetic perception. In *Handbook of Perception, Vol. VIB: Feeling and Hurting.* (E. C. Carterette and M. P. Frieddman, eds), pp.105-155, Academic Press, New York and London.

CORKIN, S. (1979). Hidden figures test performance: lasting effects of unilateral penetrating head injury and transient effects of bilateral cingulotomy. *Neuropsychologia* **17**, 585-605.

CRITCHLEY, M. (1953). *The Parietal Lobes.* Arnold, London.

DANTA, G., HILTON, R. C. and O'BOYLE, D. J. (1978). Hemispheric function and binocular depth perception. *Brain* **101**, 569-590.

DAVIDOFF, J. B. (1975). Hemispheric differences in the perception of lightness. *Neuropsychologia* **13**, 121-124.

DAVIDOFF, J. B. (1976). Hemispheric sensitivity differences in the perception of colour. *Quarterly Journal of Experimental Psychology* **28**, 381-394.

DAVIDOFF, J. B. (1977). Hemispheric differences in dot detection. *Cortex* **13**, 434-444.

DAVIDOFF, J. (1982). Studies with non-verbal stimuli. In *Divided Visual Field Studies of Cerebral Organisation* (J. G. Beaumont, ed.), pp.29-55. Academic Press, London and New York.

DE RENZI, E. (1982). *Disorders of Space Exploration and Cognition.* Wiley, Chichester.

DE RENZI, E. and SPINNLER, H. (1966a). Facial recognition in brain damaged patients. *Neurology* **16**, 145-152.

DE RENZI, E. and SPINNLER, H. (1966b). Visual recognition in patients with unilateral cerebral disease. *Journal of Nervous and Mental Disease* **142**, 515-525.

DE RENZI, E. and SPINNLER, H. (1967). Impaired performance on colour tasks in patients with hemispheric damage. *Cortex* **3**, 194-217.

DE RENZI, E., FAGLIONI, P. and SCOTTI, G. (1970). Hemispheric contribution to the exploration of space through the visual and tactile modality. *Cortex* **6**, 191-203.

DE RENZI, E., FAGLIONI, P. and SCOTTI, G. (1971). Judgement of spatial orientation in patients with focal brain damage. *Journal of Neurology, Neurosurgery and Psychiatry* **34**, 489-495.

DE RENZI, E., FAGLIONI, P. and PREVIDI, P. (1977a). Spatial memory and hemispheric locus of lesion. *Cortex* **13**, 424-433.

DE RENZI, E. FAGLIONI, P. and VILLA, P. (1977b). Topographical amnesia. *Journal of Neurology, Neurosurgery and Psychiatry* **40**, 498-505.

DIMOND, S. J. and BEAUMONT, J. G. (1972a). Hemisphere function and colour naming. *Journal of Experimental Psychology* **96**, 87-92.

DIMOND, S. J. and BEAUMONT, J. G. (1972b). Perceptual integration between and within the cerebral hemispheres. *British Journal of Psychology* **63**, 509-514.

DODDS, A. G. (1978). Hemispheric differences in tactuo-spatial processing. *Neuropsychologia* **16**, 247-250.

DURNFORD, M. and KIMURA, D. (1971). Right hemisphere specialization for depth perception reflected in visual field differences. *Nature, Lond.* **231**, 394-395.

DYER, F. N. (1973). Interference and facilitation for color naming with separate bilateral presentations of the word and color. *Journal of Experimental Psychology* **99**, 314-317.

ELMAN, J. L., TAKAHASHI, K. and TOHSAKU, Y. H. (1981a). Asymmetries for the categorization of Kanji nouns, adjectives, and verbs presented to the left and right visual fields. *Brain and Language* **13**, 290-300.

ELMAN, J. L., TAKAHASHI, K. and TOHSAKU, Y. H. (1981b). Lateral asymmetries for the identification of concrete and abstract Kanji. *Neuropsychologia* **19**, 407-412.

ENDO, L. M., SHIMIZU, A. and HORI, T. (1978). Functional asymmetry of visual fields for Japanese words in Kana (syllable-based) writing and random-shape recognition in Japanese subjects. *Neuropsychologia* **16**, 291-297.

ETTLINGER, G., WARRINGTON, E. K. and ZANGWILL, O. L. (1957). A further study of visual-spatial agnosia. *Brain* **80**, 335-361.

FENNEL, E., SATZ, P. and WISE, R. (1967). Laterality differences in the perception of pressure. *Journal of Neurology, Neurosurgery and Psychiatry* **30**, 337-340.

FILBEY, R. A. and GAZZANIGA, M. S. (1969). Splitting the normal brain with reaction time. *Psychonomic Science* **17**, 335-336.

FLANERY, R. C. and BALLING, J. D. (1979). Developmental changes in hemispheric specialization for tactile spatial ability. *Developmental Psychology* **15**, 364-372.

FONTENOT, D. J. (1974). Visual field differences in the recognition of verbal and nonverbal stimuli in man. *Journal of Comparative and Physiological Psychology* **85**, 564-569.

FONTENOT, D. J. and BENTON, A. L. (1971). Tactile perception of direction in relation to hemispheric locus of lesion. *Neuropsychologia* **9**, 83-88.

FONTENOT, D. J. and BENTON, A. L. (1972). Perception of direction in the right and left visual fields. *Neuropsychologia* **10**, 447-452.

FRANCO, L. and SPERRY, R. W. (1977). Hemispheric lateralization for cognitive processing of geometry. *Neuropsychologia* **15**, 107-114.

GARDNER, E. B., ENGLISH, A. G., FLANNERY, B. M., HARTNETT, M. B., McCORMICK, J. K. and WILHELMY, B. B. (1977). Shape-recognition accuracy and response latency in a bilateral tactile task. *Neuropsychologia* **15**, 607-616.

GESCHWIND, N. (1965). Disconnexion syndromes in animals and man. *Brain* **88**, 237-294; 585-644.

GIBSON, J. J. (1962). Observations on active touch. *Psychological Review* **69**, 477-491.

GOFF, G. D., ROSNER, B. S., DETRE, T. and KENNARD, D. (1965). Vibration perception in normal man and medical patients. *Journal of Neurology, Neurosurgery and Psychiatry* **28**, 503-509.

GRANT, D. W. (1980). Visual asymmetry on a colour naming task: a developmental perspective. *Perceptual and Motor Skills* **50**, 475-480.

GRANT, D. W. (1981). Visual asymmetry on a colour naming task: a longitudinal study with primary school children. *Child Development* **52**, 370-372.

GROSS, M. M. (1972). Hemispheric specialisation for processing of visually presented verbal and spatial stimuli. *Perception and Psychophysics* **12**, 357-363.

HAMSHER, K. de S. (1978a). Stereopsis and unilateral brain disease. *Investigative Ophthalmology* **17**, 336-343.

HAMSHER, K. de S. (1978b). Stereopsis and the perception of anomalous contours. *Neuropsychologia* **16**, 453-459.

HANNAY, H. J. (1979). Asymmetry in reception and retention of colours. *Brain and Language* **8**, 191-201.

HANNAY, H. J., VARNEY, N. R. and BENTON, A. L. (1976). Visual localization in patients with unilateral brain disease. *Journal of Neurology, Neurosurgery and Psychiatry* **39**, 307-313.

HARRIMAN, J. and CASTELL, L. (1979). Manual asymmetry for tactile discrimination. *Perceptual and Motor Skills* **48**, 290.

HATTA, T. (1977a). Recognition of Japanese Kanji in the left and right visual fields. *Neuropsychologia* **15**, 685-688.

HATTA, T. (1977b). Lateral recognition of abstract and concrete Kanji in Japanese. *Perceptual and Motor Skills* **45**, 731-734.

HATTA, T. and DIMOND, S. J. (1980). Comparison of lateral differences for digit and random form recognition in Japanese and Westerners. *Journal of Experimental Psychology: Human Perception and Performance* **6**, 368-374.

HÉCAEN, H. and ANGELERGUES, R. (1963). *La Cécité Psychique*. Masson, Paris.

HÉCAEN, H., TZORTZIS, C. and MASURE, M. C. (1972). Troubles de l'orientation spatiale dans une épreuve de recherche d'itinéraire lors des lésions corticales unilaterales. *Perception* **1**, 325-330.

HEILMAN, K. M. (1979). Neglect and related disorders. In *Clinical Neuropsychology* (K. M. Heilman and E. Valenstein, eds). Oxford University Press, London.

HELLIGE, J. B. (1978). Visual laterality patterns for pure versus mixed-list presentation. *Journal of Experimental Psychology: Human Perception and Performance* **4**, 121-131.

HELLIGE, J. B. and COX, P. J. (1976). Effects of concurrent verbal memory on recognition of stimuli from the left and right visual fields. *Journal of Experimental Psychology: Human Perception and Performance* **2**, 210-221.

HERMELIN, B. and O'CONNOR, N. (1971). Functional asymmetry in the reading of Braille. *Neuropsychologia* **9**, 431-435.

HOLMES, G. (1918). Disturbances of visual orientation. *British Journal of Ophthalmology* **2**, 449-469 and 506-516.

HOLMES, G. (1919). Disturbances of visual space perception. *British Medical Journal* **2**, 230-233.

HOLMES, G. and HORRAX, G. (1919). Disturbances of spatial orientation and visual attention with loss of stereoscopic vision. *Archives of Neurology and Psychiatry* **1**, 385-407.

HOWES, D. and BOLLER, F. (1975). Simple reaction time: Evidence for focal impairment from lesions of the right hemisphere. *Brain* **98**, 317-322.

JEEVES, M. A. and DIXON, N. F. (1970). Hemisphere differences in response rates to visual stimuli. *Psychonomic Science* **20**, 249-251.

JOYNT, R. J. and GOLDSTEIN, M. N. (1975). Minor cerebral hemisphere. In *Advances in Neurology*, Vol. 7 (W. J. Friedlander, ed.), pp.147-183. Raven Press, New York.

JULESZ, B. (1971). *Foundations of Cyclopean Perception*. Chicago University Press, Chicago.

KIMURA, D. (1963). Right temporal lobe damage. Perception of unfamiliar stimuli after damage. *Archives of Neurology* **8**, 264-271.

KIMURA, D. (1966). Dual functional asymmetry of the brain in visual perception. *Neuropsychologia* **4**, 275-285.

KIMURA, D. (1969). Spatial localisation in left and right visual fields. *Canadian Journal of Psychology* **23**, 445-458.

KIMURA, D. and DURNFORD, M. (1974). Normal studies on the function of the right hemisphere in vision. In *Hemisphere Function in the Human Brain* (S. J. Dimond and J. G. Beaumont, eds), pp.25-47. Elek, London.

KLATZKY, R. L. (1972). Visual and verbal coding of laterally presented pictures. *Journal of Experimental Psychology* **96**, 439-448.

LAWLER, K. (1982). Aspects of spatial vision. Unpublished doctoral thesis, University of Oxford.

LEHMAN, D. and WALCHLI, P. (1975). Depth perception and location of brain lesion. *Journal of Neurology* **209**, 157-164.

LENZ, H. (1944). Raumsinnstörungen bei Himverletzungen. *Deutsche Zeitschrift für Nervenheilk* **157**, 22-64.

LEVY, J. and REID, M. (1976). Variations in writing posture and cerebral organization. *Science* **194**, 337-339.

LEVY-AGRESTI, J. and SPERRY, R. W. (1968). Differential perceptual capacities in the major and minor hemispheres. *Proceedings of the National Academy of Sciences* **61**, 1151.

MALONE, D. R. and HANNAY, H. J. (1978). Hemispheric dominance and normal color memory. *Neuropsychologia* **16**, 51-59.

MARR, D. (1980). Visual information processing: the structure and creation of visual representations. *Phil. Trans. of the Royal Society, London,* **B290** 199-218.

MARR, D. and NISHIHARA, H. K. (1978a). Representation and recognition of the spatial organisation of three-dimensional shapes. *Proceedings of the Royal Society of London, Series B* **200**, 269-294.

MARR, D. and NISHIHARA, H. K. (1978b). Visual information processing: artificial intelligence and the sensorium of sight. *Technology Review* **81**, 2-23.

McFIE, J. and ZANGWILL, O. L. (1960). Visual-constructive disabilities associated with lesions of the left cerebral hemisphere. *Brain* **83**, 243-260.

McFIE, J. PIERCY, M. F. and ZANGWILL, O. L. (1950). Visual spatial agnosia associated with lesions of the right cerebral hemisphere. *Brain* **73**, 167-190.

McGLONE, J. and DAVIDSON, W. (1973). The relation between cerebral speech laterality and spatial ability with special reference to sex and hand preference. *Neuropsychologia* **11**, 105-113.

McKEEVER, W. F. and JACKSON, T. L. (1979). Cerebral dominance assessed by object- and color-naming latencies: sex and familial sinistrality effects. *Brain and Language* **7**, 175-190.

McKEEVER, W. F., HOEMANN, H. W., FLORIAN, V. A. and VAN DEVENTER, A. D. (1976). Evidence of minimal cerebral asymmetries for the processing of English words and American sign language in the congenitally deaf. *Neuropsychologia* **14**, 413-423.

MILNER, B. (1965). Visually guided maze learning in man: effects of bilateral hippocampal, bilateral frontal, and unilateral cerebral lesions. *Neuropsychologia* **3**, 317-338.

MILNER, B. (1971). Interhemispheric differences in the localization of psychological processes in man. *British Medical Bulletin* **27**, 272-277.

MOSCOVITCH, M. (1979). Information processing and the cerebral hemispheres. In *Handbook of Behavioral Neurobiology, Vol. 2: Neuropsychology* (M. S. Gazzaniga, ed.), pp.379-446. Plenum Press, New York.

NEBES, R. D. (1971). Superiority of the minor hemisphere in commissurotomized man for the perception of part-whole relations. *Cortex* **7**, 333-349.

NEBES, R. D. (1972). Dominance of the minor hemisphere in commissurotomized man on a test of figural unification. *Brain* **95**, 633-638.

NEBES, R. D. (1973). Perception of spatial relationships by the right and left hemispheres in commissurotomized man. *Neuropsychologia* **11**, 285-290.

NEWCOMBE, F. (1969). *Missile Wounds of the Brain.* Oxford University Press, London.

NEWCOMBE, F. and RATCLIFF, G. (1979). Long term psychological consequences of cerebral lesions. In *Handbook of Behavioural Neurobiology, Vol. 2: Neuropsychology* (M. S. Gazzaniga, ed.). Plenum Press, New York.

NEWCOMBE, F. and RUSSELL, W. R. (1969). Dissociated visual perceptual and spatial deficits in focal lesions of the right hemisphere. *Journal of Neurology, Neurosurgery and Psychiatry* **32**, 73-81.

OSCAR-BERMAN, M., GOODGLASS, H. and CHERLOW, D. G. (1973). Perceptual laterality and iconic recognition of visual material by Korsakoff patients and normal adults. *Journal of Comparative and Physiological Psychology* **82**, 316-321.

OSCAR-BERMAN, M., REHBEIN, L., PORFERT, A. and GOODGLASS, H. (1978). Dichhaptic hand-order effects with verbal and nonverbal tactile stimulation. *Brain and Language* **6**, 323-333.

OXBURY, J. M., CAMPBELL, D. C. and OXBURY, S. M. (1974). Unilateral spatial neglect and impairments of spatial and analysis and visual perception. *Brain* **97**, 551-564.

PAIVIO, A. and ERNEST, C. H. (1971). Imagery ability and visual perception of verbal and nonverbal stimuli. *Perception and Psychophysics* **10**, 429-432.

PENNAL, B. E. (1977). Human cerebral asymmetry in color discrimination. *Neuropsychologia* **15**, 563-568.

PERRET, E. and REGLI, F. (1970). Age and the perceptual threshold for vibratory stimuli. *European Neurology* **4**, 65-76.

PHIPPARD, D. (1977). Hemifield differences in visual perception in deaf and hearing subjects. *Neuropsychologia* **15**, 555-561.

POHL, W., BUTTERS, N. and GOODGLASS, H. (1972). Spatial discrimination systems and cerebral lateralization. *Cortex* **8**, 305-314.

POIZNER, H. and LANE, H. (1979). Cerebral asymmetry in the perception of American sign language. *Brain and Language* **7**, 210-226.

POLICH, J. M. (1978). Hemispheric differences in stimulus identification. *Perception and Psychophysics* **24**, 49-57.

RATCLIFF, G. (1979). Spatial thought, mental rotation and the right cerebral hemisphere. *Neuropsychologia* **17**, 49-54.

RATCLIFF, G. (1982). Disturbances of spatial orientation associated with cerebral lesions. In *Spatial Abilities: Development and Physiological Foundations* (M. Potegal, ed.). Academic Press, New York and London.

RATCLIFF, G. and DAVIES-JONES, G. A. B. (1972). Defective visual localization in focal brain wounds. *Brain* **95**, 46-60.

RATCLIFF, G. and NEWCOMBE, F. (1973). Spatial orientation in man: effects of left, right and bilateral posterior cerebral lesions. *Journal of Neurology, Neurosurgery and Psychiatry* **36**, 448-454.

RATCLIFF, G. and NEWCOMBE, F. (1982). Object recognition: some deductions from the clinical evidence. In *Normality and Pathology in Cognitive Function* (A. W. Ellis, ed.), pp.147-171. Academic Press, London and New York.

RISSE, G. L., LE DOUX, J., SPRINGER, S. P., WILSON, D. H. and GAZZANIGA, M. S. (1978). The anterior commissure in man: functional variation in a multi-sensory system. *Neuropsychologia* **16**, 23-31.

ROBERTSHAW, S. and SHELDON, M. (1976). Laterality effects in judgement of the identity and position of letters: a signal detection analysis. *Quarterly Journal of Experimental Psychology* **28**, 115-121.

RONDOT, P., RECONDO, J. and RIBADEAU-DUMAS, J. L. (1977). Visuomotor ataxia. *Brain* **100**, 355-376.

ROSS, J. E. (in press). Disturbance of stereoscopic vision in patients with unilateral stroke. *Behavioural Brain Research*.

ROTHSTEIN, T. B. and SACKS, J. (1972). Defective stereopsis in lesions of the parietal lobe. *American Journal of Ophthalmology* **73**, 281-284.

RUBENS, A. B. (1979). Agnosia. In *Clinical Neuropsychology* (K. M. Heilman and E. Valenstein, eds). Oxford University Press, New York.

RUDEL, R. G., DENCKLA, M. B. and SPALTEN, E. (1974). The functional asymmetry of Braille letter learning in normal, sighted children. *Neurology* **24**, 733-738.

RUDEL, R. G., DENCKLA, M. B. and HIRSCH, S. (1977). The development of left-hand superiority for discriminating Braille configurations. *Neurology* **27**, 160-164.

SASANUMA, S. and KOBAYASHI, Y. (1978). Tachistoscopic recognition of line orientation. *Neuropsychologia* **16**, 239-242.

SASANUMA, S., ITOH, M., MORI, K. and KOBAYASHI, Y. (1977). Tachistoscopic recognition of Kana and Kanji words. *Neuropsychologia* **15**, 547-553.

SCHMULLER, J. and GOODMAN, B. (1980). Bilateral tachistoscopic perception, handedness and laterality, II: Nonverbal stimuli. *Brain and Language* **11**, 12-18.

SEMMES, J., WEINSTEIN, S., GHENT, L. and TEUBER, H. L. (1955). Spatial orientation in man: I. Analyses by locus of lesion. *Journal of Psychology* **39**, 227-244.

SEMMES, J., WEINSTEIN, S., GHENT, L. and TEUBER, H. L. (1960). *Somatosensory Changes after Penetrating Brain Wounds in Man*. Harvard University Press, Cambridge Mass.

SEMMES, J., WEINSTEIN, S., GHENT, L. and TEUBER, H. L. (1963). Correlates of impaired orientation in personal and extra-personal space. *Brain* **86**, 742-772.

SHALLICE, T. (1979). Case study approach in neuropsychological research. *Journal of Clinical Neuropsychology* **1**, 183-211.

SHALLICE, T. (1981). The neurological impairment of cognitive processes. *British Medical Bulletin* **37**, 187-192.

SPERRY, R. W. (1974). Lateral specialization in the surgically separated hemispheres. In *The Neurosciences: Third Study Program*. (F. O. Schmidt and F. G. Worden, eds). MIT Press, Cambridge, Mass.

TUEBER, H.-L. and MISHKIN, M. (1954). Judgement of visual and postural vertical after brain injury. *Journal of Psychology* **38**, 161-175.

UMILTA, C., RIZZOLATTI, G., MARZI, C. A., ZAMBONI, G., FRANZINI, C., CAMARDA, R. and BERLUCCHI, G. (1974). Hemispheric differences in the discrimination of line orientation. *Neuropsychologia* **12**, 165-174.

UMILTA, C., BAGNARA, S. and SIMION, F. (1978). Laterality effects for simple and complex geometrical figures, and nonsense patterns. *Neuropsychologia* **16**, 43-49.

UMILTA, C., SALMASO, D., BAGNARA, S. and SIMION, F. (1979). Evidence for a right hemisphere superiority and for a serial search strategy in a dot detection task. *Cortex* **15**, 597-608.

VAN DEN ABELL, T. and HEILMAN, K. M. (unpub.). Lateralized warning stimuli, phasic hemispheric arousal and reaction time. Paper presented to the International Neuropsychological Society, Minneapolis, February, 1978.

VANDERPLAS, J. M. and GARVIN, E. A. (1959). The association value of random shapes. *Journal of Experimental Psychology* **57**, 147-154.

VARNEY, N. R. and BENTON, A. L. (1975). Tactile perception of direction in relation to handedness and familial handedness. *Neuropsychologia* **13**, 449-454.

WALL, P. D. (1975). The somatosensory system. In *Handbook of Psychobiology* (M. S. Gazzaniga and C. Blakemore, eds), pp.373-392. Academic Press, New York and London.

WARRINGTON, E. K. (1975). The selective impairment of semantic memory. *Quarterly Journal of Experimental Psychology* **27**, 635-658.

WARRINGTON, E. K. and JAMES, M. (1967a). Tachistoscopic number estimation in patients with unilateral cerebral lesions. *Journal of Neurology, Neurosurgery and Psychiatry* **30**, 468-474.

WARRINGTON, E. K. and JAMES, M. (1967b). Disorders of visual perception in patients with unilateral cerebral lesions. *Neuropsychologia* **5**, 253-266.

WARRINGTON, E. K. and RABIN, P. (1970). Perceptual matching in patients with cerebral lesions. *Neuropsychologia* **8**, 475-487.

WARRINGTON, E. K. and SHALLICE, T. (1979). Semantic access dyslexia. *Brain* **102**, 43-64.

WARRINGTON, E. K. and TAYLOR, A. M. (1973). The contribution of the right parietal lobe to object recognition. *Cortex* **9**, 152-164.

WARRINGTON, E. K. and TAYLOR, A. M. (1978). Two categorical stages of object recognition. *Perception* **7**, 695-705.

WEBSTER, W. G. and THURBER, A. D., (1978). Problem-solving strategies and manifest brain asymmetry. *Cortex* **14**, 474-484.

WEINSTEIN, S. (1968). Intensive and extensive aspects of tactile sensitivity as a function of body part, sex and laterality. In *The Skin Senses* (D. R. Kenshalo, ed.), pp.195-222. Thomas, Springfield, Ill.

WHITE, M. J. (1972). Hemispheric asymmetries in tachistoscopic information processing. *British Journal of Psychology* **63**, 497-508.

WILKINS, A. and MOSCOVITCH, M. (1978). Selective impairment of semantic memory after temporal lobectomy. *Neuropsychologia* **16**, 73-79.

WILSON, D. H., REEVES, A., CULVER, C. and GAZZANIGA, M. S. (1977). Cerebral commissurotomy for control of intractable seizures. *Neurology* **27**, 708-715.

WITELSON, S. F. (1974). Hemispheric specialization for linguistic and nonlinguistic tactual perception using a dichotomous stimulation technique. *Cortex* **10**, 3-17.

WYKE, M. and ETTLINGER, G. (1961). Efficiency of recognition in left and right visual fields: its relation to the phenomenon of visual extinction. *Archives of Neurology* **5**, 659-665.

YOUNG, A. W. (1982). Methodological and theoretical bases of visual hemifield studies. In *Divided Visual Field Studies of Cerebral Organisation* (J. G. Beaumont, ed.), pp.11-27. Academic Press, London and New York.

YOUNG, A. W. and BION, P. J. (1979). Hemispheric laterality effects in the enumeration of visually presented collections of dots by children. *Neuropsychologia* **17**, 99-102.

YOUNG, A. W. and BION, P. J. (1981). Identification and storage of line drawings presented to the left and right cerebral hemispheres of adults and children. *Cortex* **17**, 459-463.

YOUNG, A. W. and ELLIS, A. W. (1979). Perception of numerical stimuli felt by fingers of the left and right hands. *Quarterly Journal of Experimental Psychology* **31**, 263-272.

YOUNG, A. W., BION, P. J. and ELLIS, A. W. (1980). Studies toward a model of laterality effects for picture and word naming. *Brain and Language* **11**, 54-65.

ZAIDEL, D. and SPERRY, R. W. (1974). Memory impairment after commissurotomy in man. *Brain* **97**, 263-272.

ZAIDEL, E. (1975). A technique for presenting lateralized visual input with prolonged exposure. *Vision Research* **15**, 283-289.

ZAIDEL, E. (1976). Auditory vocabulary of the right hemisphere following brain bisection or hemidecortication. *Cortex* **12**, 191-211.

ZAIDEL, E. (1977). Unilateral auditory language comprehension in the Token Test following cerebral commissurotomy and hemispherectomy. *Neuropsychologia* **15**, 1-18.

ZAIDEL, E. (1978). Auditory language comprehension in the right hemisphere following cerebral commissurotomy and hemispherectomy: a comparison with child language and aphasia. In *Acquisition and Breakdown of Language, Parallels and Divergences* (A. Caramazza and E. Zurif, eds). John Hopkins Press, Baltimore.

ZAIDEL, D. and SPERRY, R. W. (1974). Memory impairment after commissurotomy in man. *Brain* **97**, 263-272.

2

THE ROLE OF THE RIGHT HEMISPHERE IN FACE PERCEPTION

Hadyn D. Ellis

Introduction

THE LAST decade has witnessed a decided upsurge of interest in the face as a psychological stimulus. Basically interest has concerned the three main functions of a face, which are: 1) to serve as the principal means of discriminating among individuals; (2) to act as the chief source of information concerning a person's emotional state; and 3) to provide other, non-verbal communications which may or may not concord with the verbal message. Experiments exploring the many aspects of perceiving and remembering facial differences are reviewed by Ellis (1975, 1981), Clifford and Bull (1978), Baddeley (1979), Davies (1979), Yarmey (1979) and Hay and Young (1982). Reviews of the equally fascinating expressive functions of faces may be found in Frijda (1970), Izard (1971), Ekman *et al.*, (1972), and Salzen (1981). Argyle and Cook (1976) discuss the face as a non-verbal source of communication.

Many theoretical positions have been adopted regarding particularly the discrimination of faces and the interpretations made of the expressions they convey; these involve a range of approaches from the biological to the cognitive. The present chapter is concerned with general neuro-psychological aspects of face research, and, in particular, it is devoted to reviewing the evidence linking the more efficient processing of facial information, both physical and emotional, to the right hemisphere.

As we shall see, the literature in this field is not entirely consistent; there are

FUNCTIONS OF THE RIGHT CEREBRAL HEMISPHERE
0-12-773250-0 *Copyright © 1983 by Academic Press, London.
All rights of reproduction in any form reserved.*

apparent discrepancies, sometimes among similar kinds of studies and sometimes between the different kinds of evidence that arise from clinical and laboratory investigations. In many instances it is possible to resolve what appear to be contradictory results, but inevitably some conflicting findings remain unresolved.

Any discussion of the fact that normally the two cortical hemispheres of the brain act in a concerted, integrated fashion will largely be postponed until the end of the chapter. In the meantime much of the discussion will ignore this important consideration; instead, the right and left hemispheres will be treated provisionally as if they were separate and independent processors of information.

The argument of the main portion of the chapter takes a dialectical form in which the *thesis* that the right hemisphere is unequivocally superior to the left hemisphere in perceiving and remembering faces will be examined; the *antithesis* (though strictly intermediate position) that there is no unequivocal hemisphere asymmetry in face-processing capabilities will then be presented; and finally a *synthesis* will be attempted whereby the particular superiorities of the right hemisphere in dealing with facial stimuli will be discussed and evaluated.

Evidence for Right Hemisphere Superiority

Prosopagnosia

One of the earliest observations of right hemisphere involvement in perceiving and remembering faces was made by Hughlings Jackson: he cited the case of a woman with a right hemisphere tumour who displayed difficulties in recognising people (Levy, 1980). A subsequent report by Wilbrand (1892) confirmed the suspicion that the right hemisphere might specialise in memory for faces, as well as in the processing of other non-verbal material.

This connection was largely ignored until comparatively recently when interest developed in the clinical condition which Bodamer (1947) labelled as *prosopagnosia*. This is a rare symptom usually following brain damage in which the patient loses the ability to recognise familiar people on the basis of physiognomic information; instead he has to rely on other visual cues such as dress, gait and distinguishing marks, or to recognise someone from his or her voice (Charcot, 1883; Hoff and Potzl, 1937; Bodamer, 1947; Bornstein, 1963). In one reported case, however, prosopagnosia followed a developmental course and there was some evidence for it being a familial characteristic (McConachie, 1976). Hécaen (1981) has recently argued that there are at least three distinct types of prosopagnosia involving: 1) perceptual difficulties; 2) perceptual distortions (metamorphosia); or 3) disturbance of face memory. Most investigators, however, have treated it as a unitary condition requiring a single explanation. Unfortunately, there is insufficient opportunity in this review to explore prosopagnosia in its various forms, but it is worth bearing in mind that the syndrome should properly be treated as a plural rather than a singular condition.

Divisions exist not only over the symptoms of prosopagnosia, but also concerning its likely causes. Some have argued that it arises from damage to a mechanism that has evolved specifically to process faces (Tzavaras et al., 1970; Whiteley and Warrington, 1977; Geschwind, 1979). Others, on the other hand, have pointed out that prosopagnosia rarely occurs without other symptoms, such as colour agnosia or loss of topographical memory, (Pallis, 1955; Beyn and Knyazeva, 1962; Cole and Perez-Cruet, 1964; Cohn et al., 1974). Additionally, prosopagnosic patients sometimes display difficulties in distinguishing individual exemplars among complex visual objects other than faces, which suggests that the condition may be a manifestation of damage to a more general, higher-order visual recognition system (Faust, 1947; De Renzi et al., 1969; Bornstein et al., 1969; Lhermitte et al., 1972). The latter view avoids the notion of there being an area of the brain with the specific and sole function of processing faces. This debate is discussed more fully elsewhere (Meadows, 1974; Ellis, 1975, 1981; Yin, 1978; Benton, 1980; Kolb and Wishaw, 1980; Hay and Young, 1982).

The present significance of the issue as to whether prosopagnosia is a symptom of damage to a face-specific area of the brain arises in connection with a retrospective survey of 22 prosopagnosic patients conducted by Hécaen and Angelergues (1962). They discovered that 73% of these cases involved unilateral right hemisphere lesions; 17% of the patients had bilateral lesions; and in only 10% of the cases was unilateral left hemisphere damage suspected. This survey indicates fairly strong evidence for right hemisphere involvement in face recognition.

Brain Damage

Further support for the suggestion of a particular role for the right hemisphere in processing faces came from a number of studies in which patients with left and right unilateral brain lesions were compared on face memory tasks. Milner (1968) examined post-operative patients, 26 following left-sided temporal lobectomy and 21 following right-sided temporal lobectomy, and discovered that, provided a short delay occurred between presentation and test, there was a small but significant advantage to the left impaired groups. With no intervening interval the right lobectomy patients were significantly poorer at recognising faces than were control-subjects, but not significantly worse than the left temporal lobectomy patients. Similar results were reported by De Renzi and his associates in their various studies of patients with unilateral brain injury

(De Renzi and Spinnler, 1966; De Renzi et al., 1968, 1969). Benton and Van Allan (1968) also noted that right hemisphere disease was more closely related than left hemisphere disease to impairment in facial recognition. Yin (1970) then claimed that this relative impairment is only true for upright face tests. His right hemisphere damaged group was unimpaired relative to controls on a test involving inverted faces. By contrast the left damaged group was markedly impaired at the inverted-faces task. The ability of unilaterally damaged patients to cope with more usual facial transformations (e.g. changes in expression, disguise, lighting) was examined by Tzavaras et al. (1970). In contrast to Yin, they found that their right-damaged patients had considerably more difficulty than the controls and left-damaged groups in picking out a face transformed in such natural or everyday fashions.

Commissurotomy Studies

Another source of evidence for a right hemisphere superiority at recognising faces comes from that special category of commissurotomised patients studied by Sperry and his associates. Levy et al. (1972) presented chimaeric faces (i.e. left half of one face and the right half of another face) tachistoscopically. This ensured that the left 'face' went to the patient's right hemisphere and the right 'face' to the left hemisphere. When asked to select, by pointing, which face had been presented from a small array of faces, the overwhelming choice was for the one shown to the right hemisphere. Milner and Dunne (1977) and Schwartz and Smith (1980) found similar, though less dramatic effects, when chimaeric face stimuli were briefly presented to normal subjects. In both studies there was a tendency for subjects to report that they had seen the 'face' appearing in the left visual field (LVF), that is, the face that arrived initially at the right hemisphere (provided subjects fixated the mid-line of the two face halves). There was also a comparative failure to acknowledge the right hand face.

Tachistoscopic Studies

During the last decade cerebral asymmetries in face identification have been extensively investigated using tachistoscopic exposures to normal subjects, who are usually required to make a binary discrimination response. Many of these studies have revealed a LVF advantage both for speed of response (Rizzolatti et al., 1971; Geffen et al., 1971, 1972; St. John 1979) and for accuracy of response (Hilliard, 1973; Ellis and Shepherd, 1975; Klein et al., 1976; Hines, 1978).

The speed or accuracy superiority for processing face stimuli falling in the LVF has been considered fairly robust, being evident despite variations among studies in: the total number of stimuli used; the use of bilateral or unilateral presentation; the types of facial representation employed (photographs or drawings, colour or monochrome); presentation duration (8 ms to 400 ms); interstimulus interval (500 ms to 20 s); subject variables (age and sex); and diversities in the size of stimuli used, their eccentricity (or distance from the fixation point), and the luminance levels in the tachistoscope; as well as variations in instructions to subjects, etc. that are almost bound to exist from one study to the next. Some of these are discussed more fully in a recent review of this area by Sergent and Bindra (1981).

The LVF advantage has also been reported when long-term memory mechanisms are assumed to be involved. Both Jones (1979a) and Finlay and French (1978) adopted a procedure whereby subjects first saw a long series of faces, then much later observed them individually along with new faces presented in a tachistoscope and reported as to whether or not each was familiar. In both studies a significant LVF superiority was found. As Jones (1979a) points out, this experimental paradigm is rather more like the ones employed with brain-damaged patients than are those involving short-term storage of facial images for comparison with a test face.

All of the studies reviewed so far have favoured the view that the right hemisphere has an advantage over the left hemisphere in the reception and/or storage of faces. As I mentioned earlier, some researchers would go further and argue that this superiority arises from the location of a specific facial processing system in the right hemisphere. Others, however, would prefer to view the asymmetry as arising from a more general right hemisphere superiority in analysing visuospatial information. Right hemisphere damage also impairs recognition of objects other than faces (De Renzi and Spinnler, 1966; Kolb and Wishaw, 1980). Commissurotomised patients also manually select the left half of other non-verbal stimuli (Levy et al., 1972). As for tachistoscopic studies using normal subjects, again there is an abundance of evidence that tasks such as dot detection (Davidoff, 1977), dot localisation (Bryden, 1976), telling time from a clock face (Brizzolara et al., 1975), discriminating between pictures of shoes (St. John, 1979), and discriminating complex and geometrical figures (Umilta et al., 1978a) all display a LVF advantage. Furthermore, depth perception (Kimura and Durnford, 1974), and simple sensory discrimination (Davidoff, 1975) have been found to be better carried out when stimuli are presented in the LVF.

Studies using non-facial visual stimuli, however, have always been less consistent in their findings, especially where verbal labels are easily supplied for the stimuli. Similarly, inconsistency has arisen when inverted faces have been presented tachistoscopically. Ellis and Shepherd (1975) found a LVF advantage for both upright and inverted faces, but a later experiment by Leehey et al. (1978) failed to replicate the asymmetry for inverted faces; and studies reported by Young and Bion (1980; 1981) also found the LVF advantgage only for upright faces. Leehey et al. (1978) have suggested that, because in the Ellis and Shepherd experiment the presentation duration was very brief (15 ms), the faces may have been processed as patterns rather than faces. This explanation, however, is unlikely: many studies have employed equally brief presentations simply in order to make the test reasonably difficult. Discriminability is also a function of size, illumination and eccentricity of stimuli, and so it is usually not possible for one investigator to comment meaningfully on the identifiability of the stimuli used by another. It seems to me that a more likely explanation for the discrepancy in results lies in the observation that the recognition of inverted faces is very much dependent on how similar they are to one another. Bradshaw *et al.* (1980) have shown that, when discriminations are easy, recognition tasks are faster for stimuli presented in the LVF, regardless as to stimulus category (schematic faces *v* schematic houses) or orientation (upright faces *v* inverted faces). It is probably significant that Ellis and Shepherd did not find the usual overall superior performance on upright compared with inverted faces — perhaps because the faces employed were rather dissimilar and therefore equivalent to Bradshaw *et al.*'s easily discriminated schematic stimuli. The lack of any metric for evaluating and comparing across studies the difficulty of the face recognition tasks employed is a stumbling block to progress in the whole area, not least in the field of asymmetry. This problem is discussed and one possible solution to it presented by Davies, *et al.* (1979).

Evidence Against Right Hemisphere Superiority

If research on cerebral asymmetry in processing faces had stopped in the early-to-mid 1970s, we would probably all happily accept that the right hemisphere is better adapted for processing complex patterns, such as faces. This belief is attractive because such an advantage could easily be seen as compensation for the left hemisphere's dominance in linguistic processing (see Gazzaniga and Le Doux, 1978).

However, research did not stop. Instead there was an increase in activity and occasionally people reported that they had failed to demonstrate a LVF/right hemisphere superiority in perceiving or remembering faces. How many others also could not replicate the effect we shall never know accurately, but we can assume that there are a number of negative results gathering dust in laboratories throughout the world. I must confess that I was only alerted to this possibility when two postgraduate students working with me found persistent difficulty in replicating some of my own results (Hay, 1978; Freeman, 1980). I will have more to say about their work shortly. In the meantime let us examine other results that are inconsistent with the simple asymmetry for face processing detailed in the previous section.

Prosopagnosia and Other Brain Disorders

One of the most significant investigations on this topic was published by Meadows (1974) in which he reviewed much of the evidence on prosopagnosia, with particular emphasis on post-mortem findings. According to his analysis, in all seven cases that came to necropsy, there was evidence for damage to the right occipitotemporal area, and in most cases there was an approximately symmetrical lesion in the left hemisphere. He further argues that in every case there was evidence of bilateral disease.

The presence of left hemisphere damage is easily overlooked. Newcombe (1979) reports a case in which unilateral right posterior damage was first diagnosed; left parietal damage was only later found, however, when, on the basis of Meadows' review, it was carefully looked for in a brain scan. There are also other cases where bilateral damage has either been noted or suspected in patients showing prosopagnosia (Pallis, 1955; Beyn and Knyazeva, 1962; Gloning et al., 1966). An additional consideration worth noting is that, in a few cases, prosopagnosia has been found in right handed patients with apparent unilateral left hemisphere pathology (Cole and Perez-Cruet, 1964; Agnetti et al., 1978). Thus the earlier belief that prosopagnosia results exclusively from right hemisphere damage must now be questioned.

It should be noted that there are no reported studies relating general left hemisphere damage to a specific impairment in face memory greater than that found for those with comparable right hemisphere damage. There is work of marginal relevance, however, involving temporary hemisphere impairment. Berent (1977) investigated face memory among patients undergoing unilateral electroconvulsive therapy (ECT). He found in one experiment that left sided ECT led to an increase both in errors and response latency when patients were required to select a face for its similarity to a target face in terms of emotional expression. In a second experiment, though, Berent required his patients to identify a face shown before ECT from an array of three faces. Here right ECT proved detrimental to performance. Berent (1981) argues that these results indicate bilateral involvement in face processing, with any asymmetry dependent upon the particular task and processing strategies employed. He mentions the possibility of the left hemisphere using verbal mediation in encoding, say, facial expression. This is interesting in view of the fact that, although Hamsher et al. (1979) found the usual association between right hemisphere damage and face processing tasks, they also observed left-damaged patients with aphasia to show equally poor performance. Benton (1980) argues that verbal strategies in face processing may be important and that this is one possible explanation of the Hamsher et al. results. It should be said, however, that there is little evidence to favour verbal mediation in face processing (Ellis, 1975; Sergent and Bindra, 1981).

Levy *et al.* (1972) in their experiments on patients with sectioned corpora callosa mentioned earlier also observed that, when the task involved naming chimaeric faces, there was a strong tendency to identify the one falling in the right visual field (RVF). Interestingly, they also found that these patients had great difficulty in learning to associate names and faces. Gazzaniga *et al.* (1977) insist that all one can rightfully conclude from these data is that the two cerebral hemispheres perform equally well at recognising faces. This view is shared by Sergent and Bindra (1981) who conclude that while there may be differences in processing strategies, the left and right hemispheres are more or less equivalent in their abilities to process faces, provided the input is not too degraded or briefly presented. Interestingly, Sperry *et al.* (1979) have demonstrated in split-brain patients equivalent capabilities of the two hemispheres both in person identification and in attachment of appropriate emotional responses to particular faces. This work involved a novel technique using a semi-occluded contact lens for allowing prolonged inspection of the faces while restricting input to one hemiretina and, therefore, to a single hemisphere.

Tachistoscopic Studies

A number of investigators have recently reported difficulty in replicating the tachistoscopic LVF superiority for face processing reviewed earlier. Generally, they have found no VF differences (Bradshaw *et al.*, 1976; Hay, 1978; Hannay and Rogers, 1979; Berteleson *et al.*, 1979; Freeman, 1980; Galper and Costa, 1980; McKeever and Dixon, 1981).

In some circumstances, however, a RVF advantage has been observed. Patterson and Bradshaw (1975), using schematic faces, found that whereas 'easy' discriminations revealed a LVF advantage, 'difficult' discriminations (i.e. only one facial feature different in each case) were more easily made when stimuli fell in the RVF. This effect is modified somewhat when 'easy' and 'difficult' trials are randomly mixed (Bradshaw *et al.*, 1980).

Marzi and Berlucchi (1977) found a RVF advantage in recognising famous faces. This study will be considered at length later on but its relevance to the present discussion is that the authors explain their finding by suggesting that under impoverished viewing conditions subjects may make identifications based on a single feature—a process they see as parallel to that in the Patterson and Bradshaw (1975) 'difficult' discrimination condition. Sergent and Bindra (1981) give an excellent analysis of these kinds of observations. They conclude that only under impoverished viewing conditions does a LVF advantage occur at all. They further claim that in most tachistoscopic studies, in order to allow the necessary brief exposures, faces are chosen so as to be highly discriminable which favours a wholistic right hemisphere strategy; this is a debatable observation in the light of our earlier discussion on the recognition of inverted faces, but it underlines the need for some kind of universally accepted face metric. The views of Sergent and Bindra will be further considered in the next section.

In a rather different type of experiment from the ones reviewed so far, Jones (1979b) found a RVF advantage for male subjects only in discriminating faces into the categories male and female. The question of sex differences in VF effects has generally attracted much interest (see McGlone, 1980). In research using face stimuli some have observed a LVF effect for male subjects only (Rizzolatti and Buchtel, 1977), while others have found no sex differences (e.g. Hannay and Rogers, 1979; Freeman, 1980). Moreover, Hilliard (1973) who was one of the first investigators to publish a LVF accuracy superiority, used only female subjects. In view of the inconsistent nature of the sex by VF interaction no more will be made of the matter: to attempt to resolve it would require a digression into methodological issues that are outwith the scope of this chapter. It is sufficient to note, in the present context, that the traditional view of a LVF superiority in processing faces may not obtain for both sexes under all testing situations (Rizzolatti and Buchtel, 1977). This caveat will be encountered again when I later discuss laterality for the perception of emotional expressions.

The problem of individual differences in the phenomenon of asymmetry in face processing has been looked at in a variety of other ways. Benton (1980), for example, simply observes that examination of reported LVF effects reveals some heterogeneity among subjects. For example, in Hilliard's (1973) study, despite a significant overall LVF superiority, five of his 20 strongly right-handed subjects showed a RVF advantage in face recognition. This suggests that a sizeable minority of subjects adopt a very different strategy for processing faces from that favoured by most subjects.

Galper and Costa (1980) examined such individual differences in some detail. They presented subjects with a series of faces that were either described in social terms (personality, main qualities and colour preferences) or in physical terms (hair, eyes, shape of face). Later the faces were mixed with new faces and presented tachistoscopically in either the LVF or RVF. Galper and Costa found that their subjects could be divided into two groups: those who displayed more accurate LVF performance following 'social' information about the face, and better RVF performance following physical information; and those subjects who showed the reverse pattern of performance. It would seem that individual strategies can be an important factor in facial VF effects. If subjects *implicitly* adopt idiosyncratic strategies, the net effect in any particular experiment would be no VF differences because some may adopt 'LVF strategies' and some 'RVF strategies'. Further work confirming the lability of asymmetry for face processing, depending on instructions etc., has recently been published by Proudfoot (1982).

In summary, the work reviewed in this section has been selected to show just how erroneous it is simply to ascribe superior facial processing to the minor hemisphere. The dominant hemisphere may equal or even supercede it, particularly when the task requires fine or analytic discriminations or, perhaps less persuasively where verbal mediation is involved. Additionally, individual strategies must be considered, and, when possible, exposed for analysis. This is not necessarily to deny completely the earlier thesis that the right hemisphere may under most circumstances display superior performance, but the argument requires clarification and modification. After all, as Teuber (1978) pointed out, even following complete removal of the right hemisphere, face recognition is still possible. And according to Strauss and Verity (personal communication) there is no difference in face recognition ability between patients who have undergone right hemispherectomy and those who have undergone left hemispherectomy.

Nonetheless, in the next section I will attempt to identify more specifically the distinctive role of the right hemisphere in perceiving and remembering facial identity and expression. In a sense this will constitute a process of synthesis in which two alternative views, that the right hemisphere is unequivocally superior in processing faces and that the two hemispheres are equipotential in this respect, will be qualified. There will also be a slight shift in emphasis of evidence: the bulk of the work now to be considered has been accomplished using tachistoscopic procedures on normal subjects.

Synthesis

It should be clear by now that one cannot talk in terms of an absolute superiority for right hemisphere processing of faces. However, despite the undoubted ability of the left hemisphere to deal with physiognomic configurations, most of the hemisphere differences reported have favoured the right hemisphere (or left visual field of presentation). In the remainder of this chapter I shall explore the various factors that might underly any such hemispheric asymmetry.

Model of Face Processing

Figure 1 illustrates a simple flow-diagram model of the processes that may underlie face processing. It is offered as a heuristic model; it may not be entirely accurate, but it does serve conceptually to isolate certain stages that I believe are essential to any successful face-recognition system. Furthermore, the model is drawn so as to indicate, roughly, which of the subprocesses are likely to be better conducted in the right hemisphere; those for which the cerebral hemispheres may be equipotential (though not necessarily qualitatively identical); and the one stage, naming, for which there may be a left hemisphere superiority. The present model is an elaboration of the two-stage model suggested in my previous reviews of face memory (Ellis, 1975, 1981), and owes much to the models recently

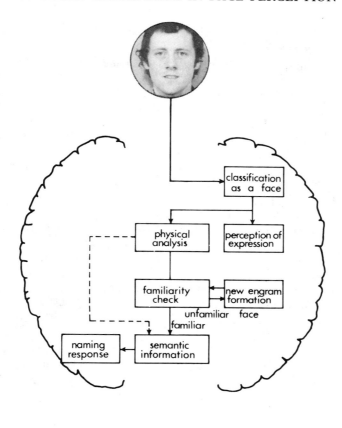

LEFT   HEMISPHERE   RIGHT   HEMISPHERE

Fig 1. Heuristic model of face processing roughly indicating: the subprocesses for which there may be a right hemisphere advantage; the subprocesses equally well conducted by both hemispheres (though, probably involving rather different strategies); and the one response process, naming, for which there is relatively unequivocal evidence of a left hemisphere superiority.

suggested by Bruce (1979) and Hay and Young (1982). It also takes account of the suggestion made by Ellis *et al.* (1979) that familiar and unfamiliar faces are processed in rather different ways, with the central or expressive facial features being more salient for familiar faces whereas peripheral features are equally important for the identification of relatively unfamiliar faces.

A. Classification

For a pattern to be processed as a face, it must first be classified as such—a process which Rosch *et al.* (1976) describe as assignment to a basic level category. The input may then proceed to a subordinate level of processing. Failure to gain appropriate initial assignment means that the input will not benefit from the existing schemata, or cognitive structures, that enable a deep level of processing to take place. The richness of the schemata will vary according to the significance of the material. It is not clear whether every object category enjoys distinctive classification or whether, as Konorski (1967) has suggested, objects are grouped by certain shared characteristics and are handled by a correspondingly smaller number of what he terms 'gnostic units'.

The importance of initial categorisation is illustrated by an experiment performed by Wiseman and Neisser (1974). They presented subjects with the patterns devised by Mooney (1957), which are sometimes quite difficult to perceive as faces, and subsequently found a high rate of recognition only for those patterns in which the subjects could perceive a face.

No one has yet employed the Mooney faces in laterality experiments, but Newcombe (1974) in a study of patients with unilateral penetration wounds, did find that those with right hemisphere damage had greater difficulty than those with left hemisphere damage at perceiving faces in the patterns.

Hay (1981) has also performed an experiment of relevance to the question of classification. He tachistoscopically displayed line-drawings of 'faces' in the LVF or RVF. The 'faces' were either normal or had the position of internal features scrambled. Subjects were required to classify as rapidly as possible each input either as a face or as a non-face. While there was no apparent asymmetry in accuracy, Hay found a significant LVF advantage in speed of response. This result, together with Newcombe's observations suggests that the right hemisphere has an advantage in the early classification of patterns to the category faces.

B. Physical analysis

Following the successful allocation of a pattern to the face category, it is hypothesised that the next stages involve analyses of its physical attributes and emotional expression. The latter process will be subsequently examined in a separate section.

The physical analysis stage might involve a number of separate processes and could be conducted differently by the two hemispheres. It has been conventional to argue that the left hemisphere performs an analytic type of processing in which facial features are checked separately. The right hemisphere, on the other hand, is thought to analyse faces in a wholistic manner (Patterson and Bradshaw, 1975; Bradshaw *et al.*, 1980). Attractive though they are, there is no good reason either to accept or to reject these suggestions. Indeed, the related dichotomy put forward by Cohen (1973), to the effect that the left hemisphere is a serial processor and the right hemisphere a parallel processor of information, has run into some difficulty. Polich (1978) concluded that both hemispheres analysed input serially; and White and White (1975) decided that both favoured a parallel mode of processing. These and other empirical inconsistencies make it difficult to accept unequivocally Cohen's suggested dichotomy. Whether the hemispheres do differ in the ways that they analyse the physical properties of a face must remain an open question, though, as we have already seen and will see again, the idea helps to explain many apparently inconsistent or contradictory data.

Some as yet unpublished work by Freeman (1980) may be of relevance to the issue. She compared VF asymmetries for photographs of faces, highly detailed line tracings of the same faces, and low-detailed tracings of the faces, examples of which are shown in Fig. 2. Twenty-four subjects were presented with a face in one of the three modes from a set of 20 faces randomly falling in either VF for 15 ms. This was followed 3 s later by a comparison face in the same mode shown

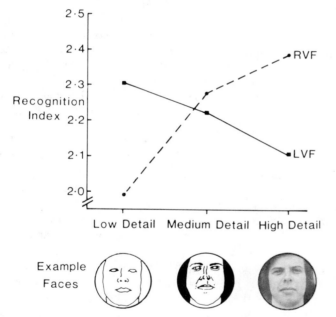

FIG. 2. Data from a study by Freeman (1980). The recognition index is an arc sine transformation of A prime scores (a non-parametric detection sensitivity measure).

for 3 s in centre field. The accuracy of subjects' same/different vocal responses revealed the interesting pattern also shown in Fig. 2. There was a significant interaction between VF and mode caused by a) photographs being better matched following RVF presentation; and b) the low information, outline faces being more accurately discriminated following LVF presentation. The finding that low information faces are better processed when falling in the LVF was replicated no less than three times by Freemand and thus must be considered a robust phenomenon. The finding of a RVF advantage for photographed faces, however, did not emerge in Freeman's other experiments and, consequently, will not be considered further.

One possible explanation for Freeman's results is that faces containing low detail or minimal information lend themselves more readily to analysis as a whole and are less easily fragmented into separate features. There is no obvious way that this suggestion can be verified but it has the merit of fitting the rather general notions of hemispheric processing strategies for faces mentioned earlier (Levy *et al.*, 1972; Patterson and Bradshaw, 1975). It is also in keeping with the questionable idea that the right hemisphere specialises in wholistic or gestalt perceptual analysis (Nebes, 1971). Furthermore, it corresponds to the ideas subsequently advanced by Sergent and Bindra (1981) that have already been mentioned. They are firmly of the opinion that the right hemisphere can make rapid, wholistic analyses of faces seen under impoverished viewing conditions, and argue that when stimuli are such as to favour this type of processing a LVF advantage will be found. It may be worth adding that Matthews (1978) has provided some evidence that face perception may involve a rapid general analysis of the outline followed by a serial analysis of the internal features. The possibility that those two processes are dominated in turn by the right and left hemispheres merits further exploration.

A slightly different explanation of Freeman's data is that the LVF/right hemisphere combination is superior only when the faces used in an experiment are difficult to discriminate. Reducing facial detail certainly appears to increase the similarity among the set of faces used by Freeman, and it is quite possible that her results arose from a right hemisphere advantage only evident under conditions where the faces to be discriminated are highly similar.

Freeman herself tested this idea by arranging pairs of photographed faces to be either very similar or dissimilar. Judgements of the similarity of the faces were obtained in another experiment (for details see Davies *et al.*, 1979). In Freeman's experiment pairs of faces randomly occurred which were either identical or different; when different, the decision was either fairly easy or quite difficult.

The results indicated no VF difference in accuracy for 'different' decisions regardless of whether the discriminations were easy or difficult. Overall, the former were more accurate than the latter but this did not interact with VF. Similar results have also been reported by Young and Bion (1980), and it would seem therefore that the difficulty of discriminating among faces is not a useful basis for distinguishing the contribution of the left and right hemispheres in processing faces. Moreover, the stimulus-mode effect found by Freeman cannot be simply explained by appealing to a superior right hemisphere capacity for discerning differences between similar pairs of faces. This conclusion is somewhat at variance with that reached by Sergent and Bindra (1981). They argue that the right hemisphere may have an advantage on easy discriminations because it can employ a fast wholistic analysis. They are less precise as to the processing mechanism of the left hemisphere, except to deny that it involves any linguistic mediation. The corollary to their argument, however, is that decisions involving pairs of dissimilar faces should yield a LVF superiority. In Freeman's experiment using photographs of real faces this result was not found. Perhaps Sergent and Bindra's ideas arise from considering experiments where artificial faces have been used that, under some circumstances, lend themselves more easily to piecemeal analysis. The problem of drawing inferences from studies employing such artificial stimuli is explored more fully elsewhere (Ellis, 1981).

C. Representation

The mental representation of a face varies over time, with internal features fading more rapidly than external ones (Walker-Smith, 1978). According to Moscovitch et al. (1976) any right hemisphere advantage in face processing occurs only if memory is involved. They found that simultaneous pairs of photographed faces were compared equally well when presented together in either visual field. When one member of the pair had to be retained longer than 50 ms, however, a LVF advantage was observed. Moscovitch et al. argue that this is due to the right hemisphere being more able to form an abstract representation of a face and thus functioning better in the memory situation. The two hemispheres, they claim, are equally capable of making decisions on the basis of early, precategorical information. This explanation is challenged by Sergent and Bindra (1981), however, and it is worth noting that Strauss and Moscovitch (unpub.) themselves found a LVF advantage for simultaneously presented pairs of faces, as did St John (1979).

The significance of longer term memory factors in asymmetry for processing faces may be seen from work completed by Hay (1978, see also Hay and Ellis, 1981). Hay used a Sternberg-type task, in which 10 subjects were given a fixed positive set of one, two or four faces and had then to decide whether or not a given test face, randomly presented in one or other visual field, was a member of the positive set. The findings were quite interesting; when test faces occurred in the LVF there was a significant latency advantage over RVF presentation for positive judgements only. Negative decisions (i.e. target not a member of the set) were made equally quickly following presentation in either visual field.

However, when the procedure was changed so that the positive set was variable and thus had to be learned afresh before each trial, Hay found much faster responses when targets occurred in the LVF, regardless as to whether the decision was positive or negative. Furthermore, analysis of the first experiment, involving a fixed positive set, indicated a LVF advantage for both positive and negative decisions in the first half of the trials, arguably before the left hemisphere had developed as robust a representation of this positive set. Together these observations have been interpreted by Hay and Ellis (1981) as indicating that the right hemisphere is faster than the left hemisphere at constructing mental representations of faces that can be accessed when making decisions concerning facial familiarity. The left hemisphere is slower to achieve these; and it may be particularly slow to establish representations that assist identity matches rather than those which favour the detection of differences (cf. Bradshaw *et al.*, 1980).

Memory factors in cerebral asymmetries for processing faces are probably quite important. Prosopagnosic patients often appear to have little difficulty matching simultaneously presented faces (Benton and Van Allen, 1972); instead their problems arise when trying to match a face to one held in long-term memory. This deficit has also been observed in right hemisphere damaged patients not diagnosed as suffering from prosopagnosia (Warrington and James, 1967; Milner, 1968).

Elsewhere I have discussed the fact that any mental representation of another person's face is unlikely to be of a simple, static view (Ellis, 1981). Rather our knowledge of each face is the result of experiencing it from a variety of angles, in a number of contexts, and, particularly in the case of celebrities, via different media. Each of these inputs can ultimately lead to a feeling of familiarity and be followed by the relevant semantic information about the person.

The stage labelled 'familiarity check' in Fig. 1 is here conceived as analogous to the logogen model of word recognition proposed by Morton (1969) and also adopted by Hay and Young (1982) in their model of face recognition. The units corresponding to known faces are able to respond to their appropriate inputs despite the uniqueness of each encounter. The units may be pre-set for lowered thresholds by contextual cues or other relevant information, and they are probably tuned by experience so as to make correct familiarity discriminations on less and less sensory evidence.

Novel faces are not just discarded as unknown; rather a new unit is established which is incorporated into the corpus of known faces, albeit in a relatively raw or unsophisticated form. Should the same picture of the new person be encountered, there is a reasonable chance that it will be recognised as being familiar. The greater the delay, or the less similar the circumstances of the second encounter, the more likely the input will be incorrectly assigned to the 'unfamiliar' category. We are actually quite good at retaining information about photographs of strangers' faces, and can successfully cope with certain changes in pose between first and second encounters (Ellis, 1981). This facility does not extend to other-race faces (Ellis and Deregowski, 1981).

Bertelson and his associates investigated the idea that there may be a hemisphere asymmetry in the ability to deal with faces transformed by pose or expression between presentation and test (Bertelson and Vanhaelen, unpub.;

Bertelson *et al.*, 1979). They performed two experiments which are well worth considering in detail. In one experiment they gave a group of eight subjects the usual task of making speeded 'same' or 'different' judgements of pairs of faces that were either identical pictures of the same face or pictures of two different individuals; the first face of each pair was presented centrally and the second occurred randomly in the LVF or RVF. The second group of eight subjects were required to make 'same' judgements when the test picture was of the same person but taken from a different angle. The only significant VF effect was observed for the latencies of subjects in the second group. Here a small but consistent advantage in processing time was found when the test face occurred in the LVF.

In another experiment Bertelson and Vanhaelen (unpub.) examined both change in pose and change in expression (smiling first, neutral second). Both conditions produced faster LVF responses, with the expression change causing a significantly larger effect. The inference drawn by the authors from these data is that there is a left hemifield advantage in the extraction of feature invariants from faces. This becomes evident under conditions of some change between target and test and, as we have also seen in this chapter (p.40) when two identical pictures of a person have to be matched, there may be no difference between the VFs.

In terms of the face-processing model shown in Fig. 1, the right hemisphere is either more adept at constructing a robust internal representation capable of recognising a variation in the input, or it is quicker at transforming the novel picture into a form that enables a successful search in the face memory store to be achieved.

D. Familiar faces

So far we have largely concentrated on the recognition of faces that a subject encounters for the first time in the laboratory. The results of Hay and Ellis (1981) suggest that, in experiments where subjects rapidly attempt to match a probe face to any one of a fixed set of faces held in memory, a LVF advantage may occur initially. Once the set of faces used becomes relatively familiar, however, the VF asymmetry appears to become modified so that it is evident only for positive decisions. Negative decisions (i.e. probe not found in the memory set) are made equally quickly from either VF. Indeed, in an experiment reported by Umilta *et al.* (1978b) subjects were given photographs of the four faces to be used in a laterality study four days later. Some subjects were urged to look at the pictures regularly in order to become familiar with them; others were also given names to assign to the faces. Both procedures led to a reversal in the usual asymmetry, with shorter latencies in assigning two faces to one response button and two faces to another button being found following RVF presentations. Two further groups of subjects were tested who were not shown the face prior to the practice session for the experiment. Overall, both displayed the usual LVF superiority, despite the fact that one group learned to associate names with the faces. Curiously, these groups did not change laterality over the four experimental sessions when it would be expected that the 40 encounters with each face every day would lead to the development of an increased sense of familiarity with the four faces. Another surprising feature of the data was that there was no difference in VF effects between the group who learned to name the faces and the group who simply became familiar with their features.

Marzi and Berlucchi (1977) found a similar reversal in the usual VF asymmetry in a study using faces of famous people. Here half the subjects saw a set of 40 faces each occurring for (an unusually long) 400ms in the LVF, followed by another set of 40 faces in the RVF; and the other half of the subjects had RVF followed by LVF presentation. Both groups then saw the 80 faces presented in centre field. In all conditions the response requirement was naming or describing the person. There was a small, but significant, RVF advantage (35·5% correct) over the LVF (30·2% correct). Interestingly, these scores for peripheral presentation were markedly lower than for central presentation (73·2%).

The inference drawn from these studies by Marzi and Berlucchi and by Umilta *et al.* is that, under certain circumstances, particularly when viewing conditions are impoverished and perhaps only one or two features can be discerned, the left hemisphere is superior in identifying well-known faces. They were aware of the earlier work of Warrington and James (1967), however, which apparently pointed to the opposite conclusion. Briefly, Warrington and James gave unilateral brain damaged subjects and controls two tests of face memory: identification of 10 famous faces; and immediate selection of an unknown face seen for 10 s from an array of 16 faces. The group with right hemisphere damage tended to perform less well than the left hemisphere damaged group on both tests, although for some reason, perhaps connected with testing dates, the right hemisphere group were no worse than the control group at the test using famous faces. Warrington and James further discovered that there was no association between memory for unknown faces and famous faces. There was a significant relationship between the incidence of right parietal damage and low scores on the unknown faces test, together with a non-significant trend for poor identification of famous faces being associated with right temporal lobe damage. Overall, however, error rates in both tasks were low, suggesting that neither was a very sensitive test of face memory. This may account for the lack of association between the two tests. Phillips and Rawles (1979), for example, have reported a small but significantly positive correlation between recognition of unknown faces and identification of famous faces.

The discrepancy between the results of Marzi and Berlucchi, and Warrington and James, though, may not be as large as at first sight seems. Warrington and James also noted that the greatest incidence of naming errors in their famous faces test was found among their left hemisphere subjects, particularly those with temporal damage and showing some dysphasia. These errors were defined as occurring when the patient was clearly able to identify the face by giving the celebrity's profession, nationality, etc. but could not provide his name. In Marzi and Berlucchi's study naming was the principal means of identifying the faces shown, which may account for the RVF superiority under impoverished viewing conditions.

Young and Bion (1981) gave the issue of naming particularly close attention. In one experiment they bilaterally presented faces of famous men and required a naming response from one group of subjects. Under these conditions no VF asymmetry emerged. Another group of subjects, given identical presentation conditions, were allowed, before responding freely, to consult a list containing the names of all the celebrities used in the experiment. Under these response conditions a LVF superiority was observed, which was the result of a doubling in accuracy for stimuli falling in the LVF when the list of names were provided to subjects, whereas this assistance to recall did not improve accuracy for stimuli presented in the RVF.

Young and Bion also investigated the abilities of subjects from age 7 years to adult to identify pictures of people they knew personally (classmates, colleagues). In this experiment both bilateral and random unilateral presentation conditions were employed. The results were unequivocal, a LVF accuracy advantage was observed for naming the faces in both the bilateral and unilateral condition at all ages.

The results of Young and Bion are generally in conflict with those of Marzi and Berlucchi. They are in agreement, however, with those arising from a study by Leehey and Cahn (1979). These particular experiments were an extremely careful attempt to test Marzi and Berlucchi's conclusions. In the first experiment Leehey and Cahn used faces that were likely to be known to one group of subjects, but were not known by another group. Bilateral presentation was used, followed by selection of the faces shown from an array of 12 faces. Both groups of subjects displayed a significant LVF superiority. In the second experiment, another group of subjects, who also knew the people depicted in the photographs, were required to name the faces shown. Again, a significant LVF advantage was found, although the absolute performance level was lower than that found for Experiment 1, in which subjects simply had to select the faces shown from an array of alternatives.

Thus, the findings of Umilta et al (1978b) and Marzi and Berlucchi (1977) have not been supported by other workers. The reason for such discrepancies in the literature are difficult to discover, though one odd aspect of both studies was the use of blocked trials. In Marzi and Berlucchi's experiment 40 stimuli occurred in one VF followed by another 40 in the opposite VF. Although subjects' eye movements were monitored in an attempt to ensure that fixations were not made to the stimulated field during the long exposure duration, it is possible that some kind of strategy of icon scanning might have operated in favour of the RVF. Marzi and Berlucchi do not give any reason for choosing this rather unusual form of blocked presentation. Umilta *et al.* too, employed a procedure in which the field in which a face was shown was blocked (also for 40 trials). They did not find any interaction between naming the face and VF asymmetry, however, which led them to dismiss any explanation for the RVF advantage in terms of the use of verbal labels. Naming did cause an overall reduction in latency, but this was evident for stimuli falling in either VF.

The various discrepancies among the results from experiments involving familiar faces are impossible to resolve unequivocally. Consequently, although Fig. 1 does show naming as a task with a left hemisphere advantage the suggestion should be accepted with caution—except of course that the motor control of speech output is usually found in the left hemisphere.

E. Interaction between the hemispheres

One aspect of cerebral asymmetry in face recognition that it is not possible to show in Fig. 1 is the interaction between the hemispheres. Klein *et al.* (1976) point out that 'functional asymmetry need not remain constant but can vary with the level of activity and interaction of the two hemispheres' (p.64). They argue that, for example, left hemisphere verbal coding may affect any manifestation of right hemisphere superiority in processing faces. This idea was also addressed by Freeman (1980). She compared subjects' performance on a same/different task involving faces of medium-level information (see Fig. 2) with the performance of other subjects who performed the same test with the additional, simultaneous task of remembering words. A six-word list was given a few seconds before a face was briefly shown. Three seconds after the first face a comparison face was shown and subjects decided whether or not the two faces were identical. They then reported the word list. Figure 3 illustrates the results. As mentioned earlier, there was no VF asymmetry under normal conditions. When a concurrent verbal task was given, however, a clear and significant LVF superiority emerged. Accuracy for faces initially shown in the RVF was the same as in the control condition: what changed was the LVF score. Freeman argues that these observations may indicate that normally right hemisphere activity is inhibited by the left hemisphere. When the left hemisphere is active, however, there is a release of inhibitory control. Notice that these observations are quite at variance with the ideas of Kinsbourne (1970) whose model of attentional selectivity would have predicted the opposite result. Freeman's results must be replicated before too much is made of them, but they do illustrate possible interactions between the hemispheres and serve to support the work of Klein *et al.*

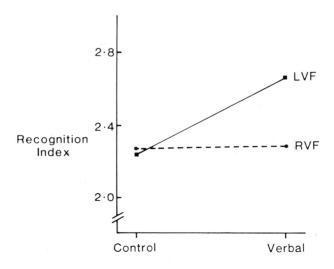

FIG. 3. Results of a study by Freeman (1980) showing that, compared with a control condition, a concurrent verbal task leads to a significant improvement in recognition of LVF faces. The recognition index used was an arc sine transformation of A prime.

Emotion

Any model of face processing must take account of the fact that faces are not simply the paramount emblems of individuality but that they also directly convey emotional expression. Indeed, Hochberg (1972) suggested that the expressive functions of faces are the principal reason for their being so well remembered. In a similar vein, Yin (1970) argued that the disability shown by right hemisphere damaged patients for remembering faces might be the result of an underlying failure to appreciate their emotional content. It is also true that some prosopagnosic patients have complained that faces appear expressionless or bland (Bodamer, 1947), though usually expressions can be identified by them (Hécaen, 1981).

Not surprisingly, therefore, the model under consideration here incorporates a distinct and separate unit for the analysis of facial expression. It is shown in Fig. 1 as one of the mechanisms for which there is a right hemisphere perceptual superiority. The relative roles of the two cerebral hemispheres in controlling facial indices of emotion will not be considered in any detail. The particular role of the right hemisphere in generating slightly asymmetrical bilateral facial expression is discussed in two papers by Campbell (1978, 1979); and related work may be found in Sackeim et al. (1978) and Heller and Levy (1981). The interested reader should also consult a recent critique by Ekman et al. (1981).

These authors claim that asymmetrical facial expressions occur only for deliberate gestures; according to them spontaneous emotional expressions are controlled by different neural pathways which do not produce consistent asymmetries.

Before addressing the particular issue of emotional perception, however, I ought at least to mention some of the background information on asymmetries in the cerebral representation of emotion. For example, Gainotti (1972) studied patients with either left or right hemisphere damage and concluded that the left hemisphere specialises in positive emotional states, whereas the right hemisphere predominates in the control of negative emotions. Much earlier, Goldstein (1939) had noted that left hemisphere lesions are associated with 'the catastrophic reaction', characterised by signs of distress and depression. Lesions of the right hemisphere more often result in the patient displaying a flatness of affect (Walsh, 1978).

The above evidence does not suggest superiority of either cerebral hemisphere in the reception or the expression of emotions. Instead, the studies mentioned so far imply a qualitative rather than a quantitative distinction. In the remainder of this section findings will be reviewed that do lead to the tentative conclusion that there is a dominance relationship for the perception of facially expressed emotion in favour of the right hemisphere.

Perception of Emotions

There is a rather weak clinical evidence indicating that the right hemisphere may be pre-eminent in perceiving facial expressions of emotion. DeKosky *et al.* (1980) examined controls and patients with unilateral brain disease on several tasks requiring an interpretation of emotions from facial expressions. In one test patients had to name the expression depicted by an actor. In another test an emotional label (e.g. 'happy') was given and the subject was required to select which of four emotions displayed in photographs of the same actor depicted that particular emotion. In a third test the subject was presented with two pictures of the same actor with either the same or a different facial expression, and simply asked whether the emotions displayed were same or different. Additionally, both groups of subjects performed a simple face discrimination test in which they had to indicate whether two photographs were of the same person.

There were some indications in the results of DeKosky *et al.* that the right hemisphere damage group was particularly impaired at the tasks requiring extraction of emotion information from faces and also at the test requiring them to name the emotion of the scene. The effects were small, however, and did not always achieve a satisfactory level of statistical significance. Moreover, the largest difference between left and right damaged patients was found for the face discrimination test. In fact, an analysis of covariance revealed that the differences between the two hemisphere groups on the emotion tests could be accounted for by differential abilities to discriminate faces. DeKosky *et al.* still believe, however, that their data indicate some relationship between site of brain injury and ability to discern emotional expressions in faces. They point out that, apart from the ability to perceive facial differences, other factors such as dysphasia are also of importance, particularly when verbal labelling of emotional states is involved in the task.

It must be admitted that the data provided by De Kosky *et al.* do not show convincingly that there is an asymmetry in the ability to perceive emotional expression. Indeed, the study raises the question as to whether it is meaningful to separate the perception of facial structure from the perception of its emotional expression.

Some evidence that the two faculties can be dissociated has been reported, however. Kurucz and Feldmar (1979) examined a group of elderly chronic organic brain syndrome patients, with what they term 'prosopoaffective agnosia'. This diagnosis was made in a previous study by Kurucz *et al.* (1979), which revealed each patient to have great difficulty in accurately perceiving expressions in drawings and photographs of faces. The same patients were then tested by Kurucz and Feldmar on their ability to recognise famous and familiar faces. The correlation between scores on the original emotion test and recognition test was virtually zero: some of the patients with severe 'prosopoaffective agnosia' were well able to identify faces. Kurucz and Feldmar conclude that the ability to recognise faces and identify emotional expressions are quite independent.

A similar conclusion was reached following a more rigorous, tachistoscopic study of normal subjects' abilities to discriminate emotional expressions in faces carried out by Ley and Bryden (1979). Cartoon line drawings of five faces each displaying five different emotional expressions served as stimuli. Subjects were briefly shown a face in either the LVF or RVF followed by a centre-field face. Their task was to decide: a) whether the faces were of the same person; and b) whether the emotions displayed were identical. A significant LVF advantage in accuracy was found for both judgements, though the decision concerning emotional similarity was only significant for the extremely positive and the extremely negative expressions.

In order to assess the interdependence of the identity and emotional judgements Ley and Bryden employed analyses of covariance. When errors on the identity judgements were the covariate, all the significant effects were retained. When errors on the emotional judgements were the covariate the main effect for visual fields was lost, which suggests that the identity judgement effect was to some extent dependent on the emotional judgement effect. However, accuracy at reaching the two judgements was not significantly correlated, confirming the independence of the two functions found by Kurucz and Feldmar.

Ley and Bryden's results also reveal a right hemisphere superiority in perceiving both positive and negative emotions which could be interpreted as being inconsistent with the finding relating the site of brain damage to the type of emotional response mentioned in the introduction to this section (from which one tentatively might have predicted a left hemisphere superiority for discerning positive emotions and a right hemisphere superiority for negative states). There is probably not much point in pursuing this discrepancy any further since there may be so many differences between perceiving expression and actual emotional reaction. However, it is perhaps noteworthy that Ley and Bryden only examined female subjects. Strauss and Moscovitch (unpub.), tested both sexes by employing a similar design but using a latency measure and found an overall LVF superiority for all expressions. Male subjects, however, displayed a LVF advantage only in the processing of the expression of surprise: for them happy and sad expressions were handled equally well in either hemifield.

An earlier study by Suberi and McKeever (1977) had also employed only female subjects, and, like that of Ley and Bryden, it too revealed more efficient LVF processing of memorised faces, this time displaying happy, sad or angry expressions. A smaller LVF latency advantage was discovered for faces bearing neutral expressions.

A subsequent experiment by McKeever and Dixon (1981), however, did systematically examine sex differences in hemifield asymmetry for perceiving emotional expression. In essence, the results of this study confirmed those of Strauss and Moscovitch insofar as female subjects showed a LVF superiority across various orienting conditions, either involving subjects empathising with sadness while memorising the target face, or following emotionally neutral instructions; whereas male subjects showed no such asymmetry regardless of orienting condition. Similar results were reported by Ladavas *et al.* (1980), who also found a LVF speed advantage in discriminating six different facial expressions for female subjects, but found no hemifield difference for male subjects. Rather contradictory data are offered by Safer (1981) which are difficult to reconcile with the ones just reviewed. Without going into details, I should report that Safer discovered male subjects to be more accurate in discriminating emotional expression following LVF presentation, whereas female subjects were equally accurate whichever visual field contained the test face. It would seem that sex differences in asymmetry for emotional perception are no more reliable than for face recognition.

Discussion

Figure 1 illustrates the general conclusion to be drawn from this review of the literature. It indicates a right hemisphere superiority for classifying incoming patterns as faces; establishing internal representations for novel faces; and perceiving emotional expression in faces.

There are no good grounds for supposing any difference between the hemispheres for the analysis of face structure. However, they may achieve this by different procedures: the left hemisphere may rely on a serial process in which particular features may be given special analysis; the right hemisphere may instead employ a more diffuse analysis in which the spatial relationships among features are discerned and identified.

Each hemisphere may be able to categorise faces as being familiar or unfamiliar with equal facility. It would seem that they both are then able to access semantic information concerning the particular person. According to the study by Sperry *et al.* (1979), mentioned earlier, either hemisphere is able to associate a range of social and emotional responses appropriate to the particular face. Their investigation of two patients with cerebral commissurotomy revealed that the right and left hemispheres are equipotential in selecting pictures of the subjects' self, relatives, public figures and historical characters.

Figure 1 suggests only a single function, naming, in which a left hemisphere advantage may occur. Even here the evidence is equivocal, and it has even been argued on the basis of tachistoscope work that there is no asymmetry in the recognition of written names (Hay, 1978).

In the Introduction to this chapter it was explained that, for the main part, the survey of work on face recognition would treat the hemispheres as independent entities. Of course, in most people the left and right cerebral hemispheres are undamaged and are connected by various commissures which link their corresponding or homologous parts. Gazzaniga and Le Doux (1978) emphasized the fact that the mind is integrated rather than divided, and that 'the illusion of a single, complete psychological space is created from two separate neural representations of the same information' (p.17). According to these authors, any apparent differences in the ways the two hemispheres operate reflect variations in degrees of expertise, and thus it would be misleading to consider them as exclusively specialising in a particular process. That is not to deny any greater facility either in depositing or accessing a particular class of information, such as faces; and it is clear from earlier discussions in this chapter that, on balance, the right hemisphere does possess the slight advantage in certain aspects of face processing.

The practical advantage of this scheme is that it allows verbal processing and face processing to occur concurrently with little or no mutual interference (Kellogg, 1980). This is because the two hemispheres may simultaneously handle different types of information. Evidence from tachistoscopic studies confirms this notion. Words and faces can be recognised when one occurs in the RVF and one in the LVF—especially if the word falls in the RVF and the face in the LVF (Hines, 1975; Hay, 1978).

These observations on hemisphere complementarity lead me, finally, to consider whether any right hemisphere advantage in processing faces has evolved because of the left hemisphere dominance for language. Perhaps the most productive approach to this question is to search for evidence of any asymmetry in face recognition within non-human primates. It is already known that squirrel monkeys can reliably recognise pictures of human faces (Marriott, 1976), and that rhesus monkeys can recognise photographs of other monkeys transformed in size, pose, colour and illumination (Rosenfeldt and Van Hoesen, 1979). Perrett *et al.* (1982) have actually recorded from single cells within the temporal lobes of rhesus monkeys that respond vigorously to the sight of monkey or human faces. Although as yet no systematic study of the distribution of such cells across the left and right hemispheres has been undertaken, Perrett (personal communication) noted that more of them were found in the left hemisphere. This observation was made in just three animals and may have arisen because more attention was paid to left hemisphere sites. The recent work of Overman and Doty (1982), however, indicates that, unlike humans, macaques show no asymmetry in the processing of left-left or right-right facial composites. This suggests that lower primates may be entirely bilateral in their processing of faces, and provides circumstantial evidence for the idea that any asymmetry found in human subjects may have arisen as a result of language development in the dominant hemisphere. The evolution of a language processor situated usually in the left hemisphere may have reduce the available space available in that hemisphere for processing visuospatial information, including faces. This, perhaps together with the right hemisphere's particular involvement in emotional interpretation, may underly the slight asymmetry in perceiving and remembering faces that has been reported over the years.

Acknowledgements

I am indebted to Janice Freeman and Dennis Hay for allowing me to cite work from their Ph.D theses. I should also like to thank the following for reading and commenting upon earlier drafts of this chapter, Graham Davies, Colin Gray, Denis Parker and Andrew Young.

References

AGNETTI, V., CARRERAS, M., PINNA, L. and ROSATI, G. (1978). Ictal prosopagnosia and epileptogenic damage of the dominant hemisphere. A case history. *Cortex* **14**, 50-57.
ARGYLE, M. and COOK, M. (1976). *Gaze and Mutual Gaze.* Cambridge University Press, Cambridge.

BADDELEY, A. D. (1979). Applied cognitive and cognitive applied psychology: the case of face recognition. In *Perspectives On Memory Research* (L. G. Nilsson, ed.). L. Erlbaum, New Jersey.

BENTON, A. L. (1980). The neuropsychology of face recognition. *American Psychologist* **35**, 176-186.

BENTON, A. L. and VAN ALLEN, M. W. (1968). Impairment in facial recognition in patients with cerebral disease. *Cortex* **4**, 344-358.

BENTON, A. L. and VAN ALLEN, M. W. (1972). Prosopagnosia and facial discrimination. *Journal of Neurological Science* **15**, 167-172.

BERENT, S. (1977). Functional asymmetry of the human brain in the recognition of faces. *Neuropsychologia* **15**, 829-851.

BERENT, S. (1981) Lateralization of brain functions. In *Handbook of Clinical Neuropsychology* (S. Filskov and T. J. Boll. eds). Wiley, New York.

BERTELSON, P. and VANHAELEN, H. (unpub.). Extracting physiognomic invariants in the two hemifields. Paper presented at the Experimental Psychology Society, Cambridge, 1978.

BERTELSON, P., VANHAELEN, H. and MORAIS, J. (1979). Left hemifield superiority and the extraction of physiognomic information. In *Structure and Function of Cerebral Commissures* (I. Steele-Russell, M. W. Van Hof and G. Berlucchi, eds). Macmillan, Woking.

BEYN, E. S. and KNYAZEVA, G. R. (1962). The problem of prosopagnosia. *Journal of Neurology, Neurosurgery and Psychiatry* **25**, 154-158.

BODAMER, J. (1947). Die Prosop-Agnosie. *Archiv für Psychiatrie und Nervenkrankheiten* **179**, 6-53.

BORNSTEIN, B. (1963). Prosopagnosia. In *Problems of Dynamic Neurology* (L. Halpern, ed.). Hadessah Medical Organization, Jerusalem.

BORNSTEIN, B., SROKA, H. and MUNITZ, H. (1969). Prosopagnosia with animal face agnosia. *Cortex* **5**, 164-169.

BRADSHAW, J., GATES, A. and PATTERSON, K. (1976). Hemisphere differences in processing visual patterns. *Quaterly Journal of Experimental Psychology* **28**, 667-681.

BRADSHAW, J. L., TAYLOR, M. J., PATTERSON, K. and NETTLETON, N. C. (1980). Upright and inverted faces, and housefronts, in two visual fields: a right and left hemisphere contribution. *Journal of Clinical Neuropsychology* **2**, 245-257.

BRIZZOLARA, D., UMILTA, C., MARZI, C., BERLUCCHI, G. and RIZZOLATTI, G. (1975). A verbal response in a discriminative reaction time task with lateralized visual stimuli is compatible with a right-hemisphere superiority. *Brain Research* **85**, 185.

BRYDEN, P. M. (1976). Response bias and hemispheric differences in dot localization. *Perception and Psychophysics* **19**, 23-28.

BRUCE, V. (1979). Searching for politicians: an information-processing approach to face recognition. *Quarterly Journal of Experimental Psychology* **31**, 373-395.

CAMPBELL, R. (1978). Asymmetries in interpreting and expressing a posed facial expression. *Cortex* **14**, 327-342.

CAMPBELL, R. (1979). Left handers' smiles: asymmetries in the projection of a posed facial expression. *Cortex* **15**, 571-579.

CHARCOT, J. M. (1883). Un cas de suppression brusque et isolée de la vision mentale des signes et des objets (formes et couleurs). *Le Progres Medical* **88**, 568-571.

CLIFFORD, B. R. and BULL, R. (1978). *The Psychology of Person Identification*. Routledge and Kegan Paul, London.

COHEN, G. (1973). Hemispheric differences in serial versus parallel processing. *Journal of Experimental Psychology* **97**, 349-356.

COHN, R., NEUMANN, M. and WOOD, D. (1974). Prosopagnosia: a clinicopathalogic study. *Transactions of the American Neurological Association* **99**, 201-203.

COLE, M. and PEREZ-CRUET, J. (1964). Prosopagnosia. *Neuropsychologia* **2**, 237-245.

DAVIDOFF, J. (1975). Hemispheric differences in the perception of lightness. *Neuropsychologia* **13**, 121-124.

DAVIDOFF, J. (1977). Hemispheric differences in dot detection. *Cortex* **13**, 434-444.

DAVIES, G. M. (1979). Face recognition: issues and theories. In *Practical Aspects of Memory* (M. M. Gruneberg, P. E. Morris and R. N. Sykes, eds.). Academic Press, London and New York.

DAVIES, G. M., SHEPHERD, J. W. and ELLIS, H. D. (1979). Similarity effects in face recognition. *American Journal of Psychology* **92**, 507-523.

DE KOSKY, S., HEILMAN, K., BOWERS, D. and VALENSTEIN, E. (1980). Recognition and discrimination of emotional faces and pictures. *Brain and Language* **9**, 206-214.

DE RENZI, E. and SPINNLER, H. (1966). Visual recognition in patients with unilateral cerebral disease. *Journal of Nervous and Mental Disease* **142**, 513-525.

DE RENZI, E., FAGLIONI, P. and SPINNLER, H. (1968). The performance of patients with unilateral brain damage on face recognition tasks. *Cortex* **4**, 17-34.

DE RENZI, E., SCOTTI, G. and SPINNLER, H. (1969). Perceptual and associative disorders of visual recognition. *Neurology* **19**, 634-642.

EKMAN, P., FRIESEN, W. and ELLSWORTH, P. (1972). *Emotion in the Human Face: Guidelines for Research and an Integration of Findings.* Pergamon Press, New York.

EKMAN, P., HAGER, J. and FRIESEN, W. (1981). The symmetry of emotional and deliberate facial actions. *Psychophysiology* **18**, 101-106.

ELLIS, H. D. (1975). Recognizing faces. *British Journal of Psychology* **66**, 409-426.

ELLIS, H. D. (1981). Theories of face recognition. In *Perceiving and Remembering Faces* (G. M. Davies, H. D. Ellis and J. W. Shepherd, eds). Academic Press, London and New York.

ELLIS, H. D. and DEREGOWSKI, J. B. (1981). Within-race and between-race recognition of transformed and untransformed faces. *American Journal of Psychology* **94**, 27-35.

ELLIS, H. D. and SHEPHERD, J. W. (1975). Recognition of upright and inverted faces presented in the left and right visual fields. *Cortex* **11**, 3-7.

ELLIS, H. D., SHEPHERD, J. W. and DAVIES, G. M. (1979). Identification of familiar and unfamiliar faces from internal and external features: some implications for theories of face recognition. *Perception* **8**, 431-439.

FAUST, C. (1947). Partielle Seelenblindheit nach Occipitalverletzung mit besonder Beeintrachtigung des Physiognomieer Kennens. *Nervenartz.*, **18**, 294-297.

FINLAY, D. C. and FRENCH, J. (1978). Visual field differences in a facial recognition task using signal detection theory. *Neuropsychologia* **16**, 103-107.

FREEMAN, J. (1980). Cerebral asymmetries in the processing of faces. Ph.D. thesis, University of Aberdeen.

FRIJDA, N. H. (1970). Emotion and recognition of emotion. In *Feelings and Emotion, The Loyola Symposium* (M. B. Arnold, ed.). Academic Press, New York and London.

GAINOTTI, D. (1972). Emotional behavior and hemispheric side of lesion. *Cortex* **8**, 41-55.

GALPER, R. E. and COSTA, L. (1980). Hemispheric superiority for recognizing faces depends upon how they are learned. *Cortex* **16**, 21-38.

GAZZANIGA, M. S. and LE DOUX, J. E. (1978). *The Integrated Mind.* Plenum Press, New York.

GAZZANIGA, M., LE DOUX, J. and WILSON, D. (1977). Right hemisphere clues to some mechanisms of consciousness. *Neurology* **27**, 1140-1147.

GEFFEN, G., BRADSHAW, J. and WALLACE, G. (1971). Interhemispheric effects on reaction time to verbal and nonverbal visual stimuli. *Journal of Experimental Psychology* **87**, 415-422.

GEFFEN, G., BRADSHAW, J. and NETTLETON, N. (1972). Hemispheric asymmetry: verbal and spatial encoding of visual stimuli. *Journal of Experimental Psychology* **95**, 25-31.

GESCHWIND, N. (1979). Specializations of the human brain. *Scientific American* **241**, 158-168.

GLONING, I., GLONING, K., HOFF, H. and TSCHABITSCHER, H. (1966). Zur Prosopagnosie. *Neuropsychologia* **4**, 113-131.

GOLDSTEIN, K., (1939). *The Organism: A Holistic Approach to Biology, Derived from Pathological Data in Man.* American Book, New York.

HANNAY, H. J. and ROGERS, J. P. (1979). Individual differences and asymmetry effects in memory for unfamiliar faces. *Cortex* **15**, 257-267.

HAMSHER, K., LEVIN, H. and BENTON, A. (1979). Facial recognition in patients with focal brain lesions. *Archives of Neurology* **36**, 837-839.

HAY, D. C. (1978). An information processing analysis of cerebral asymmetries. Ph.D. thesis, University of Aberdeen.

HAY, D. C. (1981). Asymmetries in face processing: evidence for a right hemisphere perceptual advantage. *Quarterly Journal of Experimental Psychology* **33A**, 267-274.

HAY, D. C. and ELLIS, H. D. (1981). Asymmetries in facial recognition: Evidence for a memory component. *Cortex* **17**, 357-368.

HAY, D. C. and YOUNG, A. W. (1982). The human face, In *Normality and Pathology in Cognitive Functions* (A. Ellis, ed.), pp.173-202. Academic Press, London and New York.

HÉCAEN, H. (1981). Neuropsychology of face recognition. In *Perceiving and Remembering Faces* (G. M. Davies, H. D. Ellis and J. W. Shepherd, eds). Academic Press, London and New York.

HÉCAEN, H. and ANGELERGUES, R. (1962). Agnosia for faces (prosopagnosia). *Archives of Neurology* **7**, 92-100.

HELLER, W. and LEVY, J. (1981). Perception and expression of emotion in right handers and left handers. *Neuropsychologia* **19**, 263-272.

HILLIARD, R. D. (1973). Hemispheric laterality effects on a facial recognition task in normal subjects. *Cortex* **9**, 246-258.

HINES, D. (1975). Independent functioning of the two cerebral hemispheres for recognizing bilaterally presented tachistoscopic visual half-field stimuli. *Cortex* **11**, 132-143.

HINES, D. (1978). Visual information processing in the left and right hemispheres *Neuropsychologia* **16**, 593-600.

HOCHBERG, J. (1972). The representation of things and people. In *Art, Perception and Reality* (E. Gombrich, J. Hochberg and M. Black eds). The John Hopkins University Press, Baltimore.

HOFF, H. and POTZL, O. (1937). Über eine optisch-agnosische Störung des "Physiognomie-Gedachtnisses". *Zeitschrift für die Gesamte Neurologie und Psychiatrie* **159**, 367-395.

IZARD, C. E. (1971). *The Face of Emotion.* Appleton-Century Crofts, New York.

JONES, B. (1979a). Lateral asymmetry in testing long-term memory for faces. *Cortex* **15**, 183-186.

JONES, B. (1979b). Sex and visual field effects on accuracy and decision making when subjects classify male and female faces. *Cortex* **15**, 551-560.

KELLOGG, R. T. (1980). Is conscious attention necessary for long-term storage? *Journal of Experimental Psychology (Human Learning and Memory)* **4**, 379-390.

KIMURA, D. and DURNFORD, M. (1974). Normal studies on the function of the right hemisphere in vision. In *Hemisphere Function in the Human Brain* (S. J. Dimond and J. G. Beaumont, eds). Elek, London.

KINSBOURNE, M. (1970). The cerebral basis of lateral asymmetries in attention. *Acta Psychologica* **33**, 193-201.

KLEIN, D., MOSCOVITCH, M. and VIGNA, C. (1976). Attentional mechanisms and perceptual asymmetries in tachistoscopic recognition of words and faces. *Neuropsychologia* **14**, 55-66.

KOLB, B. and WISHAW, I. Q. (1980). *Fundamentals of Human Neuropsychology.* Freeman and Co., San Francisco.

KONORSKI, J. (1967). *Integrative Activity of the Brain.* University of Chicago Press, Chicago.

KURUCZ, J. and FELDMAR, G. (1979). Prosopo-affective agnosia as a symptom of cerebral organic disease. *Journal of the American Geriatric Society* **27**, 225-230.

KURUCZ, J., FELDMAR, G. and WERNER, W. (1979). Prosopo-affective agnosia associated with chronic organic brain syndrome. *Journal of the American Geriatric Society* **27**, 91-95.

LADAVAS, E., UMILTA, C. and RICCI-BITTI, P. (1980). Evidence for sex differences in right hemisphere dominance for emotions. *Neuropsychologia* **18**, 361-366.

LEEHEY, S. C. and CAHN, A. (1979). Lateral asymmetries in the recognition of words, familiar faces and unfamiliar faces. *Neuropsychologia* **17**, 619-635.

LEEHEY, S., CAREY, S., DIAMOND, R. and CAHN, A. (1978). Upright and inverted faces: the right hemisphere knows the difference. *Cortex* **14**, 411-419.

LEVY, J. (1980). Cerebral asymmetry and the psychology of man. In *The Brain and Psychology* (M. C. Wittrock, ed.). Academic Press, New York and London.

LEVY, J., SPERRY, R. and TREVARTHEN, C. (1972). Perception of bilateral chimeric figures following hemispheric deconnection. *Brain* **95**, 61-78.

LEY, R. G. and BRYDEN, M. P. (1979). Hemispheric differences in processing emotions and faces. *Brain and Language* **7**, 127-138.

LHERMITTE, F., CHAIN, F., ESCOUROLLE, R., DUCARNE, B. and PILLON, B. (1972). Étude anatomo-clinique d'un cas de prosopagnosie. *Revue Neurologique* **126**, 329-346.

MARRIOTT, B. M. (1976). Picture perception in squirrel monkeys. Ph.D. thesis, University of Aberdeen.

MARZI, C. A. and BERLUCCHI, G. (1977). Right visual field superiority for accuracy of recognition of famous faces in normals. *Neuropsychologia* **15**, 751-756.

MATTHEWS, M. L. (1978). Discrimination of Identi-Kit constructions of faces: evidence for a dual processing strategy. *Perception and Psychophysics* **23**, 153-161.

MCCONACHIE, H. R. (1976). Developmental prosopagnosia. A single case report. *Cortex* **12**, 76-82.

MCGLONE, J. (1980). Sex differences in human brain asymmetry. A critical review. *The Behavioral and Brain Sciences* **3**, 215-227.

MCKEEVER, W. F. and DIXON, M. S. (1981). Right hemisphere superiority for discriminating memorized from nonmemorized faces: affective imagery, sex, and perceived emotionality effects. *Brain and Language* **12**, 246-260.

MEADOWS, J. C. (1974). The anatomical basis of prosopagnosia. *Journal of Neurology, Neurosurgery and Psychiatry* **37**, 489-501.

MILNER, A. D. and DUNNE, J. J. (1977). Lateralised perception of bilateral chimaeric faces by normal subjects. *Nature*, Lond. **268**, No. 5616, 175-176.

MILNER, B. (1968). Visual recognition and recall after right temporal lobe excision in man. *Neuropsychologia* **6**, 191-209.

MOONEY, C. M. (1957). Age in the development of closure ability in children. *Canadian Journal of Psychology* **11**, 219-226.

MORTON, J. (1969). Interaction and information in word recognition. *Psychological Review* **76**, 165-178.

MOSCOVITCH, M., SCULLION, D. and CHRISTIE, D. (1976). Early versus late stages of processing and their relation to functional hemispheric asymmetries in face recognition. *Journal of Experimental Psychology (Human Perception and Performance)* **2**, 401-406.

NEBES, R. (1971). Handedness and the perception of part-whole relationships. *Cortex* **7**, 350-356.

NEWCOMBE, F. (1974). Selective deficits after focal cerebral injury. In *Hemisphere Function in the Human Brain* (S. J. Dimond and J. G. Beaumont, eds). Elek, London.

NEWCOMBE, F. (1979). The processing of visual information in prosopagnosia and acquired dyslexia: Functional versus physiological interpretations. In *Research in Psychology and Medicine* (D. J. Osborne, M. M. Gruneberg and J. R. Eiser, eds). Academic Press, London and New York.

OVERMAN, W. H., and DOTY, R. W. (1982). Hemispheric specialization displayed by man but not macaques for analysis of faces. *Neuropsychologia* **20**, 113-128.

PALLIS, C. A. (1955). Impaired identification of faces and places with agnosia for colours. *Journal of Neurology, Neurosurgery and Psychiatry* **18**, 218-224.

PERRETT, D., ROLLS, E. and CAAN, W. (1982). Visual neurones responsive to faces in the monkey temporal cortex. *Experimental Brain Research* **47**, 329-342.

PATTERSON, K. and BRADSHAW, J. L. (1975). Differential hemispheric mediation of non-verbal visual stimuli. *Journal of Experimental Psychology (Human Learning and Memory)* **3**, 406-417.

PHILLIPS, R. J. and RAWLES, R. E. (1979). Recognition of upright and inverted faces: a correlational study. *Perception* **8**, 577-583.

POLICH, J. M. (1978). Hemispheric differences in stimulus identification. *Perception and Psychophysics* **24**, 49-57.

PROUDFOOT, R. E. (1982). Hemispheric asymmetry for face recognition: Some effects of visual masking, hemiretinal stimulation and learning task. *Neuropsychologia* **20**, 129-144.

RIZZOLATTI, G. and BUCHTEL, H. A. (1977). Hemispheric superiority in reaction time to faces: A sex difference. *Cortex* **13**, 300-305.

RIZZOLATTI, G., UMILTA, C. and BERLUCCHI, G. (1971). Opposite superiorities of the left and right cerebral hemispheres in discriminative reaction time to physiognomical and alphabetical material. *Brain* **94**, 431-442.

ROSCH, E., SIMPSON, C. and MILLER, R. (1976). Structural bases of typicality effects. *Journal of Experimental Psychology (Human Perception and Performance)* **2**, 491-502.

ROSENFELDT, S. A. and VAN HOESEN, G. W. (1979). Face recognition in the rhesus monkey. *Neuropsychologia* **17**, 503-509.

SACKEIM, H., GUR, R. and SAUCY, M. (1978). Emotions are expressed more strongly on the left side of the face. *Science* **202**, 434-435.

SAFER, M. A. (1981). Sex and hemisphere differences in access to codes for processing emotional expressions and faces. *Journal of Experimental Psychology (General)* **110**, 86-100.

SALZEN, E. A. (1981). Perception of emotion in faces. In *Perceiving and Remembering Faces* (G. M. Davies, H. D. Ellis and J. W. Shepherd, eds). Academic Press, London and New York.

SCHWARTZ, M. and SMITH, M. L. (1980). Visual asymmetries with chimeric stimuli. *Neuropsychologia* **18**, 103-106.

SERGENT, J. and BINDRA, D. (1981). Differential hemispheric processing of faces: Methodological considerations and reinterpretation. *Psychological Bulletin* **89**, 541-554.

SPERRY, R., ZAIDEL, E. and ZAIDEL, D. (1979). Self recognition and social awareness in the deconnected minor hemisphere. *Neuropsychologia* **17**, 153-166.

ST JOHN, R. C. (1979). Lateral asymmetry in face perception. Research Bulletin 495, Department of Psychology, University of Western Ontario.

STRAUSS, E., and MOSCOVITCH, M. (unpub.). Perception of facial expressions. MS (1981).

SUBERI, M. and MCKEEVER, W. F. (1977). Differential right hemispheric memory storage of emotional and non-emotional faces. *Neuropsychologia* **15**, 757-768.

TEUBER, H.-L. (1978). The brain and human behavior. In *Handbook of Sensory Physiology* Vol. 8 (R. Held, H. W. Leibowitz and H.-L. Teuber, eds). Springer-Verlag, Berlin.

TZAVARAS, A., HÉCAEN, H. and LE BRAS, H. (1970). Le probleme de la specificité de la reconnaissance du visage humaine lors des lesions hemispheriques unilaterales. *Neuropsychologia* **8**, 403-416.

UMILTA, C., BAGNARA, S. and SIMION, F. (1978a). Laterality effects for simple and complex geometrical figures and nonsense patterns. *Neuropsychologia* **16**, 43-49.

UMILTA, C., BRIZZOLARA, D., TABOSSI, P. and FAIRWEATHER, H. (1978b). Factors affecting face recognition in the cerebral hemispheres—familiarity and naming. In *Attention and Performance*, Vol. 7 (J. Requin, ed.). L. Erlbaum, New Jersey.

WALKER-SMITH, G. J. (1978). The effects of delay and exposure duration in a face recognition task. *Perception and Psychophysics* **24**, 63-70.

WALSH, K. (1978). *Neuropsychology: A Clinical Approach*. Churchill Livingstone, Edinburgh.

WARRINGTON, E. K. and JAMES, M. (1967). An experimental investigation of facial recognition in patients with unilateral cerebral lesions. *Cortex* **3**, 317-326.

WHITE, M. J. and WHITE, K. G. (1975). Parallel-serial processing and hemispheric function. *Neuropsychologia* **13**, 377-381.

WHITELEY, A. M. and WARRINGTON, E. K. (1977). Prosopagnosia: A clinical psychological and anatomical study of three patients. *Journal of Neurology, Neurosurgery and Psychiatry* **40**, 395-403.

WILBRAND, H. (1892). Ein Fall von Seelenblindheit und Hemianopsie mit Sections Befund. *Deutsche Zeitschrift für Nervenheilkunde* **2**, 361-387.

WISEMAN, S. and NEISSER, U. (1974). Perceptual organization as a determinant of visual recognition memory. *American Journal of Psychology* **87**, 675-681.

YARMEY, A. D. (1979). *The Psychology of Eyewitness Testimony*. The Free Press, New York.

YIN, R. K. (1970). Face recognition by brain-injured patients: A dissociable ability. *Neuropsychologia* **8**, 395-402.

YIN, R. K. (1978). Face perception: a review of experiments with infants, normal adults, and brain-injured persons. In *Handbook of Sensory Physiology*, Vol. 8 (R. Held, H. W. Leibowitz and H.-L. Teuber, eds). Springer-Verlag, Berlin.

YOUNG, A. W. and BION, P. J. (1980). Absence of any developmental trend in right hemisphere superiority for face recognition. *Cortex* **16**, 213-221.

YOUNG, A. W. and BION, P. J. (1981). Accuracy of naming laterally presented known faces by children and adults. *Cortex* **17**, 97-106.

3

MUSIC AND THE
RIGHT HEMISPHERE

Harold W. Gordon

Introduction and Clinical Studies

ALMOST AS doctrinaire as the notion that speech is lateralised to the left
hemisphere is the counter notion that music is in the right. The universality of
the public's belief in this is best illustrated by the fact that a major stereo
headphone manufacturer has seen fit to advertise in the following manner:

> Give your right hemisphere a break! While your left hemisphere goes out every day
> and discusses, analyzes, or manipulates reality for the sake of earning a living, the
> right hemisphere nags and complains about being dragged along on mundane
> errands. Stop that right brain ennui!! Give the right side of your brain its favourite
> treat — music.

Whereas belief in left lateralisation for speech has been entrenched for more
than a century, belief in right lateralisation for music is only recent history.
Earlier descriptions of amusia — broadly defined as musical dysfunction —
attributed most musical function to the left hemisphere, thus sharing the same
cortical half-brain as language functions. In order to account for the misfit cases
where left hemisphere lesions caused relatively minor disturbances in musical
ability, the consensus was that the right hemisphere had a greater capacity to
compensate for music than it did for speech (Henschen, 1926). This is
tantamount to localising these functions in the right hemisphere since
development of a cognitive function in a new cortical area following injury is not
likely — at least, not for an adult. What can be extracted from the bulk of the

FUNCTIONS OF THE RIGHT HEMISPHERE
0-12-773250-0

Copyright © 1983 by Academic Press, London.
All rights of reproduction in any form reserved.

historical literature is that language and musical abilities are differentially affected by cortical lesions wherever they may be located in the brain. (For contrast, it may be pointed out that different languages in multilinguals have, in some cases, also suffered differential dysfunction following unilateral left lesions (Paradis, 1977; Albert and Obler, 1978).)

A number of exhaustive reviews have reported that patients, especially those with high degrees of musical sophistication, have had major or minor defects in their musical ability, with or without accompanying deficits in language (see Wertheim, 1969; Benton, 1977; Brust, 1980). However, to summarise the range of reports is hardly helpful to our perspective: we find aphasia occurs without effect on musical ability, with limited effect in certain functions of music, or with severe effect in virtually all musical functions. Amusia has been described following lesions of the left hemisphere, right hemisphere, and both hemispheres. Clearly, any effort to localise musical ability in one or the other hemisphere with this kind of background is futile. Confusion has been precipitated not only by imprecise case descriptions but also by lack of agreement on what constitutes musical ability. Thus, the bulk of the case reports since the first quarter of this century have not contributed much more than the original notion that the two cognitive functions, music and language, have *separate* cortical locations although even this point was proposed by the phrenologists early in the last century and has been perpetrated throughout the neurological literature ever since. The present-day acceptance that music and language functions may be attributed, respectively, to right and left hemispheres has been derived from the much more recent results of empirical studies. And even so, the issue is not considered settled.

Left hemisphere association with musical ability was a reasonable deduction from the oft-reported concurrence of language and music disturbances following damage to the left hemisphere even though the extent of damage to the two functions was not consistent. Often, there was little effect on music in the face of more severe language disturbances following left hemisphere damage, or severe deficits following right damage with little or no language difficulties. Had the early researchers been more aware of the cognitive differences between left and right hemispheric function, they may have been more inclined to observe whether deficits in musical abilities following left or right hemisphere lesions were qualitatively different from each other. For example, it might have been expected that patients with speech disturbances and other indications of left hemisphere pathology could recognise and even hum songs or entire passages of songs. On the other hand, patients with evidence of right hemisphere pathology may have lost an appreciation for overall musical quality while preserving some technical skills. Also there may have been qualitative differences in the kind of music most preserved (or disturbed) following unilateral lesions. Atemporal, chordal, pastoral passages may have been better preserved following left hemisphere lesions than right, while rhythmic or tempo features may have been more disturbed.

In retrospect, some case reports do indicate differences. Following damage to the left hemisphere, there was relatively better preservation of appreciation, perception, and recognition of musical passages together with nearly correct production of songs or melodies, especially in regard to emotionality and tonality. By contrast, there were severe deficits in rhythm or time sense, reading musical notation, and in performing detailed musical analyses (Forster, cited by Henschen and Schaller, 1925; Brain, 1941; Jellinek, 1956; Brust, 1980). Conversely patients with right hemisphere lesions (without aphasia) were often described as having lost the sense of musical feeling or integrity of well known melodies (Botez and Wertheim, 1959; Jellinek, 1956), as well as limited insight to errors (Würtzen, 1903). Of course, not all reports lend themselves to this dichotomy. One left lesion patient could not produce (or recognise?) a well known melody while rhythm was intact (Souques and Baruk, 1926), and another patient with a right hemisphere lesion had lost his time sense (Würtzen, 1903).

One of the most important criticisms that can be levied against such case reports is that they are selective. For example, the majority of patients were musicians or persons known to have premorbid musical ability. It was probably for this reason that the cases had been published in the first place. As shall be seen later, it is just those individuals—musicians—that appear to manifest a reversed lateralisation of music function, thus representing the worst group from which to have derived general conclusions about the organisation of musical function in the brain. Had musical function been tested in brain damaged cases unselected for musical ability, the picture may have been quite different. A recent study supports this claim. The ability to sing, usually with good melody, was preserved in 21 out of 24 patients with Broca's aphasia (Yamadori et al., 1977). These patients did not have special musical skills yet were able to sing in spite of severe speech handicaps. While this was the first demonstration of intact singing following left lesions in an unselected series of patients, intact singing had already been described following complete dominant hemispherectomy in an adult (Smith, 1966) and in a young adolescent (Gordon, 1974). Further, singing was found to be more intact in patients receiving a left carotid injection of sodium amylobarbitone (prior to surgical procedures) than in those receiving right carotid injections (Gordon and Bogen, 1974). Right intracarotid injections reduced the patient's ability to sing to almost nil while speech was largely intact. However, singing alone was never produced after left carotid injection until the production of at least one word. Nevertheless, when singing was produced, it was considerably better than speech during the early recovery from the drug.

The strongest statement that can be made from these data is that the right hemisphere is 'more responsible' than the left for singing. This is a far cry from saying that singing is 'lateralised' to the right hemisphere in the same sense that we say speech is 'lateralised' to the left. With a slightly different emphasis we observe that functions of the right hemisphere *contribute* more to singing than do functions of the left hemisphere. This formulation can be generalised to characterise hemisphericity (functions of the right and left hemisphere) for any of the higher functions. Differential deficits in language, spatial construction (e.g. block design), or perception following either left or right lesions are explained by the qualitatively different contributions to these abilities by the left and right hemispheres. As it will turn out from chasing the various functions of music throughout the right and left halves of the brain, we shall learn more about the functions of the brain than about localisation of music.

The first serious blow to the clinical impression that the left hemisphere supported most musical activity was the now classic experiment in which left or right temporal patients were compared on a standard test of musical ability (Saetveit *et al.*, 1940) before and after undergoing unilateral lobectomies (Milner, 1962). No performance differences were found between the two groups prior to surgery, but following surgery, patients with right temporal lobectomies performed significantly worse than those with left temporal lobectomies. Accordingly, there were virtually no post-surgery changes in performance on any of the tests for the left temporal group, while performances declined on all tests—four of them significantly—for the right temporal group. It was concluded that removal of the right temporal lobe was specifically detrimental for processing these musical stimuli. In particular, it appeared that the right hemisphere was specialised for distinguishing tones of different timbre, loudness, and melodic patterning. However, these claims about hemispheric specialisation for music were made only in retrospect; the strongest conclusion at the time was a reference to right hemisphere superiority for 'non-verbal' stimuli. The paradox is that there is no *a priori* reason to suppose that comparing pitch qualities, tone strengths or even three- to five-note 'melodies' is the same as processing music. Whereas mental processes required for these tasks may be the same or similar to those required for music, it is a fallacy to consider these elements to be synonymous with music. Music is an entity far greater than the sum of its parts.

Studies of Normal Subjects

More direct assessment of music activation in the right hemisphere has been achieved by measurement of alpha ratios between the left and right hemispheres. Alpha frequencies (8–12 Hz) are those that are produced by the cerebral cortex when it is not actively processing information. Typically there is more alpha produced by the right hemisphere during rest so that the resting ratio, R:L, would be greater than 1.0 while L:R would be less than 1.0. If cognitive function predominates in one cerebral hemisphere, alpha frequences are 'blocked' (i.e. they occur less often) in that hemisphere, thus reflecting the increased activity. The R:L (or L:R) ratios would change accordingly.

The most striking and most consistent blocking occurs in the left hemisphere during mental arithmetic (Butler and Glass, 1974). While these and other verbal tasks produce left hemisphere blocking (Galin and Ornstein, 1972; Morrell and Salamy, 1971), spatial tasks are more apt to produce right hemisphere blocking (Galin and Ornstein, 1972; Morgan et al., 1971).

In one of the first studies of alpha blocking for music, a L:R ratio approached the value of 1.0 in a mental music task in which the subject remembered short musical segments and compared them to longer segments (McKee et al., 1973). In addition, it was shown that the ratio of alpha power (amount of alpha) for the music task was significantly greater than the ratios obtained for any one of three linguistic tasks in which the subject monitored a prose passage for the presence of a word or word form. As validation of the technique, it was further observed that the ratio (L:R) became smaller as the verbal task became more difficult. Similarly, whistling and singing also produced less alpha in the right hemisphere relative to the left than did talking the lyrics of the same song (Davidson and Schwartz, 1977). As before, this implies relatively more activity in the right hemisphere during whistling and singing than during talking. However, it was pointed out that the relative difference in alpha blocking was not due to changes in the right hemisphere for music but to a relatively greater activation in the left hemisphere during talking than during the other tasks.

A more convincing demonstration of right hemisphere activation for music was found by alpha blocking in musical and other cognitive tasks where no motor output was required. The right hemisphere was significantly more active while passively listening to Baroque concerti than during silent reading of word lists, solving mathematical problems, or while looking at paintings (Osborne and Gale, 1976). By contrast, words and maths produced significantly more activity in the left hemisphere than did pictures but not significantly more than music. However, greater left activation was seen in the immediate post-stimulus period for both words and maths relative to music (but not relative to pictures).

Right hemisphere dominance was further confirmed by increased blood flow to the right hemisphere in subjects listening to a classical guitar concerto (Carmon et al., 1975). This technique of measuring regional cerebral blood flow, rCBF, is accomplished by injecting an inert radioactive substance (Xenon 133) into the internal carotid artery* and measuring the decay curve, reflective of the rate at which blood is pumped through different areas of the cerebral cortex. Increases in blood volumes relative to rest imply activation, decreases indicate deactivation. Most of the patients undergoing this procedure (to determine blood

---

* The current technique is to administer Xenon by inhalation rather than by injection.

flow abnormalities prior to surgery) were observed to have increases in blood flow in the right hemisphere during passive listening to predominately chordal guitar music and decreases while listening to a prose passage. Conversely, blood flow increased only slightly in the left hemisphere during music but greatly during the prose (see Fig. 1).

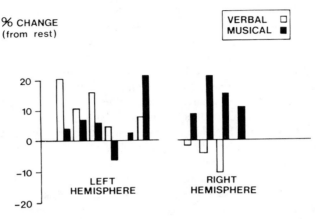

FIG. 1. Changes in regional cerebral blood flow observed in subjects listening to musical or verbal stimuli.

The bulk of experimentation in hemispheric lateralisation of music has been carried out with the dichotic listening technique in which two auditory stimuli are presented simultaneously, one to each ear. The result is a binaural competition that has been maintained to functionally block the ipsilateral ear-to-cortex pathways in favour of the contralateral pathways. Therefore, an index of left and right hemisphere performance is obtained by virtue of relative performances between the respective (contralateral) right and left ears. An auditory stimulus producing right ear dominance would imply left hemisphere superiority; left ear dominance, right hemisphere superiority; no ear dominance, no hemispheric superiority. The dominance of the contralateral over the ipsilateral pathways was shown initially by ear deficits contralateral to temporal lobe damage with greater losses in the right ear following left lobe damage (Kimura, 1961a) and confirmed by complete extinction in the left ear by patients with complete forebrain commissurotomy (Milner *et al.*, 1968). Subsequently, subjects without brain damage also had consistent right ear dominances for dichotically-presented digits (Kimura, 1961b). Later other verbal stimuli were rigorously tested resulting in the same right ear bias (Studdert-Kennedy and Shankweiler, 1970). Thus an experimental tool was established based on the findings that contralateral pathways were stronger, even in non-neurological subjects, and ear asymmetries of performance reflected hemispheric asymmetries of function.

Almost immediately, the technique was employed for musical stimuli (Kimura, 1964; Shankweiler, 1966). Instead of verbal items the two stimuli were brief melodies played on solo, orchestral instruments. To report what they heard, subjects selected the two melodies from among four played binaurally in succession following the dichotic pair. The results were opposite to those for verbal stimuli: more correct responses were obtained from the left ear. The reliability of the technique has been found to be fairly good, although less so for musical stimuli (Blumstein et al., 1975). In no case was the technique good enough to fulfill the initial high expectations that dichotic listening could be used clinically as a non-invasive technique to localise the speech centre and/or other hemispheric functions in normal subjects. Nevertheless, the conclusion was undeniable. The dichotic results substantiated the experimental reports on neurological patients—music was better processed by the right hemisphere. This conclusion had theoretical appeal as well. It was made to fit one of the major dichotomies of hemispheric function that had been derived from visual stimuli in which right and left hemisphere function were characterised by 'non-verbal' and 'verbal' processing, respectively.

The non-verbal/verbal dichotomy has had tremendous impact on subsequent considerations of right and left hemisphere function. For one thing, it is simple, a factor which is always appealing. Secondly, it is 'logical': if language is in the left, the most efficient arrangement would be that non-verbal characteristics (music included) would be in the right, if nothing else to reduce processing interference (Levy, 1976). But there are some rather unsettling aspects. In the first place, strict localisation of music in the right hemisphere denies most of the historical observations in which music was associated with the left hemisphere. As naïve as the early reports might appear in light of modern evidence, they cannot be so easily dismissed as examples of poor observation, testing, or reporting. It would appear that the music/language dichotomy needs to allow for these observations.

A second unsettling aspect in reference to the non-verbal/verbal dichotomy is the characterisation of hemispheric function as 'non-' something. One cannot help but ask whether the right hemisphere is 'pro-' anything. Certainly, the right hemisphere has some verbal skills (Zaidel, 1976), but it would be far more useful to find a characterisation of right hemisphere function that gave more insight into its specialisation. Continued inquiry into the cerebral contributions to musical function has brought forth partial resolution of these issues and, more importantly, has provided some insight into brain organisation, as well.

One of the key findings that helps explain the early reports of left hemisphere involvement is that right hemispheric dominance for music is not absolute and must be qualified by stimulus characteristics as well as task requirements.

Although the majority of musical tasks have resulted in right hemisphere dominance, some musical stimuli have evoked either left hemisphere dominance or have failed to be lateralised to one side or the other. One of the first failures to replicate left ear dominance for melodic stimuli (Gordon, 1970) nevertheless showed the expected left ear dominance for chordal stimuli (as well as the well entrenched right ear superiority for digits). It was difficult to reject the lack of asymmetry for melodies as artifactual experimental design because of the presence of left ear dominance for chords, and thus a challenge to the hypothesis was offered in which right hemisphere dominance for melodies (or music, *per se*) was too simple a concept. The explanation offered for the apparently negative results was that only the non-temporal, wholistic aspects of music are better processed by the right hemisphere. The melodies had been played on a recorder, an instrument devoid of orchestral quality such as timbre—a musical element showing strong right hemisphere dominance in the neurological patients (Milner, 1962). Presumably, the temporal or pitch qualities of the melody were more salient than the melodic entity, itself, forcing the bilateral contributions of the two hemispheres. Music as an entity is probably not localised in any one area, and is lateralised according to which elements are being assessed.

This point was tested explicitly in a later study where the same melodies were modified so that they differed either by pitch or pitch patterns (rhythms held constant), or by rhythm (pitch or pitch patterns held constant) (Gordon, 1978a). As before, no left ear superiority was obtained for either test. In fact, for the melodies differing on the rhythm dimension, a significant *right* ear superiority was obtained. Unfortunately, this study did not add much to the understanding of right hemisphere specialisation, but the results nevertheless demonstrated that the music-in-the-right-hemisphere concept needed revision. Clearly, the left hemisphere could also be superior for musical items even though they were not, in any way, verbal in nature.

In support of right hemisphere superiority for perception of orchestral melodies, a left ear dominance was obtained for dichotic presentation of brief, unfamiliar melodies played on a violin (Spellacy, 1970), although in an attempt to break music into elements, there was failure to achieve a left ear superiority for four-tone frequency patterns, for temporal patterns, and for timbre. In fact, there were trends for right ear dominance for the temporal patterns while there was a slight left ear dominance for the frequency patterns. None of these trends reached significance.

In the case of singing, verbal elements are added to melodic ones and the natural question is whether the combined musical/verbal skills influence, or are influenced by, cognitive processes. Two dichotic listening studies directly compared tonal, melodic aspects of a combined vocal/musical stimulus with verbal aspects. In the first study, letter sequences were sung to different melodies; the subject was asked to identify either the letter sequences or the melodies (Bartholomeus, 1974). A double dissociation resulted. There was a right ear dominance when the letter sequence was to be recalled and a left ear dominance when the melody was to be recalled. Thus it was shown that hemispheric dominance could be manipulated for the same stimulus depending on task requirements. Both hemispheres processed the information simultaneously and each was capable of control, depending on the one most needed to perform the task. This principle of dynamic hemispheric participation has been shown quite dramatically in patients with complete forebrain commissurotomy for split-half (chimæric) faces or patterns (Levy et al., 1972; Levy and Trevarthen, 1976). When the two half-patterns were recombined at the midline but flashed separately to opposite hemispheres each hemisphere completed its pattern-half into the scotoma and imagined it saw a complete figure. The pattern arriving in the right hemisphere was 'reported' (non-verbally by pointing) when simple recognition was required but the left hemisphere reported its pattern out loud when a verbal description was required. There were rare double reports indicating the right hemisphere dominated for the recognition task; the left for the verbal task.

The same double dissociation for vocal/musical components was shown in another dichotic task in which digits were either sung to three-tone patterns or were spoken together with a piano-generated, three-tone pattern (Goodglass and Calderon, 1977). In either condition, recall of tonal patterns whether sung or played produced left ear dominance; recall of digits whether spoken or sung produced right ear dominance. Again, the hemisphere that specialised for the required task was the one that controlled the resultant asymmetry. It is clear that the two processes were carried out simultaneously in separate hemispheres, each of which could be accessed independently, and presumably with little interference. Thus, lateralisation of musical stimuli is not only dependent on which elements are tested, but also on conditions of hemispheric control.

The results of dichotic listening experiments have been equivocal in proving right hemisphere dominance for music and music elements. Left ear superiority does appear for melodies, globally perceived, but such results are less likely when single musical elements such as tones or musical sounds are used as stimuli. However, in the case of these single, simpler stimuli, there is some evidence that the results may have been affected by artifacts of the dichotic listening technique rather than by (lack of) hemispheric differences. For example, contrary to results reported for the dichotic technique, left ear superiority for elemental stimuli was found when measured by response time techniques.

In one response time study, subjects were required to push a button when they heard a target word or a target tone. A double dissociation between the ears and stimuli was observed in which response times were faster to verbal stimuli presented to the right ear, but to tonal stimuli presented to the left (Kallman,

1977; 1978). The importance of methodology can be more clearly seen in another study in which accuracy and speed of response produced opposite asymmetries with the same stimuli. Left ear dominance was found for detecting rhythm changes in a well known melody when the ears were compared by response times; but a right ear dominance was found when ears were compared by accuracy (Gates and Bradshaw, 1977). For detecting pitch changes, the right ear was again more accurate but there was no difference between the ears when measured by response times. However task requirements in this experiment differed from most studies in an important way. Rather than detect a target or make an affirmative match, the subject was required to detect a difference — a change from the target — in successive repetitions of the same melody. The task requirement to detect a change may evoke hemispheric functions different from those required to detect a similarity. In a response time study where chord matches were required, a left ear superiority was obtained (Taub *et al.*, 1976). As it happened, alpha blocking was also assessed, thus confirming the results of the behavioural technique with psychophysiological evidence.

Right hemisphere dominance for brief musical or tonal stimuli has also been demonstrated by the technique of auditory evoked potentials (Taub *et al.*, 1976; Shucard *et al.*, 1979). Since high level cognitive processing is unlikely during the relatively short latencies, emergence of right hemisphere dominance implies some natural proclivity for music-like stimuli. This idea is supported by the finding in infants of right hemisphere dominance in the evoked potential from musical tones where verbal stimuli had produced a left hemisphere dominance (Molfese *et al.*, 1975). Can it be that at least part of the right hemisphere superiority for music is due to an innate cortical structure conductive to receiving simple, less structured stimuli? Another infant study supports this view. Cardiac habituation was measured in 3-month-old infants for verbal or musical stimuli when either was played to the left or right ear (Glanville *et al.*, 1977). Greater habituation occurred to speech stimuli when presented to the right ear and to music stimuli when presented to the left. The auditory system is the last of the special senses to develop and it is unlikely that infants are 'processing' these stimuli in a 'cognitive' way. Yet, these ontogenetically early asymmetries are real and must be considered in an hypothesis of brain function. It may be that cerebral asymmetries are made up of simpler, innate, 'hard-wired' systems which are the substructures on which develop the more complex cognitive systems.

The evolutionary importance of inborn musical systems seems diminished with respect to the historical role of language, even in light of the history of song and dance in more primitive societies. If anything, rhythmic elements played the larger role in tribal music and not infrequently in communication. Rhythm, as has been discussed, is attributed to the language hemisphere perhaps not coincidentally. In a dichotic experiment using Morse Code signals (Papçun *et al.*, 1974), experienced operators had a right ear preference while inexperienced non-operators had a left ear preference. In other words, a 'non-verbal' stimulus that had a verbal meaning to some people evoked the expected left hemisphere (right ear) advantage. Presumably, the inexperienced subjects recognised the rhythm patterns as perceptual wholes evoking right hemisphere processes. In another study, a right ear advantage was found in native speakers of Thai (a tone language) where the members of each dichotic word pair differed only on the basis of tone (Van Lancker and Fromkin, 1973). By contrast, a left ear advantage was observed for non-speakers of Thai for whom the pitch differences of the words had no semantic meaning.

In search of a reason for evolutionary dominance of the right hemisphere for non-verbal sounds, the current interest in emotion may be relevant. Right hemisphere dominance has been shown for perception and production of emotional expression which may be related to the right hemisphere dominance for facial recognition (see Chapter 2). The same right hemisphere dominance is found for vocal stimuli in dichotic presentation where there is a left ear preference for perception of emotional voices (King and Kimura, 1972; Carmon and Nachshon, 1973). However, as in the case of the visual stimuli where faces without emotional expression still evoke right hemisphere dominance, so do environmental sounds without apparent emotional content (Curry, 1967, 1968; Knox and Kimura, 1970).

It is left to speculation whether the development of right hemisphere superiority is an evolution of the emotional apparatus which is also conducive to perception of stimuli of non-linguistic, non-emotional content. In other words, right hemisphere superiority for processing non-emotional, non-linguistic stimuli may be an 'artifact' of hemisphere development of a cortical system for processing emotional stimuli. The critical experiments for this line of inquiry have yet to be done, although there is one study (Beaton, 1979) in which subjects reported that music was more pleasant and soothing when heard in the left ear. Fortunately, music is probably a good stimulus medium not only because of its extensive use in previous studies but also because its emotional tone can be rather conveniently manipulated. As an example, most would judge a minor musical mode to be 'sadder' than a major mode. If hemisphere asymmetries changed according to musical mode, where modes of greater emotion evoked greater right hemisphere participation, support could be claimed for the emotional hypothesis.

The evolutionary influence on higher cognitive functions such as language, music, and certain aspects of emotion is likely to be different from the influence on simpler stimuli like pure tones, clicks, noise bursts and so on. Evidence of a subsystem of innate auditory asymmetries has been highlighted by a striking auditory illusion (Deutsch, 1974). Subjects were presented (through stereo headphones) with an octave pair of pure tones (400, 800 Hz) rapidly alternating (at the rate of 2 Hz) between the ears. The left ear would receive the sequence,

400, 800, 400, . . ., while the right would receive the sequence, 800, 400, 800, ... What the subjects reported was a repeated series of 800 Hz tones in their right ear, alternating with a repeated 400 Hz tone in the left ear. The right ear presumably heard only the high tones when played to it, while the left only heard the low tones, *but at the time when it was receiving the high tones.* This phenomenon has been explained as a right ear dominance for pitch, since the reported pitches were the correct ones for the right ear, and dominance for location that varied according to the location of the high tone. That is, the location of the tone (low or high) was referred to the ear receiving the high pitch. The phenomenon was consistent for most subjects, even when the subjects knew beforehand what the actual stimuli were to be. One is forced to conclude that the phenomenon is based on some 'hard-wired' brain circuitry that is asymmetrically distributed in the brain. It is not clear what role the phenomenon may have for the other asymmetries that are reported for tone-like or musical stimuli, but it should be kept in mind when drawing conclusions from other experimental data.

Musicians and Non-musicians

The message that seems to filter down so far through most reports on patients with lesions and on normals where hemispheric activation is measured or where perceptual strategies are assessed, is that songs or melodic excerpts that can be processed as entities or non-time-dependent, musical elements are best handled by the right hemisphere. Temporal comparisons or step-by-step analyses are better handled by the left hemisphere, and these along with more elemental stimuli may generate no asymmetries depending on the task. This dichotomy fits reasonably well with what is generally accepted as typical of right and left hemisphere function. The caveats are that some musical elements are not conducive to the basic processing in one hemisphere or the other and thus fail to lateralise consistently, and secondly, that lateral dominance may also be governed by hemispheric control which is dependent on task characteristics or on cognitive functions that are different and at least partially independent of the stimulus elements themselves.

Paradoxically the one group for which the 'accepted' right/left relationships do not hold are musicians or those with extensive musical training. Where right hemisphere dominance is obtained for non-musicians, reversed or no hemisphere dominance has been obtained for musicians. The explanation used to account for these observations points out that musicians are trained to use analytic procedures, and thus invoke processes generally found in the left cerebral hemisphere. However, the argument is circular and begs the question of cerebral dominance. What is cerebral dominance for music if dominance depends on which cognitive functions are being used for processing? It makes little sense to first obtain right hemisphere dominance for melodies in non-musicians concluding that the right hemisphere is dominant for melodies, and then obtain left hemisphere dominance for musicians concluding that analytic processes in these subjects caused a reversal. Either an experiment is performed to determine hemispheric lateralisation for musical stimuli, in which case an hypothesis must be consistent with both sets of (opposing) data, or additional validation is required to substantiate the claim that musicians are using their left hemisphere and non-musicians are using their right. A number of studies have attempted to resolve this paradox, but they have yet to provide a definitive answer.

The first reported difference between musicians and non-musicians was for a task in which monaurally-presented, two-note sequences had to be detected in a 12–18 note 'melody' (Bever and Chiarello, 1974). A secondary task was to indicate whether or not the 'melody', itself, had been heard on a previous trial. No ear asymmetries were found for the primary task, presumably because of the task difficulty. (The non-musicians had chance-level performance.) For recognition, a right ear superiority was found for musicians; a left ear superiority was found for non-musicians. The group difference was due to the good right ear performance of the musicians since the left ear score of the non-musicians was not much different from the left ear of the musicians. The interpretation was that musicians had learned to use more analytically-oriented strategies and, since the task was conducive to such strategies, the left hemisphere of the musicians took the dominant role in performing the task. Support for this conclusion came from reanalysis of data from a dichotic study previously showing no ear difference for recognition of melodies (Gordon, 1970) in which a significant (positive) correlation was found between performance (musicianship?) and the right ear bias (Gordon, 1975).

Full support of the musician/non-musician dichotomy has also been reported in one study using dichotic listening and another using electrocortical measurements. In the dichotic study (Johnson, 1977), two-second melodic segments played on a violin were used since these had already produced a left ear dominance in an earlier study (Spellacy, 1970). The dichotic pair was followed by a binaural foil which was or was not one of the stimulus melodies. Musicians were defined as individuals having four years of lessons and maintaining daily practice schedules. (Non-musicians were not defined.) As expected, the ear asymmetry was in favour of the right hemisphere for non-musicians and in favour of the left hemisphere for musicians. However, the difference between groups was due to changes in the right ear score alone. The scores for left ears did not differ; the right ear was worse than the left for non-musicians and better than the left for musicians. It is unfortunate that verbal stimuli were not also included to see if the effect was stimulus-specific, but it was clear that musicians and non-musicians differed on this task. The conclusion seems warranted that the left hemisphere is more involved in making (correct) melodic matches for musicians than for non-musicians.

The same conclusion was reached following two studies using the alpha blocking technique. In one study (Davidson and Schwartz, 1977), whistling well known melodies produced a relatively greater right hemisphere activation than did talking in a non-musician group. There was no difference in alpha blocking between the whistling and talking tasks for the musician group. Investigation of alpha blocking in each hemisphere alone revealed that differences were due to changes in the amount of left hemisphere alpha only. Alpha levels did not vary in the right hemisphere among the tasks in either group. So again, differences between groups were the result of greater left hemisphere activation for music (whistling, in this case) in the musician group.

A similar finding was reported during passive musical and verbal tasks (Hirshkowitz *et al.*, 1978). Subjects listened to a newscast, noise, or the singing of a popular song. Relative to baseline, the right hemisphere of the non-musicians was more active while listening to the song; for the musicians, the left hemisphere was relatively more active. Both groups had relatively greater left hemisphere activation for both of the other tasks. What is perhaps most interesting is that non-musicians ranged from relatively strong left hemisphere activation for verbal material and essentially no asymmetry for noise, to relatively strong right hemisphere activation for song. Musicians, on the other hand, varied much less among the stimuli ranging from a slightly left hemisphere activation for verbal material, to somewhat more left activation for noise; left activation for song was somewhere in between. Unfortunately, only *relative* hemisphere activation is reported, so it is not possible to see how each hemisphere alone changed during the tasks. But it is apparent that relative to each other the left and right hemispheres of musicians are less variable. This is consistent with a conclusion that for musicians both hemispheres are more likely to be used in processing musical stimuli. This could account for the initial hypothesis that there is more left hemispheric activation rather than decreased right hemisphere activation, relative to non-musicians.

More recent behavioural studies failed to substantiate the musician/non-musician dichotomy. In one study (Zatorre, 1979), melodic and amelodic tone sequences and speech syllables (/ba, da, ga, . . . /) were presented dichotically to trained musicians and to non-musicians. The results were 'unremarkable' and harked back to the early viewpoint: melodies produce left ear dominance, speech produces right ear dominance, and in addition, there are no differences between musicians and non-musicians. Both groups had the same asymmetry on each test; there was not even a trend. Of the eight subjects (18% of the total) who obtained right ear dominance for *both* speech and music, only two were musicians.

In another study (Gaede, *et al.*, 1978), a chord analysis (how many notes in a chord) and a melody sequence analysis (which note of a sequence was changed) were each presented monaurally to four groups of subjects, divided according to high and low experience, and to high and low aptitude (judged empirically). The two tasks produced opposite ear asymmetries—chords, a greater left ear dominance; melodies, a greater right ear dominance. However, this dissociation was due to performance differences by the subjects with low aptitude *regardless of experience*; high aptitude subjects had little ear difference for either of the tasks. It should be pointed out that all subjects were non-music-major students and, like the subjects in the original musician/non-musician study (Bever and Chiarello, 1974), they would probably be classed as 'amateur' musicians at best. The question raised by this study is whether the determinant of hemispheric contribution to musical analysis is really aptitude rather than experience or training.

The results of this experiment seem to be in opposition to what one might logically suppose. With most of the evidence pointing to the right hemisphere for functional support of music processing, increased development of innate musical tendencies should actually produce greater right hemisphere superiorities. Preliminary evidence in support of this hypothesis was found in a repeat of the dichotic chords study (Gordon, 1970) where there was no ear asymmetry in non-musicians and the usual left ear asymmetry for another group of amateur musicians (Gordon, 1978b). Though many of these amateur musicians were taking or had taken music lessons, it is not likely they reached the stage of formal training in analytic procedures claimed for more advanced musician groups. It is also likely that chord stimuli are not as conducive to analytic procedures as melody-like stimuli, and thus are less influenced by training and more reflective of innate development especially in musicians. Since the passive listening studies showed alpha blocking to differ in the left hemisphere only, it is not inconsistent to suppose that right hemisphere superiority may yet increase with musical aptitude (and/or experience) if the task placed special demands on right hemisphere functions.

Accordingly, the dichotic chord stimuli were administered to more than 200 subjects drawn from five levels of musical experience (Gordon, 1980a). Aptitude was not measured. The 'lowest' group consisted of students in two special high schools whose curricula are expanded to include musical education and instrumental ensembles. The 'highest' group consisted of professional musicians employed by major orchestras. Intermediate groups were, in ascending order, a semi-professional orchestra, music teachers, and students in a (college-level) conservatory of music.

The results were puzzling. Overall left ear (right hemisphere) superiority decreased for the two highest level groups, but the effect was not due to a gradual reversal or even reduction in ear asymmetry. Instead, the professional and conservatory groups produced bimodal distributions of ear dominances. Approximately half the subjects had strong left ear superiorities while half had strong right ear superiorities; no one in these two groups (of more than 50 subjects) had equal ear scores. The high school students had the expected unimodal distribution peaking in favour of the left ear. The distributions of the other groups fell in between. Ear asymmetries for a verbal task of dichotically-presented words tended to have the same pattern: bimodal for the better musician groups, unimodal for the high school students (but this time peaking in favour of the right ear as expected). These results straddle those of all previous studies implying that musicians depend on *either* their right or left hemisphere, at least for this presumably non-analytic task. In other words, they are more polarised—more laterally dependent—than the lesser musician groups.

A secondary study with some of these same groups supported the polarity observations. In deference to the aforementioned auditory illusion for high and low tones (Deutsch, 1974), the musicians and a new group of non-musicians were requested to indicate the ear in which the lower (or higher) chord was played. Although lower and higher chords were presented an equal number of times to each ear, subjects reporting low chords indicated their left ear most often, while subjects reporting high chords indicated their right ear, as predicted by the illusion. But the illusion was most successful for the better musician groups, reduced for the non-professional groups, and nearly non-existent for the non-musician group. The bipolar distribution was confirmed in yet another dichotic chord study where subjects judged 'same' or 'different' between a monaural chord and a pair of dichotic chords (Morais *et al.*, 1982). Non-musicians showed a significant left ear advantage and a unimodal distribution of scores; musicians had no asymmetry and a bimodal distribution of scores. Thus the results of these studies confirm that musicians and non-musicians do differ, possibly along a continuum, but the difference may be one of polarity—increased use of either the left *or* the right hemisphere.

Although the critical experiment—whether or not 'right' and 'left' hemisphere musicians differ in other cognitive ways—is yet to be done, there is some support for this premise. Dichotic melodies differing either in pitch patterns or in rhythm patterns (or both) and similar to those producing no asymmetries for pitch patterns and right ear preference for rhythm (Gordon, 1978a) were presented to a group of non-musicians (Peretz and Morais, 1980). The result was lack of ear asymmetry for any stimulus set. In an effort to determine whether response bias could account for these results, the subjects had been asked to describe their method of performing the tasks, resulting in classification of subjects into an 'analytic' group if they reportedly listened for note changes, or a 'non-analytic' group if they reportedly listened for changes in the whole melody. The groups differed significantly. The analytic group tended toward greater right ear superiority, while the non-analytic group had a clear left ear superiority. What is not known is whether the analytic group was inherently 'left hemispheric' in solving problems in general, and whether the 'non-analytic' was 'right hemispheric'. An independent measure of hemispheric preference of cognitive function would have been appropriate.

Hemisphericity and Music

One emerging point relevant to understanding the musician/non-musician paradox is that it is inappropriate to lateralise music to any one hemisphere. Dominance for music is dependent both on the task to be performed and the mix of specialised skills needed from the right and left hemispheres. As an illustration of differential contributions of hemispheric functions, it is instructive to digress to the phenomenon of differential aphasia, where an acquired lesion in the left hemisphere of a multilingual individual sometimes produces a different pattern of aphasia for each language (Paradis, 1977). In order to explain the multiplicity of aphasias in one individual it must be concluded that each language is organised differently. But rather than hypothesise that each language is localised in a different place, it is more plausible to presume that each language requires a different combination of basic hemispheric abilities, albeit in the same (left) hemisphere. Thus the acquired lesion will affect some of these basic abilities and the resultant differences in aphasia will be related to the different combination of these abilities required for each language (Silverberg and Gordon, 1979). For music, a number of different cognitive processes are also necessary perhaps more so than for language, and again these change according to the task. For other tasks musicians and non-musicians may use different cognitive processes, thus having different hemispheric biases. For yet other tasks, they would use the same processes, thus having the same hemispheric biases. Group differences would be reflected accordingly.

There is also no reason to assume that any two people are alike in their development of cognitive processes or in their dependence on relative functions of the right and left hemispheres. Those who are more inclined to use their left hemisphere, ought to be left hemisphere dominant for a greater number of tasks than those who are more inclined to use their right hemisphere. This is supported by the non-musician group, who had right or left ear dominance depending on whether they reported using an analytic or a non-analytic mode of processing (Peretz and Morais, 1980). The argument for musicians goes one step further implying that those with left hemisphere dominance for some music tasks had *learned* to make more use of these analytic properties in their left hemisphere. If individuals fall along a continuum from 'right hemisphere' thinking to 'left hemisphere' thinking it is apparent that lateral (right/left) biases of the subject, whether innate or learned, are a relevant factor in trying to establish the hemisphere needed in a task process or a stimulus perception.

Empirically, 'lateral biases' imply that 'right hemisphere' thinkers perform relatively better on tests of right hemisphere function while 'left hemisphere' thinkers perform relatively better on tests of left hemisphere function (Bentin and Gordon, 1979; Gordon, 1980b). In the context of the dichotomy between musicians and non-musicians, it is relevant to ask whether the hemispheric bias of musicians is left dominant as suggested by their training; right dominant as suggested by the apparent (developmental) location of music assessed by most passive listening tasks; or either right or left according to a bimodal distribution as demonstrated in the results of the large-scale dichotic chords study.

The question of hemispheric bias—hemisphericity—is relevant to other special groups such as sculptors on the one hand and attorneys on the other. Although efforts to differentiate these groups by alpha blocking have largely failed (Dumas and Morgan, 1975), the groups can be distinguished on the basis of performances on left and right tests of cognitive function. The fact that children with developmental dyslexia are found to have primarily right hemisphere profiles is a case in point (Gordon, 1980b). Not surprisingly these subjects perform poorly on tasks attributed to the left hemisphere, but it is also true that they perform above average on tasks attributed to the right hemisphere. What is more, there is a correlation of performance among right and left hemisphere abilities and reading skills where no such correlation is apparent in normal readers. The implication is that dyslexics may be 'locked in' to a single (right hemisphere) mode of thought, using it for tasks that should be performed by left hemisphere processes.

There is a lot of fine tuning still needed in empirical studies to fully understand which functions are basic and specific to the right and left hemispheres. But enough is now known—the dichotomy is well enough established—to propose that people do differ along a 'horizontal' left/right hemisphericity axis. What is in question is whether there is mobility along this scale. Musicians may be an indication of a learned leftward shift; dyslexics an indication of an innate rightward development. In spite of data which are only preliminary and techniques that lack validation, the concept of motility along the horizontal axis has been gaining popular acceptance, especially in the area of art instruction and therapy (Edwards, 1979). Considerable work is still needed to address the problem of how hemisphere-biased individuals interact with hemispheric-biased stimuli and whether these biases can be changed.

The even larger question of how hemisphericity interacts with hemispheric-biased social behaviours (Bogen *et al.*, 1972; Thompson *et al.*, 1979) is only beginning to be touched upon. Daily endeavours, learning, working, interacting with family, friends, and co-workers all derive from cognitive functions produced by brain processes. Indeed, it has been argued that the emergent consciousness of these functions is produced by, a part of, and interactive with the brain itself and must be considered along with all phenomena studied

(Sperry, 1977). The right/left axis is just one of the dimensions along which the cognitive profile varies but one of the few that has a cortical antecedent. 'Right hemisphere' thinkers—those who perform better on tests attributed to right hemisphere function—would be expected to learn, interact personally, solve problems, perform their occupations, appreciate music, art, or hobbies qualitatively differently than would 'left hemisphere' thinkers. It is for this reason that the first job is to understand the qualitatively different, cognitive functions basic to brain processes, and then to discover how they influence our education, our occupation, our culture and our interpersonal relationships. Music is a small corner of human endeavour, yet we have shown how dependent it is upon the different functions of the right as well as of the left hemisphere. Influences of right and left hemisphere function in other aspects of cognitive behaviour are outlined in other chapters of this volume.

References

ALBERT, M. L. and OBLER, L. K. (1978). *The Bilingual Brain*. Academic Press, New York and London.

BARTHOLOMEUS, B. (1974). Effects of task requirements on ear superiority for sung speech. *Cortex* **10**, 893-896.

BEATON, A. A. (1979). Hemispheric emotional asymmetry in a dichotic listening task. *Acta Psychologica* **43**, 103-109.

BENTIN, S. and GORDON, H. W. (1979). Assessment of cognitive asymmetries in brain damaged and normal subjects: validation of a test battery. *Journal of Neurology, Neurosurgy and Psychiatry* **42(8)**, 715-723.

BENTON, A. L. (1977). The amusias. In *Music and the Brain*. (M. Critchley and R. A. Henson, eds), pp.378-397. Heinemann Medical Books, London. Charles C. Thomas, Springfield, Illinois.

BEVER, T. G. and CHIARELLO, R. J. (1974). Cerebral dominance in musicians and non-musicians. *Science* **185**, 137-139.

BLUMSTEIN, S., GOODGLASS, H. and TARTTER, V. (1975). The reliability of ear advantage in dichotic listening. *Brain and Language* **2**, 226-236.

BOGEN, J. E., DEZURE, R., TENHOUTEN, W. D. and MARSH, J. M. (1972). The other side of the brain IV: the A/P ratio. *Bulletin of the Los Angeles Neurological Societies* **37**, 49-61.

BOTEZ, M. I. and WERTHEIM, N. (1959). Expressive aphasia and amusia following a right frontal lesion in a right-handed man. *Brain* **82**, 186-202.

BRAIN, W. R. (1941). Visual disorientation with special reference to lesions of the right cerebral hemisphere. *Brain* **64**, 244-272.

BRUST, J. C. M. (1980). Music and language: musical alexia and agraphia. *Brain* **103(2)**, 367-392.

BUTLER, S. R. and GLASS, A. (1974). Asymmetries in the electroencephalogram associated with cerebral dominance. *EEG and Clinical Neurophysiology* **36**, 481-491.

CARMON, A. and NACHSHON, I. (1973). Ear asymmetry in perception of emotional non-verbal stimuli. *Acta Psychologica* **37**, 351-357.

CARMON, A., LAVY, S., GORDON, H. and PORTNOY, Z. (1975). Hemispheric differences in rCBF during verbal and non-verbal tasks. In *Brain Work* (D. H. Ingvar and N. A. Lassan, eds), pp.414-423. Alfred Benzon Symposium VIII, Copenhagen, Munksgaard.

CURRY, F. K. W. (1967). A comparison of left-handed and right-handed subjects on verbal and non-verbal dichotic listening tasks. *Cortex* 3, 343-352.

CURRY, F. K. W. (1968). A comparison of the performances of a right hemispherectomized subject and 25 normal on four dichotic listening tasks. *Cortex* 4, 144-153.

DAVIDSON, R. J. and SCHWARTZ, G. E. (1977). The influence of musical training on patterns of EEG asymmetry during musical and non-musical self-generation tasks. *Psychophysiology* 14(1), 58-63.

DEUTSCH, D. (1974). An auditory illusion. *Nature*, Lond. 251, 307-309.

DUMAS, R. and MORGAN, A. (1975). EEG asymmetry as a function of occupation, task, and task difficulty. *Neuropsychologia* 13, 219-228.

EDWARDS, B. (1979). *Drawing on the Right Side of the Brain*, St. Martins Press, New York.

GAEDE, S. E., PARSONS, O. A. and BERTERA, J. H. (1978). Hemispheric differences in music perception aptitude vs. experience. *Neuropsychologia* 16, 369-373.

GALIN, D. and ORNSTEIN, R. (1972). Lateral specialization of cognitive mode: an EEG study. *Psychophysiology* 9, 412-418.

GATES, A. and BRADSHAW, J. L. (1977). The role of the cerebral hemispheres in music. *Brain and Language* 4, 403-431.

GLANVILLE, B. B., BEST, C. T. and LEVENSON, R. (1977). A cardiac measure of cerebral asymmetries in infant auditory perception. *Developmental Psychology* 23(8), 54-58.

GOODGLASS, H. and CALDERON, M. (1977). Parallel processing of verbal and non-verbal musical stimuli in right and left hemisphere. *Neuropsychologia* 15, 397-407.

GORDON, H. W. (1970). Hemispheric asymmetries in the perception of musical chords. *Cortex* 6, 387-398.

GORDON, H. W. (1974). Auditory specialization of the right and left hemispheres. In *Hemispheric Disconnection and Cerebral Function*. (M. Kinsbourne and W. L. Smith, eds), pp.126-136. Charles C. Thomas, Springfield, Illinois.

GORDON, H. W. (1975). Hemispheric asymmetry and musical performance. *Science* 189, 68-69.

GORDON, H. W. (1978a). Left hemisphere dominance for rhythmic elements in dichotically presented melodies. *Cortex* 14, 58-70.

GORDON, H. W. (1978b). Hemispheric asymmetry for dichotically presented chords in musicians and non-musicians, males and females. *Acta Psychologia* 42, 383-395.

GORDON, H. W. (1980a). Degree of ear asymmetries for perception of dichotic chords and for illusory chord localization in musicians of different levels of competence. *Journal of Experimental Psychology: Human Perception and Performance* 6(3), 516-527.

GORDON, H. W. (1980b). Cognitive asymmetry in dyslexic families. *Neuropsychologia* 18, 645-653.

GORDON, H. W. and BOGEN, J. E. (1974). Hemispheric lateralization of singing after intracarotid sodium amylobarbitone. *Journal of Neurology, Neurosurgery and Psychiatry* 37, 727-738.

HENSCHEN, S. E. (1926). On the function of the right hemisphere of the brain in relation to the left in speech, music and calculation. *Brain* 49, 110-123.

HENSCHEN, S. E. and SCHALLER, W. F. (1925). Clinical and anatomical contributions on brain pathology. *Archives of Neurological Psychiatry* 13, 226-249.

HIRSHKOWITZ, M., EARLE, J. and PALEY, B. (1978). EEG Alpha asymmetry in musicians and non-musicians: a study of hemispheric specialization. *Neuropsychologia* 16, 125-128.

JELLINEK, A. (1956). Amusia. *Folia Phoniatrica* 8, 124-149.

JOHNSON, P. R. (1977). Dichotically stimulated ear differences in musicians and non-musicians. *Cortex* **13**, 385-389.

KALLMAN, H. J. (1977). Ear asymmetries with monaurally-presented sounds. *Neuropsychologia* **15(6)**, 833-835.

KALLMAN, H. J. (1978). Can expectancy explain reaction time ear asymmetries. *Neuropsychologia* **16(2)**, 225-228.

KIMURA, D. (1961a). Some effects of temporal-lobe damage on auditory perception. *Canadian Journal of Psychology* **15**, 156-165.

KIMURA, D. (1961b). Cerebral dominance and the perception of verbal stimuli. *Canadian Journal of Psychology* **15**, 166-171.

KIMURA, D. (1964). Left-right differences in the perception of melodies. *Quarterly Journal Experimental Psychology* **16**, 355-358.

KING, F. L. and KIMURA, D. (1972). Left ear superiority in dichotic perception of vocal, non-verbal sounds. *Canadian Journal of Psychology* **26**, 111-116.

KNOX, C. and KIMURA, D. (1970). Cerebral processing of nonverbal sounds in boys and girls. *Neuropsychologia* **8**, 227-237.

LEVY, J. (1976). Cerebral lateralization and spatial ability. *Behavior Genetics* **6(2)**, 171-188.

LEVY, J. and TREVARTHEN, C. B. (1976). Metacontrol of hemispheric function in human split-brain patients. *Journal of Experimental Psychology: Human Perception and Performance* **2(3)**, 229-312.

LEVY, J., TREVARTHEN, C. and SPERRY, R. W. (1972). Perception of bilateral chimeric figures following hemispheric deconnexion. *Brain* **95**, 61-78.

McKEE, G., HUMPHREY, B. and McADAM, D. W. (1973). Scaled lateralization of alpha activity during linguistic and musical tasks. *Psychophysiology* **10(4)**, 441-443.

MILNER, B. (1962). Laterality effects in audition. In *Interhemispheric relations and cerebral dominance*. (V. B. Mountcastle, ed.). The Johns Hopkins Press, Baltimore.

MILNER, B., TAYLOR, L. and SPERRY, R. W. (1968). Lateralized suppression of dichotically presented digits after commissural section in man. *Science* **161**, 184-186.

MOLFESE, D. L., FREEMAN, R. B. and PALERMO, D. S. (1975). The ontogeny of brain lateralization for speech and non-speech stimuli. *Brain and Language* **2**, 356-368.

MORAIS, J., PERETZ, I., GUDANSKI, M. and GUIARD, Y. (1982). Ear asymmetry for chord recognition in musicians and nonmusicians. *Neuropsychologia* **20**, 351-354.

MORGAN, A. H., McDONALD, P. J. and MacDONALD, H. (1971). Differences in bilateral alpha activity as a function of experimental task, with a note on lateral eye movements and hypnotizability. *Neuropsychologia* **9**, 459-469.

MORRELL, L. K. and SALAMY, J. G. (1971). Hemispheric asymmetry of electrocortical responses to speed stimuli. *Science* **174**, 164-166.

OSBORNE, K. and GALE, O. (1976). Bilateral EEG differentiation of stimuli. *Biological Psychology* **4**, 185-196.

PAPÇUN, G., KRASHEN, S., TERBEEK, D., REMINGTON, R. and HARSHMAN, R. (1974). Is the left hemisphere specialized for speech, language, and/or something else? *Journal of The Acoustic Society of America* **55**, 319-327.

PARADIS, M. (1977). Bilingualism and Aphasia. In *Studies In Neurolinguistics* Vol. 3 (H. A. Whitaker and H. Whitaker, eds). Academic Press, New York and London.

PERETZ, I. and MORAIS, J. (1980). Modes of processing melodies and ear asymmetry in non-musicians. *Neuropsychologia* **18**, 477-489.

SAETVEIT, J. G., LEWIS, D. and SEASHORE, C. G. (1940). *Revision of the Seashore measures of musical talents. University of Iowa Student Aims Progressive Research (No. 65)*. University of Iowa Press, Iowa City.

SHANKWEILER, D. (1966). Effects of temporal-lobe damage on perception of dichotically presented melodies. *Journal of Comparative and Physiological Psychology* **62**, 115-119.

SHUCARD, D. W., SHUCARD, J. L., and THOMAS, J. G. (1979). Auditory evoked potentials as probes of hemispheric differences in cognitive processing. *Science* **197(4310)**, 1295-1298.

SILVERBERG, R. and GORDON, H. W. (1979). Differential aphasia in two bilinguals. *Neurology* **29(1)**, 51-55.

SMITH, A. (1966). Speech and other functions after left (dominant) hemisperectomy. *Journal of Neurology, Neurosurgery and Psychiatry* **29**, 467-471.

SOUQUES, A. and BARUK, H. (1926). Un cas d'amusie chez un professeur de piano. *Revue Neurologique* 179-183.

SPELLACY, F. (1970). Lateral preferences in the identification of patterned stimuli. *Journal of the Acoustic Society of America* **47(2)**, 574-578.

SPERRY, R. W. (1977). Forebrain commissurotomy and conscious awareness. *Journal of Medicine and Philosophy* **2(2)**, 101-126.

STUDDERT-KENNEDY, M. and SHANKWEILER, D. (1970). Hemispheric specialization for speech perception. *Journal of The Acoustic Society of America* **48(2)**, 579-594.

TAUB, J. M., TANGUAY, P. E. and CLARKSON, D. (1976). Electroencephalographic and reaction time asymmetries to musical chord stimuli. *Physiology and Behavior* **17(6)**, 925-930.

THOMPSON, A. L., BOGEN, J. E. and MARSH, J. F. (1979). Cultural hemisphericity: evidence from cognitive tests. *International Journal of Neuroscience* **9**, 37-43.

VAN LANCKER, D. and FROMKIN, V. A. (1973). Hemispheric specialization for pitch and "tone": evidence from Thai. *Journal of Phonetics* **1**, 101-109.

WERTHEIM, N. (1969). The amusias. In *Handbook of Clinical Neurology*, Vol. 4 (P. J. Vinken and G. W. Bruyn, eds). North-Holland Publishing Co., Amsterdam.

WÜRTZEN, C. H. (1903). Einzelve Formen der Amusie, an Beispielen erlautert. *Deutsche Zeitschrift für Nervenheilkunde* **24**, 465-473.

YAMADORI, A., OSUMI, Y., MASUHARA, S., and OKUBO, M. (1977). Preservation of singing in Broca's aphasia. *Journal of Neurology Neurosurgery and Psychiatry* **40**, 221-224.

ZAIDEL, E. (1976). Auditory vocabulary of the right hemisphere following brain bisection or hemidecortication. *Cortex* **12**, 191-211.

ZATORRE, R. J. (1979). Recognition of dichotic melodies by musicians and non-musicians. *Neuropsychologia* **17**, 607-617.

4

LANGUAGE CAPABILITIES OF THE RIGHT HEMISPHERE

Alan Searleman

Introduction

DURING THE last 150 years an enormous amount of information has been collected about the way language is processed by the brain. The bulk of this information has been obtained by clinical examination of patients who had suffered some type of brain lesion or malfunction. The prevalent view that emerged from these case studies was that in right handed people it was the left hemisphere that was responsible for linguistic functioning.

The modern view of the roles that the left and right hemispheres play in controlling linguistic abilities is much less narrow-minded. Although it is still believed, and rightfully so, that the left hemisphere is the prime mediator of language functioning in most people, researchers are now more willing to accept the fact that the right hemisphere also has some linguistic capabilities (Searleman, 1977). Much of the evidence to support this last statement has come from the development of new techniques that can more accurately assess the degree and direction of language lateralisation in clinical and normal populations.

This chapter will examine what is currently known about the linguistic abilities of the right hemisphere. Evidence for right hemisphere language skills will be amassed from both brain damaged and neurologically normal subjects. A recurring theme throughout the chapter will be that the right hemisphere's ability to comprehend language far outstrips its ability to produce language.

FUNCTIONS OF THE RIGHT CEREBRAL HEMISPHERE
0-12-773250-0
Copyright © 1983 by Academic Press, London.
All rights of reproduction in any form reserved.

Given the focus of this volume, the chapter will emphasise the linguistic abilities of the right hemisphere of right handed people. However, the effects of other subject variables on language lateralisation will be briefly considered.

Clinical Evidence of Right Hemisphere Linguistic Abilities

Although the cortex is usually considered the mediator of language functions, it is always important to remember that subcortical mechanisms may play a role in linguistic functioning. The thalamus, in particular, has received considerable attention concerning its possible participation in language processing (Brown, 1979; Ojemann, 1976, 1977; Penfield and Roberts, 1959). Since the exact role that subcortical mechanisms play in processing language is still unknown, it is not always possible to separate their contributions in terms of language functions from the contributions of the two cerebral hemispheres. This should be kept in mind while reading this chapter.

The Disconnected or Isolated Left and Right Hemispheres

The remarkable degree of functional plasticity of the developing brain during the first few years of life has been extensively documented (Basser, 1962; Lenneberg, 1967; Zangwill, 1960), though the interpretation of this data has been disputed by St James-Roberts (1981). A substantial portion of the data that supports the plasticity claim stems from the unfortunate fact that it is sometimes necessary to perform a hemispherectomy to help alleviate the symptoms of infantile hemiplegia or to destroy life-threatening tumours. The removal of a diseased or malfunctioning hemisphere can provide an excellent opportunity to examine the skills of the remaining hemisphere. Most of the post-operative examinations of these patients had indicated that following an early left hemispherectomy for the treatment of infantile hemiplegia the right hemisphere could 'take-over' the linguistic functioning that would normally have been performed by the left hemisphere (Basser, 1962; Carlson *et al.*, 1968; Krynauw, 1950; McFie, 1961; White, 1961).

More recently, however, Dennis and Whitaker (1976, 1977) have conducted a detailed examination of the linguistic abilities of three patients who each underwent a hemispherectomy soon after birth. These hemispherectomies, one right and two left, clearly showed that the language development and acquisition of isolated left and right hemispheres is not the same. Although it was discovered that phonemic and semantic abilities were similarly well developed by each hemisphere, the syntactic abilities of the right hemisphere definitely lagged behind those of the left. Specifically, when testing these children at either age 9 or 10 years it was revealed (Dennis and Whitaker, 1976) that:

in relation to the left, the right brain half is deficient in understanding auditory language, especially when meaning is conveyed by syntactic diversity; detecting and correcting errors of surface syntactic structure; repeating stylistically permuted sentences producing tag questions which match the grammatical features of a heard statement; determining sentence implication; integrating semantic and syntactic information to replace missing pronouns; and performing judgements of word interrelationships in sentences. (p.428)

As the authors pointed out, this study is unique in that it is the first examination of language acquisition in presumably healthy hemispheres isolated *before* the beginning of language development. This research certainly suggests that there are definite limits to the degree that one hemisphere can 'take-over' for another. Based on this admittedly small sample, it appears that an isolated right hemisphere charged with the task of acquiring language skills just does not do as well as an isolated left hemisphere.

The hemispherectomy literature has helped to fuel a controversy concerning how long after birth the right hemisphere retains the ability to acquire language given a grossly damaged or non-functional left hemisphere. Some researchers believe that language is predominantly lateralised to the left hemisphere by age 5 years (Krashen, 1972, 1973) while others maintain that language lateralisation, and therefore functional plasticity, will continue to occur until puberty (Basser, 1962; Lenneberg, 1967; Obrador, 1964). Therefore, it is very instructive to investigate the right hemisphere's linguistic skills in adults who have had to undergo a left hemispherectomy. Examination of such patients can provide valuable information concerning the nature and extent of the residual linguistic functions as well as the possible acquisition of new language skills by the mature right hemisphere.

Due to the high operative mortality rate and the fact that the recurrence of neoplasm is common, relatively few hemispherectomies are performed on adults for treatment of tumours (Burkland and Smith, 1977). In addition, because of the very obvious debilitating effects that a left hemispherectomy would have for most adults, only a handful have been reported in the literature (Burklund and Smith, 1977; Crockett and Estridge, 1951; French *et al.*, 1955; Hillier, 1954; Smith, 1966; Zollinger, 1935).

One of the most remarkable features concerning these patients who often differed widely in such important factors as intelligence, sex, age of onset of disease, age when the left hemisphere was removed, amount of cortical tissue removed, degree of disease infiltrating the right hemisphere, accompanying physiological and psychological disorders, and methods of testing, is that they all had certain residual linguistic abilities in common following the left hemispherectomy. Immediately after the operation, while most of these patients were severely impaired in the production of voluntary, propositional speech, they were able to produce over-learned, automatic phrases. As an example, Smith (1966) reported that:

E.C.'s attempts to reply to questions immediately after the operation were totally unsuccessful. He would open his mouth and utter isolated words, and after apparently struggling to organize words for meaningful speech, recognized his inability and would utter expletives or short emotional phrases (e.g. 'Goddamit!'). Expletives and curses were well articulated and clearly understandable. However, he could not repeat simple words on command or communicate in 'propositional' speech until 10 weeks post-operatively. (p.468)

By observing the linguistic abilities of these left hemispherectomy patients it is clear that both receptive and expressive language skills were greatly affected by the removal of the left hemisphere. However, it was found that in all cases that the patients could generally comprehend language much better than they could produce it. For example, immediately following hemispherectomy, patients were usually able to respond non-verbally to spoken command, while any form of expressive language was impossible to perform (Burklund and Smith, 1977; Smith, 1966).

Perhaps the most developed form of expressive speech in these patients was singing. This is probably due to at least two factors. First, considerable evidence has accumulated to indicate that the right hemisphere may be specialised for certain musical abilities (Bogen and Gordon, 1971; Gordon, unpub.; Henschen, 1926; Luria, 1966). Secondly, the right hemisphere has already shown a propensity to be able to produce over-learned phrases, of which well-known songs is an example. Burklund and Smith (1977) report that one month after the operation the most recent adult to have a left hemispherectomy (was able to sing (words and melody "Jingle Bells" with only occasional dysarticulation.' (p.629).

Several of the patients continued to show improvement following the removal of the left hemisphere in both verbal comprehension and in the use of voluntary, propositional speech (Burklund and Smith, 1977; Crockett and Estridge, 1951; Smith, 1966; Zollinger, 1935). Before the recurrence of neoplasm, Burklund and Smith (1977) noted that their patient showed progressive, yet erratic, improvement in his response to verbal commands, his response to written commands, his use of propositional speech, and his ability to write (which was the most severely impaired language function following the surgery).

In 1973, Gott published her findings concerning the linguistic capabilities of an unusual left hemispherectomy patient (R.S.). What makes R.S. a particularly interesting case is that although she was only 10 years old when she had her left hemisphere removed to relieve right-sided convulsions, she was already pubescent. It also appears almost certain that her left hemisphere had been her dominant language hemisphere because of evidence indicating a progressively worsening aphasia just prior to the operation and because of the profound effect that the removal of the left hemisphere had on her linguistic functioning (Zaidel, 1978a). Thus, although chronologically R.S. was not an adult when she had her hemispherectomy, and therefore was not considered with the other adult left hemispherectomy cases, she had reached puberty and she did have her language dominant hemisphere removed.

The residual linguistic skills of R.S.'s right hemisphere were very similar to the adult left hemispherectomy patients already discussed. For example, speech comprehension was markedly better than speech production and R.S.'s most well developed form of expressive speech was singing (Gott, 1973).

Zaidel (1976, 1977, 1978a, 1978b) has also extensively tested the linguistic skills of R.S.'s right hemisphere, as well as the right hemisphere of two commissurotomy patients (N.G. and L.B.) Both N.G. and L.B. had complete cerebral commissurotomies and were selected for testing because their extracallosal damage was minimal and their post-surgical recoveries were very smooth. Based upon a new contact lens procedure developed by Zaidel (1975) it is possible to lateralise stimuli for prolonged periods of time to either the right or left visual field. This new procedure permits a much greater degree of stimulus complexity and allows for free ocular scanning of the stimulus by one hemisphere at a time. Using this contact lens procedure the linguistic abilities of the disconnected hemispheres of N.G. and L.B. were also examined.

Zaidel administered a series of developmental and clinical language tests to these three patients. For instance, using the Peabody Picture Vocabulary Test it was found that the right hemispheres of N.G., L.B. and R.S. had very good auditory comprehension of single spoken words. The right hemispheres of these patients were able to understand not only concrete nouns but also abstract nouns and verbs. These results contradicted previous findings that the right hemisphere of commissurotomy patients could not process abstract nouns or verbs (Gazzaniga, 1970; Gazzaniga and Hillyard, 1971). The results of the Peabody Picture Vocabulary Test also indicated that the aural vocabulary of the right hemisphere was superior to the visual vocabulary.

Further testing revealed that while the right hemisphere has relatively little difficulty understanding single words, its comprehension is greatly reduced when it must decode whole phrases that are context-free and non-redundant. Zaidel (1977) attributes this deficit to the fact that the right hemisphere has previously been shown, by means of the Token Test, to have a severely limited short-term verbal memory. Similar to what was found with single words, aural phrases were more readily comprehended than were visually presented phrases. Based upon these findings, Zaidel (1978b) suggests that whereas the left hemisphere can utilise a phonetic code to derive meaning from words, the right hemisphere, in contrast, must rely upon a template matching or gestalt mode of processing. This less efficient mode of the right hemisphere for accessing the lexicon is usually sufficient for processing single words, but not for processing whole phrases.

In assessing the syntactical abilities of the left and right hemispheres of the two commissurotomy patients and the right hemisphere of R.S., Zaidel (1978a,

1978b) reported finding evidence of a rudimentary syntactical capability for the right hemisphere. These findings again contrast with earlier reports that the right hemisphere of commissurotomy patients possessed virtually no syntactic competence (Gazzaniga and Hillyard, 1971).

By using specially prepared chimæric stimuli (i.e., stimuli that present one scene or half-word to one visual field and a different scene or half-word to the other visual field) Levy and Trevarthen (1977) also examined some elementary language functions in a series of commissurotomy patients. In previous work, Levy and her colleagues have shown that each hemisphere in a commissurotomy patient perceives the one half of the chimæric presented to it as being perceptually complete (Levy, *et al.*, 1972).

Their most recent findings indicated that although the right hemisphere can comprehend single words it employs a qualitatively different processing strategy to do so than does the left hemisphere (Levy and Trevarthen, 1977). They propose that the left hemisphere can always analyse verbal stimuli phonetically to derive meaning, while, in contrast:

> the right hemisphere decodes written words as ideograms by direct entry to the lexicon of the visual representation, and spoken language by direct acoustic-Gestalt entry, or through a visual representation, in either case bypassing any elaborate phonetic analyser. (p.115)

These conclusions are very similar to those reached by Zaidel (1978a, 1978b), who also maintains that the right hemisphere lacks the ability to make grapheme-to-phoneme transformations and must rely upon a gestalt-template matching process to access the internal lexicon.

Before continuing to describe the linguistic abilities of the disconnected right hemisphere it is important to consider the problem of 'cross-cuing' (Gazzaniga, 1970). Cross-cuing occurs when one hemisphere has information or the correct answer to a question and some how manages to give it to the other hemisphere. As an example of cross-cuing, Gazzaniga *et al.* (1977) recently reported an interesting anecdote arising from testing the ability of a commissurotomy patient's right hemisphere to carry out verbal commands. The patient was told to 'assume the position of _____' while the word 'boxer' was tachisto-scopically presented to the left visual field. At this point

> the subject correctly assumed the pugilistic position, and when asked what the word was, said, 'boxer'. Yet on subsequent trials, when the subject was restrained, and the word 'boxer' was flashed, the left hemisphere said it saw nothing. Moments later, however, when released, he assumed the position, and said, 'O.K., it was "boxer".' (p.1146)

Clearly, the left hemisphere was only able to guess correctly the word presented to the right hemisphere when it first had the opportunity to observe the right hemisphere's response. Often, however, it is not nearly as clear-cut that cross-cuing has occurred as it was in the anecdote just cited. Given the problems associated with trying to guard against cross-cuing strategies it is absolutely essential when testing commissurotomy patients to determine whether or not the left hemisphere knows the answer that was supposedly supplied by the right hemisphere. If this is not done, or done with sufficient care, then it is likely that the right hemisphere's true linguistic abilities will be exaggerated. An example of how this procedure can be carried out in practice and at the same time illustrate the right hemisphere's ability to match objects with their verbal description comes from a study by Nebes and Sperry (1971). A commissurotomy patient was asked to blindly pick out an object with his left hand that 'makes things look bigger'. The patient picked out a magnifying glass. Since both hemispheres heard the question it was necessary to determine if the left hemisphere could possibly have influenced the right hemisphere's choice. In this particular case it seems very unlikely because when the left hemisphere was asked to guess what was in its left hand it replied a 'telescope'. Thus, there was no evidence that cross-cuing had occurred.

In terms of expressive language abilities the disconnected right hemispheres of commissurotomy patients perform poorly. There is no convincing evidence that the right hemisphere can produce speech. There is evidence, however, that some commissurotomy patients are able to spell very simple words by tactually manipulating letters with the left hand (Gazzaniga, 1970; Gazzaniga et al., 1977; Gazzaniga and LeDoux, 1978; Levy et al., 1971; Nebes and Sperry, 1971). Some are even able to write the word just completed with the left hand (Nebes, 1974). At no time during these tests were the patients able to name the word spelled or written, thus insuring that the left hemisphere had not been responsible for these achievements.

An important limiting factor that needs to be considered whenever evaluating the right hemisphere's potential for linguistic expression is that there are unmistakable instances of left hemisphere interference during right hemisphere attempts at linguistic feats (Levy et al., 1971; Levy and Trevarthen, 1977; Nebes, 1974). For example, it has sometimes been observed that a commissurotomy patient will start to write correctly the name of an object presented to the left visual field with his left hand. However, before the word is completed, the left hemisphere apparently gains control of the hand and finishes the word incorrectly. In one case, patient L.B. was given a pipe to feel with his left hand and then was instructed to write the name of the object with the same hand. Trying to comply with the instructions:

he first printed 'PI', pressing down very hard with the pencil; after completing the first two letters, he stopped, and after a delay of a second or so, gripped the pencil in a much more relaxed manner and completed the word 'Pencil'. After another pause, he then scratched out the last four letters and stated vocally that he didn't know what the object was. (Levy *et al.*, 1971, pp.53-54)

As evidence that the right hemisphere still knew what had been presented, when asked to draw the object with his left hand L.B. did in fact draw a pipe.

Undoubtedly, the commissurotomy patient who has shown the greatest amount of right hemisphere linguistic functioning has been patient P.S. When tested, P.S. was a right handed, 15-year-old boy who had had a series of severe epileptic attacks with seizure focus in the left temporal lobe when 2 years old. At age 10 intractable seizures recurred and four years later P.S. underwent complete surgical sectioning of the corpus callosum (Wilson *et al.*, 1977).

Like all the other commissurotomy patients ever tested, P.S. was unable to name objects presented exclusively to his right hemisphere. Nevertheless, by presenting lateralised stimuli to the left visual field, P.S.'s right hemisphere was capable of performing the following array of tasks (Gazzaniga *et al.*, 1977; Gazzaniga and LeDoux, 1978):

Spelling. After being presented with a lateralised line drawing or picture, P.S. was able to spell the object's name by rearranging and selecting the appropriate letters from a larger group of letters.

Writing. With his left hand P.S. was able to write the names of objects presented as lateralised line drawings or pictures.

Word-Object Matching. P.S. could correctly point to an object whose name had been lateralised.

Opposite Matching. P.S. could select from a group of words the one that was opposite in meaning to the lateralised word.

Conceptual Matching. P.S. could select from a group of words the one that was most associated with the lateralised word.

Rhyming. P.S. could select from a group of words the one that rhymed with the lateralised word.

Action Verbs. P.S. could correctly point to a picture depicting the lateralised verb.

Verbal Commands P.S. could perform a variety of actions based upon verbal commands or instructions presented to the right hemisphere.

The comprehension of language by P.S.'s right hemisphere far surpasses the right hemisphere comprehension abilities of all other commissurotomy patients. Even more impressive is the degree of linguistic expression shown by the right hemisphere of P.S. His right hemisphere is able to spell and to write with the left hand but is still not able to speak. This has led Gazzaniga and LeDoux (1978) to suggest that one expressive ability (writing) can exist in the right hemisphere in the absence of another (speech). Alternatively, as previously alluded to, the reason why there are functional differences in certain expressive modes (writing *vs* speech) may be due to varying degrees of left hemisphere interference. It is quite conceivable that the musculature controlling language production is much more under the control of the left hemisphere than is the musculature of the left hand. Thus, even if the disconnected right hemisphere was capable of verbal language production it would not be able to gain control of the necessary musculature. In contrast, the right hemisphere does have primary control over the left hand and therefore is probably able to resist left hemisphere interference more successfully. The obvious lack of any left hemisphere interference in adult left hemispherectomy patients is probably a major reason why the right hemisphere of these patients is able to produce some limited speech.

Unilateral Brain Damage and Language Functioning

It seems that whenever a right-handed adult displays any symptoms of aphasia the diagnosis is almost invariably left hemisphere damage. However, in terms of non-right-handers (NRH), a sizeable percentage are likely to become aphasic following damage to either hemisphere (Gloning *et al.*, 1969; Hardyck and Petrinovich, 1977; Hécaen and Sauguet, 1971; Humphrey and Zangwill, 1952). Likewise, there's a large body of clinical evidence to indicate that children, regardless of their preferred handedness, often become at least transiently aphasic following either left or right hemisphere injury (Alajouanine and Lhermitte, 1965; Basser, 1962; Hécaen, 1976; Moscovitch, 1977; Witelson, 1977). In addition, although its occurrence is very rare, there have been sporadic reports of crossed aphasia in right-handers (Bramwell, 1899; Brown and Wilson, 1973; Ettlinger *et al.*, 1955; Holmes and Sadoff, 1966; Trojanowski *et al.*, 1980; Wechsler, 1976; Zangwill, 1979).

Admittedly, the recovery of language skills in a right-handed aphasic who has had left hemisphere damage is often due to the transitory nature of the injury or to compensatory functioning of other undamaged left hemisphere tissue (Goldstein, 1948; Hécaen and Albert, 1978; Luria, 1970; Needles, 1942). Nevertheless, there are clear instances where a healthy right hemisphere has 'taken over' many of the linguistic chores of its damaged counterpart (Gowers, 1887, Nielsen, 1946; Russell and Espir, 1961; Zangwill, 1960). Of historical interest in this regard is the following comment made by Gowers (1887) concerning an aphasic patient:

Loss of speech due to permanent destruction of the speech region in the left hemisphere has been recovered from, and that this recovery was due to supplemental action of the corresponding right hemisphere is proved by the fact that in some cases, speech has been again lost when a fresh lesion occurred in this part of the right hemisphere. (pp.131-132)

In more recent times, Nielsen (1946) has reported similar findings.

Further evidence that the right hemisphere can sometimes be the source of aphasic speech has been obtained using the Wada Test (Czopf, 1972; Kinsbourne, 1971). The Wada Test (Wada and Rasmussen, 1960) involves the injection of sodium amobarbital into the left or right carotid arteries. This drug produces a transitory loss of functioning in the ipsilateral hemisphere that is marked by a total contralateral hemiplegia including the cessation of speech. Using the Wada Test, Kinsbourne (1971), for example, found that residual speech capabilities were not arrested following left hemisphere inactivation in two right-handed, left hemisphere damaged aphasics. However, when the right hemisphere of these aphasics was subsequently anaesthetised, all speech production ceased.

In conjunction with the evidence cited above for possible right hemisphere participation in speech production in right-handed aphasics, there has also been evidence to suggest that a shift in language perception or comprehension may occur in these patients. Several studies using either tachistoscopic tasks (Moore and Weidner, 1974) or dichotic listening tasks (Johnson *et al.*, 1977; Moore and Weidner, 1975; Pettit and Noll, 1979) have found data consistent with this hypothesis. Taken together these studies suggest that following damage to the left hemisphere the sensory field preferences for verbal stimuli shift direction in favour of the right hemisphere. These purported shifts in sensory field preference can be viewed as reflecting the increasing dependence upon the right hemisphere for speech perception in these subjects. However, it should be noted that since these studies were unable to measure the premorbid sensory field preferences for these aphasic subjects it is not possible to determine if an actual shift in preference occurred.

A word of caution that applies to all evidence that suggests that the right hemisphere plays at least a compensatory role in language recovery in left hemisphere damaged aphasics is also warranted. As was previously mentioned, the left hemisphere can disrupt or interfere with the right hemisphere. Therefore, it may not be so much that language skills shift to the right hemisphere following left hemisphere damage, but rather that the damaged left hemisphere losses some of its ability to restrain the linguistic abilities that *already* reside, and can now be utilised, in the right hemisphere.

It is well known that profound language production and comprehension deficits follow left hemisphere damage in the vast majority of right-handers. Only in the last 20 years, however, has it also become apparent that unilateral right hemisphere damage can also disrupt, although in a much milder fashion, normal language functions.

One of the first to demonstrate that subtle linguistic deficiencies can arise from right hemisphere damage was Eisenson (1962). He reported that a group of patients with unilateral right hemisphere damage performed worse than did a matched control group on a series of linguistic tasks. The linguistic deficits of these subjects was most apparent when the tasks involved the use of abstract concepts, such as when abstract words were needed to complete sentences. Contrary to the prevailing sentiment of the time, Eisenson concluded:

> that the right cerebral hemisphere might be involved with super-or extra-ordinary language function, particularly as this function calls upon the need of the individual to deal with relatively abstract established language formulations. (p.53)

Critchley (1962) also suggested that a right hemisphere injury can result in deficiencies in certain linguistically related tasks. These deficiencies were often found to be of the following types: difficulty with articulation, inability to do creative literary work, hesitations and problems in word finding, and difficulty in learning novel linguistic material.

Disturbances in writing following right hemisphere damage have also been reported (Boller, 1968; Hécaen and Marcie, 1974; Luria, 1970). Hécaen and Marcie (1974) examined the writing abilities of 30 left and 30 right hemisphere damaged patients. They found that right hemisphere lesions were associated with the iteration of strokes and letters and with the enlargement of the left hand margin, whereas left hemisphere lesions were associated with loss of continuity in writing words. Typically, the writing deficits of right hemisphere damaged patients have been attributed to perseveration tendencies and to the more general syndrome of unilateral spatial neglect that often characterises patients with right hemisphere lesions.

There is also evidence to indicate that right hemisphere damage can sometimes lead to reading difficulties. For example, Kinsbourne and Warrington (1962) examined six right-handed patients who developed a reading disorder following right hemisphere lesions. It was found that each patient made paralexic errors (misreading of words) predominantly limited to the beginning of the word. Again, similar to the writing deficits observed, the most likely reason for the errors was unilateral neglect of the left visual field because of the lesion. This is the usual explanation to account for the effects of right hemisphere damage on reading performance (Hécaen and Kremin, 1976). Coltheart (this volume) examines in detail the right hemisphere's role in the reading process.

A variety of other linguistic deficits have been reported as a result of unilateral right hemisphere damage in right-handers. Some researchers have noted that comprehension of the affective components of speech is impaired (Heilman *et al.*, 1975) following lesions of the temporo-parietal regions of the right hemisphere. Related to these findings, Ross and Mesulam (1979) report disturbances of prosody and emotional gesturing following supra-Sylvian infarctions of the right hemisphere. In an interesting study by Caramazza *et al.* (1976), it was shown that right hemisphere damage can adversely affect syllogistic reasoning. Caramazza *et al.* concluded that verbal reasoning often depends upon non-linguistic imaginal processes of the right hemisphere for full elaboration. Agrammatism, or telegraphic language, may result from right hemisphere lesions (Brown and Wilson, 1973) and finally, there is evidence that injury to the right hemisphere can cause a variety of naming difficulties (Milner, 1968; Weinstein, 1964; Weinstein and Keller, 1963).

After documenting all this assorted evidence that right hemisphere damage can affect linguistic functioning, it may be tempting to conclude from some of these studies that the right hemisphere normally plays at least a subsidiary role in the affected verbal functions. There is, however, a plausible rival explanation. It is certainly conceivable that a malfunctioning right hemisphere could be sending 'noise' over to the left hemisphere and that it is this disruption of the left hemisphere's linguistic functioning that is the actual cause of these subtle linguistic deficits.

Evidence of Right Hemisphere Linguistic Abilities in Normals

The first conclusive evidence that the right hemisphere had any linguistic abilities at all came from the clinical literature of the nineteenth century. Even today the strongest and most dramatic evidence of right hemisphere language skills is from the careful examination of brain damaged patients (especially the hemispherectomy and commissurotomy cases). Since so much of the evidence for right hemisphere linguistic capabilities is derived from clinical observations, it is always important to remember that it is often hazardous and unwarranted to try to generalise from these clinical cases to the normal population. Instead, if the goal is to determine the linguistic skills of the right hemisphere in normal right-handers, then it is better to develop techniques and procedures that directly assess these skills and to use the clinical data to guide this research and its interpretation.

Language Comprehension and Production in the Normal Right Hemisphere

The two most frequently used methods to assess the degree and direction of language lateralisation in normals have been the dichotic listening test and the tachistoscopic presentation of verbal stimuli to the visual fields. Both of these sensory field preference tests are measures of language perception or comprehension. Generally, only about 70% of right-handers show a right visual field (RVF) advantage for tachistoscopically presented verbal stimuli and only 65–85% demonstrate a right ear advantage (REA) on verbal dichotic listening tests (Kinsbourne, 1974; Levy, 1974). Even when normal right-handers do show evidence of a right sensory field preference on these tasks the overall difference between the left and right sensory fields in accuracy of recall or speed of recognition is quite small (Bryden, 1963; Krashen, 1972).

If we let the clinical evidence that shows that the right hemisphere possesses fairly well developed language comprehension abilities guide our interpretation of these findings, then some may be willing to conclude that language comprehension is largely bilaterally represented in normals. In fact, based upon such findings and the fact that a sizeable proportion of right-handers actually process left sensory field stimuli better than right field stimuli, Anderson and Jaffe (1973) have suggested that some right-handers may typically decode speech using predominantly their right hemisphere.

There's a major problem, however, in trying to interpret data from tachisto-scopic and dichotic listening tasks. If performance is worse for the left sensory field stimuli that may reflect the fact that the right hemisphere can process the verbal stimuli but just not as efficiently as can the left. Alternatively, inferior left sensory field performance could be due to the right hemisphere's total inability to process the stimuli and the right hemisphere can then best be viewed as simply being a relay station sending stimuli over the commissures to be processed by the left hemisphere.

Recently, evidence that has been accumulating from a variety of sources indicates that the right hemisphere in normals is not simply a relay situation for verbal stimuli on its way to the left hemisphere for processing. The early reports (Gazzaniga, 1970) of the linguistic capabilities of the right hemisphere of commissurotomy patients indicated that the right hemisphere was only able to process 'noun-object words' and a few adjectives, but no verbs or verb-derived nouns (e.g., 'teller' or 'locker'). These early clinical observations of the ability of the disconnected right hemisphere to process only selective classes of words, which subsequently have been considerably updated and extended by Zaidel (1978a, 1978b), stimulated a considerable amount of research with normal subjects.

Some of this research was consistent with Gazzaniga's (1970) original findings and some was not. For instance, Caplan et al. (1974) were unable to find differences in visual field superiorities in normals for recognising pure nouns, verb-derived nouns, and words that could be used as either nouns or verbs. More supportive of Gazzaniga were the findings of Ellis and Shepherd (1974). They tested 12 right-handed subjects and found that both concrete and abstract words were better recognised in the RVF than the LVF. Of particular interest, however, is their finding that while concrete and abstract words presented to the RVF did not differ significantly in terms of the probability of recognition, there was a significant difference in favour of concrete words with LVF presentations.

Hines (1976, 1977) examined the effects of familiar and unfamiliar concrete and abstract words as a function of visual field presentation. He reported that familiar abstract nouns had significantly larger RVF recognition superiorities than did familiar concrete nouns. There was no such relationship observed for the unfamiliar nouns. Similar to Ellis and Shepherd (1974), Hines concluded that the right hemisphere is able to recognise some concrete nouns (in particular, familiar nouns).

Employing a lexical decision task, in which the subject must decide whether or not a string of letters forms an English word, Day (1977) found further evidence that the right hemisphere of right-handed normals can selectively process concrete nouns but not abstract nouns. He found that there were no reaction time (RT) differences between the LVF and RVF in making lexical decisions about concrete words. In terms of abstract words, however, there were significantly faster RTs when these words were presented to the RVF. In the same article, Day described the results of two other experiments that examined each hemisphere's ability to make decisions concerning superordinate category membership for both concrete and abstract nouns. Again, the results showed that there were no RT differences between the two visual fields for concrete words, whereas abstract words were recognised significantly faster as being members of a superordinate category when presented to the RVF. This pattern of results is consistent with the hypothesis that the right hemisphere can recognise concrete category-noun associations better than abstract ones.

Day (1979) has recently replicated and extended some of his earlier findings. Using a lexical decision task, he found no difference in RT between the LVF and RVF for high imagery nouns and adjectives. However, low imagery nouns, low imagery adjectives, and both high and low imagery verbs were recognised as being words significantly faster when presented in the RVF. These findings led Day to conclude that the right hemisphere of normal right-handers can process high imagery words with the exception of verbs.

Bradshaw et al. (1977) have also investigated the right hemisphere's role in making lexical decisions. Their findings suggested that for both left- and right-handers the right hemisphere is involved in helping to reject non-words. In addition, it was noted that females generally showed more evidence of right hemisphere lexical abilities than did males. It was proposed that the right hemisphere in normal subjects has a significant role in verbal comprehension.

It is interesting to note that McFarland et al. (1978) also found that the right hemisphere is better able to process concrete than abstract words using an interference dichotic listening task. They reported that when speech was used as interference during a running memory span auditory recognition task a REA was obtained with abstract but not concrete words.

Nevertheless, there are some studies that have not found much or any evidence of selective processing of word types by the normal right hemisphere. For instance, Orenstein and Meighan (1976) failed to replicate the findings of Ellis and Shepherd (1974) using the same procedures. Also, Shanon (1979a, 1979b) has twice failed to replicate Day's (1977) original findings that concrete words are better recognised than abstract words by the right hemisphere using a similar lexical decision paradigm. In addition, Bradshaw and Gates (1978) found that only in an analysis of errors in a word naming task was there any evidence that the right hemisphere was better at processing concrete as opposed to abstract words. Unfortunately, due to these negative findings, the evidence indicating that the right hemisphere of normal right-handers can selectively process certain words classes better than others remains controversial.

There are other areas of research, however, that provide clearer evidence for language processing or comprehension abilities of the normal right hemisphere. Hellige and Webster (1979) observed that the right hemisphere appears to be superior to the left for the initial stages of letter processing. When subjects were presented with perceptually degraded letters it was observed that the LVF-right hemisphere was more efficient than the RVF-left hemisphere at extracting the relevant visual features of the letters.

Bryden and Allard (1976) also suggest that the right hemisphere is more proficient than the left for 'preprocessing' verbal stimuli. In their experiment subjects were required to name laterally presented letters printed in 10 different typefaces. They found that the perceptually difficult typefaces (i.e. most scriptlike) gave rise to LVF superiorities. From these results, it was postualted that the right hemisphere surpasses the left at global processing operations even when a verbal response is required. The notion that the right hemisphere is a global processer as opposed to being an analytical one has had many adherents (Cohen, 1973; Levy, 1974; Martin, 1979; Nebes, 1974; Semmes, 1968).

Since Coltheart (this volume) provides an in-depth account of the right hemisphere's contributions during reading, only a few further studies and observations will be necessary here. Ornstein et al. (unpublished manuscript) measured EEG alpha production differences between the two hemispheres while normal subjects read either a technical passage or a story involving metaphors and imagery. They reported finding greater right hemisphere activation during the reading of the story than during the technical material, and suggested that this may mean that some aspects of reading differentially engage the right hemisphere. Pirozzolo (1978) also suggested that the right hemisphere, particularly in children, can play an important part in the reading process. In summarising the role of the two hemispheres in reading, Pirozzolo says that

> the right hemisphere may be indispensable in beginning reading when children are learning to recognise letters and words as gestalts. (p.264)

There is also some cross-cultural evidence of right hemisphere participation in reading. In the Japanese language there are two main types of non-alphabetic symbols — *Kana* (phonetic symbols for syllables) and *Kanji* (essentially non-phonetic, logographic symbols). It has been demonstrated that normal right-handed Japanese subjects typically have a RVF advantage for *Kana* and a LVF advantage or trend for *Kanji* (Hatta, 1977; Sasanuma *et al.*, 1977). This is in keeping with the finding that left hemisphere damage in the Japanese is more likely to impair *Kana* processing while right hemisphere damage is more likely to disrupt the processing of *Kanji* (Sasanuma, 1975; Sasanuma *et al.*, 1977, 1980). It is also noteworthy that Hatta (1977) believes that:

> reading Japanese text requires the integrated action of both hemisphere processing systems to a greater extent than it would appear is required when reading French or English text. (p.687)

Finally, in terms of speech processing, there are certain speech features that appear to be processed by both hemispheres. For example, although during dichotic listening a REA is usually found for perceiving initial stop-consonants and for the articulatory features of voicing and place, no ear advantage is found for steady-state vowels (Shankweiler and Studdert-Kennedy, 1967; Studdert-Kennedy and Shankweiler, 1970). Furthermore, there is evidence that other linguistic features of speech, in particular intonation contours and pitch processing, are actually perceived better by the right hemisphere (Blumstein and Cooper, 1974; Van Lancker, 1975; Zurif, 1974; Zurif and Mendelsohn, 1972). These findings are consistent with the clinical data showing prosody disturbances following unilateral right hemisphere injury (Ross and Mesulam, 1979).

In reviewing the evidence for right hemisphere language participation in normal right-handers it is obvious that it is language comprehension abilities that are the most clearly developed. This is certainly consistent with the clinical data previously reviewed. Part of the problem, however, is in trying to assess the language production capabilities of the normal right hemisphere. There is a dearth of appropriate, non-clinical techniques available for such an evaluation.

One recently developed variant of the standard dichotic listening test, called pursuit auditory tracking, does appear to provide a way to determine hemispheric specialisation for speech production in normals (Sussman, 1971). The technique requires the subject to monitor a tone presented to one ear that varies randomly in frequency and amplitude. The subject then has to match the frequency fluctuations of the varying tone with a second tone presented to the opposite ear. This is accomplished by regulating the continuous movement of a body part.

If a speech articulator such as the jaw or tongue is used to match the varying frequency of the first tone the subject usually does better when the second tone (the cursor) is presented to the right ear rather than the left (Sussman, 1971). It was also found that a control group showed that no ear advantage occurred when the second tone was regulated by a nonspeech articulator such as the right hand. These findings take on added significance when one notes that the motor pathways involved in speech production are bilaterally represented (Berry and Eisenson, 1956; Gazzaniga, 1970; Penfield and Roberts, 1959). Taken together, this implies that the REA observed with speech articulators in the pursuit auditory tracking task is reflective of the left hemisphere's greater *functional*, but not *structural*, control of the motor pathways involved in speech production.

Perhaps the observed left hemisphere advantage in the pursuit auditory tracking task can be considered an instance of inhibitory control by the left hemisphere over the right in normal subjects. As already seen, inhibitory control of the right hemisphere's attempts at linguistic expression is a common occurrence in clinical patients (Nebes, 1974). In fact, Moscovitch (1973; 1976) has developed a model, called the functional localisation model, that explicitly posits that the left hemisphere usually inhibits or suppresses the normal right hemisphere's linguistic activities through inhibitory influences across the cerebral commissures.

The pursuit auditory tracking technique also helps to further emphasize the importance of separating speech comprehension abilities from speech production abilities when examining language lateralisation. This is because it has been shown that the magnitude of the REA in pursuit auditory tracking when using a speech articulator is unrelated to the magnitude of the REA observed in standard dichotic listening tests (Sussman and MacNeilage, 1975).

Predicting Right Hemisphere Language in Normal Subjects

One of the most active areas of current research with normal subjects involves trying to predict variations in the degree and direction of language lateralisation based upon certain subject variables. Dating from the nineteenth century, preferred handedness has often been considered an important subject variable for predicting an individual's cerebral organisation for language. Nonetheless, there is ample evidence that it is far from being a perfect predictor (Levy, 1974; Luria, 1970; Searleman, 1977).

In recent years it has been suggested that a variety of other subject variables may have predictive value for specifying cerebral language organisation. The subject variables that have received the most consideration are strength of handedness, familial sinistrality, writing hand posture, and sex. Unfortunately, for each one of these subject variables there are conflicting data concerning their role as worthwhile or useful predictors of an individual's cerebral make-up for language (Bradshaw, 1980; Briggs and Nebes, 1976; Lake and Bryden, 1976; Lishman and McMeekan, 1977; McKeever and VanDeventer, 1977; Searleman *et al.*, 1979).

In addition to these subject variables, some investigators have searched for a relationship between sighting eye dominance and hemispheric asymmetries (Bryden, 1973; Hayashi and Bryden, 1967; Sampson, 1969). There appears to be little evidence, however, that such a relationship exists (for a review see Porac and Coren, 1976). Similar to the sighting dominance findings, no direct relationship has ever been reported between preferred footedness and language lateralisation.

In an attempt to examine the usefulness of all the subject variables that have been proposed as likely predictors of cerebral organisation for language, a 240 trial consonant-vowel dichotic listening test was given to 373 college students (Searleman, 1980). On the basis of a variety of observations the 117 left-handed and 256 right-handed subjects were classified in terms of strength of handedness, familial sinistrality, writing hand posture, sex, sighting dominance, preferred footedness, and overall laterality (concordance of hand, eye, and foot dominances).

In brief, the results of the study suggested that left hemisphere language processing, at least based upon dichotic listening, is very pervasive in the normal population. Multiple regression analyses further indicated that most of the subject variables examined, either individually or in conjunction with each other, were not very useful as differential predictors of right hemisphere language comprehension abilities. In addition, surprisingly, it was found that footedness and not handedness was the single best predictor of cerebral organisation for language. Left-footedness was more likely to be associated with right hemisphere language than was left-handedness.

A possible explanation for this unexpected finding may be that although handedness is undoubtedly susceptible to cultural pressure or bias (for a review see Dawson, 1977), there is probably much less pressure or bias directed towards preferred footedness. Thus, if handedness and footedness are components of some underlying dimension that is correlated with certain hemispheric asymmetries (e.g. language), then footedness may be the more reliable and sensitive variable for predicting these asymmetries.

Conclusions

The aim of this chapter was to document and describe the linguistic abilities of the right hemisphere. Evidence was presented illustrating the remarkable ability, but not equipotentiality, of the developing right hemisphere to acquire language. Whereas it has been shown that the right hemispheres of commissurotomy and hemispherectomy patients possess some ability for comprehending written and particularly spoken language, there is little doubt that the right hemispheres of these patients are severely limited in speech production. The reasons why the right hemisphere does not typically produce propositional speech are because it cannot undertake a phonetic analysis of language, it only has a rudimentary understanding of syntax, it has a very limited short-term verbal memory, and it usually has little success in gaining access to or control of the speech musculature from the left hemisphere. These are the very skills that successful language production depend upon.

Although some of the clearest evidence for right hemisphere linguistic functioning has come from the study of clinical patients, there is considerable danger in trying to generalise these findings to normal subjects. Many of the patients who displayed the most reliable evidence of right hemisphere language abilities (N.G., L.B., R.S. and P.S.) had suffered early damage in the left hemisphere. As a consequence it is quite likely that these patients may have developed language skills in both hemispheres to a much greater degree than is typical in a normal person.

As with clinical data, the most apparent right hemisphere linguistic abilities in normal right-handers are seen in terms of language perception rather than language production. A major limiting factor in trying to evaluate the full extent of right hemisphere linguistic abilities, in both clinical and normal populations, may be the left hemisphere's tendency to suppress or interfere with right hemisphere linguistic activities. Perhaps the reason why the right hemisphere is generally more successful at language perception as opposed to production is because the left hemisphere is more successful at inhibiting the latter activities. If the left hemisphere is free to function and exert control, then it may well be impossible to ever accurately assess the full extent of the right hemisphere's linguistic capabilities.

Acknowledgement

I wish to express my gratitude to Andy Young for his helpful comments and suggestions.

References

ALAJOUANINE, T. and LHERMITTE, F. (1965). Acquired aphasia in children. *Brain* 88, 653-662.

ANDERSON, S. W. and JAFFE, J. (1973). Eye movement bias and ear preferences as indices of speech lateralization. Scientific Report, Department of Communication Science, New York State Psychiatric Institute.

BASSER, L. (1962). Hemiplegia of early onset and the faculty of speech with special reference to the effects of hemispherectomy. *Brain* **85**, 427-460.

BERRY, M. and EISENSON, J. (1956). *Speech Disorders.* Appleton-Century-Crofts, New York.

BLUMSTEIN, S. and COOPER, W. (1974). Hemispheric processing of intonation contours. *Cortex* **10**, 146-158.

BOGEN, J. and GORDON, H. (1971). Musical tests for functional lateralization with intracarotid amobarbitol. *Nature,* Lond. **230**, 524-525.

BOLLER, F. (1968). Latent aphasia: Right and left "non-aphasic" brain damaged patients compared. *Cortex* **4**, 245-256.

BRADSHAW, J. L. (1980). Right-hemisphere language: Familial and nonfamilial sinistrals, cognitive deficits and writing hand position in sinistrals, and concrete-abstract, imageable-nonimageable dimensions in word recognition. A review of interrelated issues. *Brain and Language* **10**, 172-188.

BRADSHAW, J. L. and GATES, A. (1978). Visual field differences in verbal tasks: effects of task familiarity and sex of subject. *Brain and Language* **5**, 166-187.

BRADSHAW, J. L., GATES, A. and NETTLETON, N. C. (1977). Bihemispheric involvement in lexical decisions: Handedness and a possible sex difference. *Neuropsychologia* **15**, 277-286.

BRAMWELL, B. (1899). On crossed aphasia. *Lancet* **1**, 1473-1479.

BRIGGS, G. G. and NEBES, R. D. (1976). The effects of handedness, family history and sex on the performance of a dichotic listening task. *Neuropsychologia* **14**, 129-133.

BROWN, J. W. (1979). Thalamic mechanisms in language. In *Handbook of Behavioral Neurobiology* (M. S. Gazzaniga, ed). Plenum Press, New York.

BROWN, J. W. and WILSON, F. R. (1973). Crossed aphasia in a dextral. *Neurology* **23**, 907-911.

BRYDEN, M. P. (1963). Ear preference in auditory perception. *Journal of Experimental Psychology* **65**, 103-105.

BRYDEN, M. P. (1973). Perceptual asymmetry in vision: relationship to handedness, eyedness, and speech lateralization. *Cortex* **9**, 418-432.

BRYDEN, M. P. and ALLARD, F. (1976). Visual hemifield differences depend on typeface. *Brain and Language* **3**, 191-200.

BURKLUND, C. W. and SMITH, A. (1977). Language and the cerebral hemispheres: Observations of verbal and nonverbal responses during 18 months following left ("dominant") hemispherectomy. *Neurology* **27**, 627-633.

CAPLAN, D., HOLMES, J. M. and MARSHALL, J. C. (1974). Word class and hemispheric specialization. *Neuropsychologia* **12**, 331-337.

CARAMAZZA, A., GORDON, J., ZURIF, E. B. and DELUCA, D. (1976). Right-hemispheric damage and verbal problem solving behavior. *Brain and Language* **3**, 41-46.

CARLSON, J. NETLEY, C., HENDRICK, E. B. and PRICHARD, J. S. (1968). A reexamination of intellectual disabilities in hemispherectomized patients. *Transactions of the American Neurological Association* **93**, 198-201.

COHEN, G. (1973). Hemisphere differences in serial versus parallel processing. *Journal of Experimental Psychology* **97**, 349-356.

CRITCHLEY, M. (1962). Speech and speech-loss in relation to the duality of the brain. In *Interhemispheric Relations and Cerebral Dominance* (V. B. Mountcastle, ed.) Johns Hopkins University Press, Baltimore.

CROCKETT, H. G. and ESTRIDGE, N. M. (1951). Cerebral hemispherectomy. *Bulletin of the Los Angeles Neurological Society* **16**, 71-87.

CZOPF, J. (1972). Über die Rolle der nicht dominanter Hemisphäre in der Restitution der

Sprache des Aphasischen. *Archiv für Psychiatrie und Nervenkrankheiten* **216**, 162-171.

DAWSON, J. L. M. (1977). Alaskan Eskimo hand, eye, auditory dominance and cognitive style. *Psychologia — An International Journal of Psychology in the Orient* **20**, 421-435.

● DAY, J. (1977). Right hemisphere language processing in normal right-handers. *Journal of Experimental Psychology: Human Perception and Performance* **3**, 518-528.

DAY, J. (1979). Visual half-field word recognition as a function of syntactic class and imageability. *Neuropsychologia* **17**, 515-519.

DENNIS, M. and WHITAKER, H. A. (1976). Language acquisition following hemidecortication: Linguistic superiority of the left over the right hemisphere. *Brain and Language* **3**, 404-433.

DENNIS, M. and WHITAKER, H. A. (1977). Hemispheric equipotentiality and language acquisition. In *Language Development and Neurological Theory* (S. J. Segalowitz and F. A. Gruber, eds). Academic Press, New York and London.

EISENSON, J. (1962). Language and intellectual modifications associated with right cerebral damage. *Language and Speech* **5**, 49-53.

ELLIS, H. D. and SHEPHERD, J. W. (1974). Recognition of abstract and concrete words presented in left and right visual fields. *Journal of Experimental Psychology* **103**, 1035-1036.

ETTLINGER, G., JACKSON, C. and ZANGWILL, O. L. (1955). Dysphasia following right temporal lobectomy in a right-handed man. *Journal of Neurology, Neurosurgery, and Psychiatry* **18**, 214-217.

FRENCH, L. A., JOHNSON, D. R., BROWN, I. A. and VAN BERGEN, F. B. (1955). Hemispherectomy for control of intractable convulsive seizures. *Journal of Neurosurgery* **12**, 154-164.

GAZZANIGA, M. S. (1970). *The Bisected Brain*. Appleton-Century-Crofts, New York.

● GAZZANIGA, M. S. and HILLYARD, S. (1971). Language and speech capacity of the right hemisphere. *Neuropsychologia* **9**, 273-280.

GAZZANIGA, M. S. and LEDOUX, J. E. (1978). *The Integrated Mind*. Plenum Press, New York.

GAZZANIGA, M. S., LEDOUX, J. E. and WILSON, D. H. (1977). Language, praxis, and the right hemisphere: Clues to some mechanisms of consciousness. *Neurology* **27**, 1144-1147.

GLONING, I., GLONING, K., HAUB, G. and QUATEMBER, R. (1969). Comparison of verbal behavior in right-handed and non-right-handed patients with anatomically verified lesion of one hemisphere. *Cortex* **5**, 41-52.

GOLDSTEIN, K. (1948). *Language and Language Disturbances*. Grune and Stratton, New York.

GORDON, H. (unpub.). *Verbal and Nonverbal Cerebral Processing in Man for Audition*. Unpublished doctoral dissertation, California Institute of Technology, 1973.

● GOTT, P. S. (1973). Language after dominant hemispherectomy. *Journal of Neurology, Neurosurgery, and Psychiatry* **36**, 1082-1088.

GOWERS, W. R. (1887). *Lectures on the Diagnosis of Diseases of the Brain*. Churchill, London.

HARDYCK, C. and PETRINOVICH, L. F. (1977). Left-handedness. *Psychological Bulletin* **84**, 385-404.

HATTA, T. (1977). Recognition of Japanese *Kanji* in the left and right visual fields. *Neuropsychologia* **15**, 685-688.

HAYASHI, T. and BRYDEN, M. P. (1967). Ocular dominance and perceptual asymmetry. *Perceptual and Motor Skills* **25**, 605-612.

108   *Alan Searleman*

HÉCAEN, H. (1976). Acquired aphasia in children and the ontogenesis of hemispheric functional specialization. *Brain and Language* **3**, 114-134.

HÉCAEN, H. and ALBERT, M. L. (1978). *Human Neuropsychology.* Wiley, New York.

HÉCAEN, H. and KREMIN, H. (1976). Neurolinguistic research on reading disorders resulting from left hemisphere lesions: aphasic and "pure" alexia. In *Studies in Neurolinguistics*, Vol. 2 (H. Whitaker and H. A. Whitaker, eds). Academic Press, New York and London.

HÉCAEN, H. and MARCIE, M. F. (1974). Disorders of written language following right hemisphere lesions. In *Hemisphere Function in the Human Brain* (S. J. Dimond and J. G. Beaumont, eds). Elek, London.

HÉCAEN, H. and SAUGUET, J. (1971). Cerebral dominance in left-handed subjects. *Cortex* **7**, 19-48.

HEILMAN, K. M., SCHOLES, R. and WATSON, R. T. (1975). Auditory affective agnosia. *Journal of Neurology, Neurosurgery, and Psychiatry* **38**, 69-72.

HELLIGE, J. B. and WEBSTER, R. (1979). Right hemisphere superiority for initial stages of letter processing. *Neuropsychologia* **17**, 653-660.

HENSCHEN, S. E. (1926). On the function of the right hemisphere of the brain in relation to the left in speech, music, and calculation. *Brain* **49**, 110-123.

HILLIER, W. F. (1954). Hemispherectomy for malignant glioma. *Neurology* **4**, 718-721.

HINES, D. (1976). Recognition of verbs, abstract nouns and concrete nouns from the left and right visual half-fields. *Neuropsychologia* **14**, 211-216.

HINES, D. (1977). Differences in tachistoscopic recognition between abstract and concrete words as a function of visual half-field and frequency. *Cortex* **13**, 66-73.

HOLMES, J. E. and SADOFF, R. L. (1966). Aphasia due to a right hemisphere tumour in a right-handed man. *Neurology, Minn.* **16**, 392-397.

HUMPHREY, M. E. and ZANGWILL, O. L. (1952). Dysphasia in left-handed patients with unilateral lesions. *Journal of Neurology, Neurosurgery and Psychiatry* **15**, 184-193.

JOHNSON, J. P., SOMMERS, R. K. and WEIDNER, W. E. (1977). Dichotic ear preference in aphasia. *Journal of Speech and Hearing Research* **20**, 116-129.

KINSBOURNE, M. (1971). The minor hemisphere as a source of aphasic speech. *Transactions of the American Neurological Association* **96**, 141-145.

KINSBOURNE, M. (1974). Mechanisms of hemispheric interaction in man. In *Hemispheric Disconnection and Cerebral Function* (M. Kinsbourne and W. L. Smith, eds). Charles C. Thomas, Springfield, Illinois.

KINSBOURNE, M. and WARRINGTON, E. K. (1962). A variety of reading disability associated with right hemisphere lesions. *Journal of Neurology, Neurosurgery and Psychiatry* **25**, 339-344.

KRASHEN, S. (1972). Language and the left hemisphere. *Working Papers in Phonetics* No. 24.

KRASHEN, S. (1973). Lateralization, languages, learning, and the critical period. Some new evidence. *Language Learning* **23**, 63-74.

KRYNAUW, R. A. (1950). Infantile hemiplegia treated by removing one cerebral hemisphere. *Journal of Neurology, Neurosurgery and Psychiatry* **13**, 243-267.

LAKE, D. A. and BRYDEN, M. P. (1976). Handedness and sex differences in hemispheric asymmetry. *Brain and Language* **3**, 266-282.

LENNEBERG, E. H. (1967). *Biological Foundations of Language.* Wiley, New York.

LEVY, J. (1974). Psychobiological implications of bilateral asymmetry. In *Hemisphere Function in the Human Brain* (S. J. Dimond and J. G. Beaumont, eds). Elek, London.

LEVY, J. and TREVARTHEN, C. (1977). Perceptual, semantic and phonetic aspects of elementary language processes in split-brain patients. *Brain* **100**, 105-118.

LEVY, J., NEBES, R. D. and SPERRY, R. W. (1971). Expressive language in the surgically separated minor hemisphere. *Cortex* **7**, 49-58.
LEVY, J., TREVARTHEN, C. and SPERRY, R. W. (1972). Perception of bilateral chimeric figures following hemispheric deconnection. *Brain* **95**, 61-78.
LISHMAN, W. A. and MCMEEKAN, E. R. L. (1977). Handedness in relation to direction and degree of cerebral dominance for language. *Cortex* **13**, 30-43.
LURIA, A. R. (1966). *Higher Cortical Functions in Man.* Basic Books, New York.
LURIA, A. R. (1970). *Traumatic Aphasia.* Mouton, The Hague.
MARTIN, M. (1979). Hemispheric specialization for local and global processing. *Neuropsychologia* **17**, 33-40.
MCFARLAND, K., MCFARLAND, M. L., BAIN, J. D. and ASHTON, R. (1978). Ear differences of abstract and concrete word recognition. *Neuropsychologia* **16**, 555-561.
MCFIE, J. (1961). The effects of hemispherectomy on intellectual functioning in cases of linguistic hemiplegia. *Journal of Neurology, Neurosurgery and Psychiatry* **24**, 240-249.
MCKEEVER, W. F. and VAN DEVENTER, A. D. (1977). Visual and auditory language processing asymmetries: Influences of handedness, familial sinistrality, and sex. *Cortex* **13**, 225-241.
MILNER, B. (1968). Visual recognition and recall after right temporal lobe excision in man. *Neuropsychologia* **6**, 191-209.
MOORE, W. H. and WEIDNER, W. E. (1974). Bilateral tachistoscopic word perception in aphasic and normal subjects. *Perceptual and Motor Skills* **39**, 1003-1011.
MOORE, W. H. and WEIDNER, W. E. (1975). Dichotic word-perception of aphasic and normal subjects. *Perceptual and Motor Skills* **40**, 379-386.
MOSCOVITCH, M. (1973). Language and the cerebral hemispheres: Reaction-time studies and their implications for models of cerebral dominance. In *Communication and Affect: Language and Thought* (P. Pliner, T. Alloway and L. Krames, eds). Academic Press, New York and London.
MOSCOVITCH, M. (1976). On the representation of language in the right hemisphere of right-handed people. *Brain and Languge* **3**, 47-71.
MOSCOVITCH, M. (1977). The development of lateralization of language functions and its relation to cognitive and linguistic development: A review and some theoretical speculations. In *Language Development and Neurological Theory* (S. J. Segalowitz and F. A. Gruber, eds). Academic Press, New York and London.
NEBES, R. D. (1974). Hemispheric specialization in commissurotomized man. *Psychological Bulletin* **81**, 1-14.
NEBES, R. D. and SPERRY, R. W. (1971). Hemispheric deconnection syndrome with cerebral birth injury in the dominant arm area. *Neuropsychologia* **9**, 247-259.
NEEDLES, W. (1942). Concerning transfer of cerebral dominance in the function of speech. *Journal of Nervous and Mental Disorders* **95**, 270-277.
NIELSEN, J. M. (1946). *Agnosia, Apraxia, Aphasia: Their Value in Cerebral Localization.* Hoeber, New York.
OBRADOR, S. (1964). Nervous integration after hemispherectomy in man. In *Cerebral Localization and Organization.* (G. Schaltenbrand and C. W. Woolsey, eds). University of Wisconsin Press, Madison, Wisconsin.
OJEMANN, G. A. (1976). Subcortical language mechanisms. In *Studies in Neurolinguistics*, Vol. 1 (H. Whitaker and H. A. Whitaker, eds). Academic Press, New York and London.
OJEMANN, G. A. (1977). Asymmetric function of the thalamus in man. In *Evolution and Lateralization of the Brain* (S. J. Dimond and D. A. Blizard, eds). New York Academy of Sciences, New York.

ORENSTEIN, H. B. and MEIGHAN, W. B. (1976). Recognition of bilaterally presented words varying in concreteness and frequency: Lateral dominance or sequential processing? *Bulletin of the Psychonomic Society* **7**, 179-180.

ORNSTEIN, R., HERRON, J. and JOHNSTONE, J. (unpub.). Differential right hemisphere involvement in two reading tasks. Unpublished manuscript.

PENFIELD, W. and ROBERTS, L. (1959). *Speech and Brain Mechanisms*. Princeton University Press, Princeton, N.J.

PETTIT, J. M. and NOLL, J. D. (1979). Cerebral dominance in aphasia recovery. *Brain and Language* **7**, 191-200.

PIROZZOLO, F. J. (1978). Cerebral asymmetries and reading acquisition. *Academic Therapy* **13**, 261-266.

PORAC, C. and COREN, S. (1976). The dominant eye. *Psychological Bulletin* **83**, 880-897.

ROSS, E. D. and MESULAM, M. (1979). Dominant language functions of the right hemisphere? Prosody and emotional gesturing. *Archives of Neurology* **36**, 144-148.

RUSSELL, W. R. and ESPIR, M. L. R. (1961). *Traumatic Aphasia: Its Syndromes, Psychopathology and Treatment*. Oxford University Press, London.

SAMPSON, H. (1969). Recall of digits projected to temporal and nasal hemi-retinas. *Quarterly Journal of Experimental Psychology* **21**, 39-42.

SASANUMA, S. (1975). *Kana* and *Kanji* processing in Japanese aphasics. *Brain and Language* **2**, 369-383.

SASANUMA, S., ITOH, M., MORI, K. and KOBAYASHI, Y. (1977). Tachistoscopic recognition of *Kana* and *Kanji* words. *Neuropsychologia* **15**, 547-553.

SASANUMA, S., ITOH, M., KOBAYASHI, Y. and MORI, K. (1980). The nature of the task-stimulus interaction in the tachistoscopic recognition of *Kana* and *Kanji* words. *Brain and Language* **9**, 298-306.

SEARLEMAN, A. (1977). A review of right hemisphere linguistic capabilities. *Psychological Bulletin* **84**, 503-528.

SEARLEMAN, A. (1980). Subject variables and cerebral organization for language. *Cortex* **16**, 239-254.

SEARLEMAN, A., TWEEDY, J. and SPRINGER, S. P. (1979). Interrelationships among subject variables believed to predict cerebral organization. *Brain and Language* **7**, 267-276.

SEMMES, J. (1968). Hemispheric specialization: A possible clue to mechanism. *Neuropsychologia* **6**, 11-26.

SHANKWEILER, D. and STUDDERT-KENNEDY, M. (1967). Identification of consonants and vowels presented to left and right ears. *Quarterly Journal of Experimental Psychology* **19**, 59-63.

SHANON, B. (1979a). Lateralization effects in response to words and non-words. *Cortex* **15**, 541-549.

SHANON, B. (1979b). Lateralization effects in lexical decision tasks. *Brain and Language* **8**, 380-387.

SMITH, A. (1966). Speech and other functions after left (dominant) hemispherectomy. *Journal of Neurology, Neurosurgery and Psychiatry* **29**, 467-471.

ST. JAMES-ROBERTS, I. (1981). A reinterpretation of hemispherectomy data without functional plasticity of the brain. I. Intellectual function. *Brain and Language* **13**, 31-53.

STUDDERT-KENNEDY, M. and SHANKWEILER, D. (1970). Hemispheric specialization for speech perception. *Journal of the Acoustical Society of America* **48**, 579-594.

SUSSMAN, H. (1971). The laterality effect in lingual-auditory tracking. *Journal of the Acoustical Society of America* **49**, 1874-1880.

SUSSMAN, H. and MACNEILAGE, P. (1975). Studies of hemispheric specialization for speech production. *Brain and Language* **2**, 131-151.

TROJANOWSKI, J. Q., GREEN, R. C. and LEVINE, D. N. (1980). Crossed aphasia in a dextral: A clinicopathological study. *Neurology* **30**, 709-713.

VAN LANCKER, D. (1975). Heterogeneity in language and speech. *Working Papers in Phonetics* No. 29.

WADA, J. and RASMUSSEN, T. (1960). Intracarotid injection of sodium amytal for the lateralization of cerebral speech dominance: Experimental and clinical observations. *Journal of Neurosurgery* **17**, 266-282.

WECHSLER, A. F. (1976). Crossed aphasia in an illiterate dextral. *Brain and Language* **3**, 164-172.

WEINSTEIN, E. A. (1964). Affections of speech with lesions of the non-dominant hemisphere. *Research Publications, Association for Research in Nervous and Mental Diseases* **5**, 220-225.

WEINSTEIN, E. A. and KELLER, N. J. (1963). Linguistic patterns of misnaming in brain injury. *Neuropsychologia* **1**, 79-80.

WHITE, H. H. (1961). Cerebral hemispherectomy in the treatment of infantile hemiplegia. *Confinia Neurologica* **21**, 1-50.

WILSON, D. H., REEVES, A. G. and GAZZANIGA, M. S. (1977). Cerebral commissurotomy for the control of intractable seizures. *Neurology* **27**, 708-715.

WITELSON, S. F. (1977). Early hemisphere specialization and interhemisphere plasticity: An empirical and theoretical review. In *Language and Development and Neurological Theory* (S. J. Segalowitz and F. A. Gruber, eds). Academic Press, New York and London.

ZAIDEL, E. (1975). A technique for presenting lateralized visual input with prolonged exposure. *Vision Research* **15**, 283-289.

ZAIDEL, E. (1976). Auditory vocabulary of the right hemisphere following brain bisection or hemidecortication. *Cortex* **12**, 191-211.

ZAIDEL, E. (1977). Unilateral auditory language comprehension on the Token Test following cerebral commissurotomy and hemispherectomy. *Neuropsychologia* **15**, 1-18.

ZAIDEL, E. (1978a). Auditory language comprehension in the right hemisphere following cerebral commissurotomy and hemispherectomy: A comparison with child language and aphasia. In *Language Acquisition and Language Breakdown: Parallels and Divergencies*. (A. Caramazza and E. B. Zurif, eds). Johns Hopkins Press, Baltimore.

ZAIDEL, E. (1978b). Lexical organization in the right hemisphere. In *Cerebral Correlates of Conscious Experience* (P. A. Buser and A. Rougeul-Buser, eds). North-Holland Publishing Company, New York.

ZANGWILL, O. L. (1960). *Cerebral Dominance and its Relation to Psychological Function.* Oliver and Boyd, Edinburgh.

ZANGWILL, O. L. (1979). Two cases of crossed aphasia in dextrals. *Neuropsychologia* **17**, 167-172.

ZOLLINGER, R. (1935). Removal of left cerebral hemisphere. *Archives of Neurological Psychiatry* **34**, 1055-1064.

ZURIF, E. B. (1974). Auditory lateralization: Prosodic and syntactic factors. *Brain and Language* **1**, 391-404.

ZURIF, E. B. and MENDELSOHN, M. (1972). Hemispheric specialization for the perception of speech sounds: The influence of intonation and structure. *Perception and Psychophysics* **11**, 329-332.

5

METHODS FOR
STUDYING CEREBRAL
HEMISPHERIC FUNCTION

J. Graham Beaumont

SIX APPROACHES have dominated the study of the relative specialisation of the cerebral hemispheres. Three of these, the study of the effects of lateral localised cortical lesions and the investigation of commissurotomy and hemispherectomy patients, have involved clinical subjects. The other three methods, suitable for the investigation of normal subjects, are based upon lateralised stimulus presentation: the divided visual field, dichotic listening and tactile presentation techniques. Up to about 1960, almost all the data were derived from the study of clinical lesions, but since that date, with the vogue for studies of hemisphere function, a flood of literature has appeared, resulting from the employment of the other techniques.

In addition to the six main investigative techniques, other less popular methods have also been employed to enable inferences to be drawn about the relative functional specialisation of the two hemispheres. Some of these methods warrant more attention than others. In the limited space of this chapter, most of the methods will find some mention, and an attempt will be made to indicate some of the advantages and drawbacks of each, and to form some assessment of the past and potential contribution of each to this field of study. Nevertheless, the reader will find it necessary to pursue the references cited if full justice is to be done to any of the techniques which will be examined.

The following discussion is also restricted to the study of hemisphere function in adults. Much the same considerations apply to the methods used to study children, but some aspects specific to developmental studies are discussed in

FUNCTIONS OF THE RIGHT CEREBRAL HEMISPHERE
0-12-773250-0
*Copyright © 1983 by Academic Press, London.
All rights of reproduction in any form reserved.*

Beaumont (1982a), Witelson (1977), Young (1982a), and Young (this volume).

Investigations with Clinical Subjects

Lesion Studies

Although most modern reviews remind us that the Ancient Egyptians probably knew something of lateralisation of function as early as 3,000B.C., scientific study of the behavioural effects of cerebral lesions can be considered to date from the 1860s with the publication of the work of Dax, and the studies of Broca, Wernicke and others.

The modern era of behavioural neurology, and the growth of neuropsychology to form an identifiable independent discipline, begins with the study of traumatic lesions during the Second World War. From this date, the techniques of modern experimental psychology have increasingly been employed in the study of the cognitive deficits which follow injury to the brain, with the result that increasingly sophisticated models have been generated, formulated in cognitive terms, of the functions of both the right and left cerebral hemispheres.

The logic of studies of the effects of localised cortical lesions is quite simple. It is that localised lesions in certain regions of the cortex are observed to result in particular behavioural deficits. It is therefore possible to correlate the site of a lesion as established by some physical investigation with the deficit observed, and to draw inferences about the functions served by the area which has been damaged.

There are some variations in the ways in which studies of this kind are conducted, to some extent following national 'schools', with a preference for multivariate studies of unitary cognitive functions in North America, group studies which aim to isolate and describe the functional character of the psychological deficit in Britain, and intensive study of individual cases in Eastern Europe. It is possible to overstate the differences between these schools, however, and all forms of investigation are pursued in most centres of study.

The essence of all the studies is that they are correlational in nature, and in general are based upon some rather vaguely formulated Interactionist or Associationist model of function; that is that there is a relative localisation of the basic skills upon which higher functions are founded. The effects of lesions as observed in higher functions will reflect the degree to which there has been impairment of the basic skills, or disruption of the connections between them, which cannot be compensated by the employment of alternative skills or cognitive strategies which might enable the higher function to be performed without recourse to the disabled basic skill.

There are difficulties with this approach, on two levels. The first is at a conceptual level. Neuropsychologists are rarely careful about the status of the models which they employ, and examination of these models reveals considerable conceptual problems. In particular the concept of a 'function' and its 'localisation', independent of the observed physiological changes which have occurred, is unsatisfactory. Too many models rely upon rather vague metaphors derived from other areas of science and engineering, and there has been a failure to consider the relative contribution of inhibitory and facilitatory effects which might follow from damage to cortical neurons. Most models lack validity in physiological terms, and there has been a further failure to consider their validity in cognitive terms. Neuropsychology has progressed by ignoring such issues, in the main, but it is not clear how long it may continue to do so. Further discussion of these issues is to be found in Beaumont (1983a,b), Finger (1978) and Weiskrantz (1968, 1973).

Ignoring the conceptual issues, there is a second group of difficulties on a more practical level. These concern the design of research studies, and in particular the formation of matched groups of patients with homologous left and right hemisphere lesions who can be studied on some task (or better, on two matched tasks so that double dissociation can be demonstrated: see Weiskrantz, 1968). The most important problem is in accurately matching the mass of the lesion in left and right brain lesioned subjects. It is well known that, because right hemisphere lesions (especially tumours) can grow to a larger size before they interfere to a critical degree with the individual's everyday activity, right hemisphere lesions at the time of presentation are on average larger than left hemisphere lesions. This should obviously be controlled for in any research investigation, but it naturally proves very difficult, in practical terms, to do so.

The second important problem is the degree to which it is possible to control for associated functions. If studying calculation abilities, for example, is it wise to control for general verbal competence? If this control is not introduced, then apparent lateral differences may simply reflect the presence of an aphasic deficit in some of the left hemisphere group. If the control is employed, then the resulting left hemisphere group may have less severe lesions than the right hemisphere group, or be in some way atypical of patients with lesions to the posterior left hemisphere. There is no clear solution to this problem.

A final difficulty, which has only more recently become apparent, is the vagueness with which anatomical denominations are used for areas of the cortex. Several recent studies (Bogen and Bogen, 1976; Ojemann, 1979; Ojemann and Whitaker, 1978; Whitaker and Selnes, 1976) have shown that certain cortical regions thought to be clearly defined by their association with functional losses cannot be precisely identified. This emphasises the loose way in which neuropsychologists describe cortical lesions, and the error which this may introduce into clinical and research evidence.

The evidence from brain lesioned patients should therefore be treated with a little caution, but it is nonetheless valuable, not only for its practical clinical applications, but also in validating the results of studies with normal subjects. Good reviews of the effects of right hemisphere lesions will be found in Beaumont (1983b), Dimond (1980), Hécaen and Albert (1978), Heilman and Valenstein (1979), Kinsbourne (1971, 1976, 1978), Lezak (1976), Milner and Teuber (1968), Teuber (1975), Walsh (1978).

Commissurotomy

Commissurotomy, or the 'split-brain' operation, in which the forebrain commissures are sectioned for the relief of intractible epilepsy, has been a method of importance both for the data which it has yielded and for the stimulus which it has provided for the development of laboratory techniques for the study of normal intact subjects.

The operation and its effects have been clearly described by Gazzaniga (1970), Gazzaniga and LeDoux (1978) and Dimond (1972), and further important reviews of the evidence are to be found in Beaumont (1981a, 1982b), Gazzaniga (1975a), Nebes (1974), Searleman (1977), Trevarthen (1975) and Zaidel (1978). In essence, the corpus callosum, sometimes together with the anterior commissure, is sectioned thereby severing direct cortico-cortical communication between the right and left hemispheres. By arranging for stimuli to be presented by sensory channels which arrive at a single hemisphere, the performance of that hemisphere, in relative isolation from its partner, may be studied.

Not surprisingly, such a dramatic operation has captured the imagination of many neuroscientists, who have perhaps as a result been less cautious about the interpretation of data obtained from these patients than they might have been. An example of how the evidence has been distorted and misrepresentated is with respect to the discussion of consciousness (Beaumont, 1981a), but also applies to some extent to other functions. However, on strictly methodological grounds, there are two important issues to be noted.

The first is the nature of the patient sample. This sample is small, the very extensive data in the literature being essentially derived from seven patients, of whom only two provide the majority. The variation among these patients is great, both with respect to performance and to neurological status, and many of the patients have a considerable degree of extracallosal pathology which contributes to the deficits observed. A useful discussion of this problem, with a tabulation of the patients, is provided by Whitaker and Ojemann (1977). The important point is that this evidence should not be treated as if it came from an experimental manipulation in normal subjects, and the patients should certainly not be treated as if they were a single homogeneous group.

The second difficulty is that the split-brain patients develop ingenious strategies which, despite the experimental paradigms employed, allow stimulus information to be transmitted across the midline and into both hemispheres.

Gazzaniga (1970; Gazzaniga and Hillyard, 1971) has been particularly acute at identifying some of these strategies. The strategies which have been identified, together with the remarkable lack of handicap which these patients exhibit in everyday life, suggest that the patients are adept at generating such strategies, which in turn carries implications for their performance within the laboratory. To construct an experimental paradigm which prevents all possibility of cross-cuing is a difficult task, and the possibility of its operation in any study must be actively considered.

While the opportunity must be taken to derive what information we can from commissurotomy patients, in as tight a methodological paradigm as possible, the evidence from such studies will inevitably be limited, and will present peculiar problems of interpretation, particularly because of the abnormal neurological status of the split-brain patient. Some contribution has also been made by the study of patients with partial commissurotomies (Gazzaniga, 1975b; Gazzaniga and LeDoux, 1978) and of individuals with congenital absence of the corpus callosum ('agenesis': see Chiarello, 1980; Milner and Jeeves, 1979).

Hemispherectomy

If split-brain patients pose problems for the interpretation of their performance in terms of cerebral organisation, these problems are even greater for hemispherectomy patients. In hemispherectomy one entire neocortical hemisphere is removed. The results of this operation are important in assessing the contribution of the normal hemispheres, and in discovering the degree of compensation which can be achieved by the hemisphere which remains, but the operation is rarely performed in adults, and the data is more valuable for assessing developmental aspects of cerebral organisation. Even with children, there is usually a congenital abnormality of the central nervous system which makes valid inferences to the normally developing brain difficult to draw. There are useful discussions of hemispherectomy in Kinsbourne and Smith (1974), and in both the text and commentaries of Corballis and Morgan (1978), but studies of hemispherectomy patients have yielded few clear conclusions about normal hemisphere function.

Intracarotid Sodium Amytal

Wada (1949) developed the technique of injecting sodium amytal into the common or internal carotid artery on one side of the head in order to temporarily suppress the activity of one hemisphere of the brain. The period of suppression as indexed by the appearance of a contralateral hemiplegia lasts for about 4 or 5 minutes. The method has been validated against the results of anterior temporal lobe surgery (Branch et al., 1964), and a further description with electrophysiological data is to be found in Blume *et al.* (1973). The method has been of particular value in assessing the relative frequency of unilateral left or right, or of bilateral, speech representation in groups showing different manual preferences (Rasmussen and Milner, 1975), although it has also been used to study more specific aspects of functional organisation (Gilbert and Pratt, 1977; Risse and Gazzaniga, 1978).

Although the method has been generally considered too dangerous for use in normal subjects, two papers have reported studies of lateral speech representation. in stutterers (Andrews and Quinn, 1972; Lussenhop *et al.*, 1973), although the number of subjects tested is very small.

While the method appears an elegant technique, permitting within-subject comparison of each hemisphere performing alone (given that the risks can be justified by the clinical information obtained), published reports often overlook the disadvantages of the technique. The period of suppression and the conditions of testing allow only the most superficial and poorly controlled investigations. In addition, the technique is extremely stressful for patients, in a way which undoubtedly interferes with their performance. It is also unclear how much of the drug is carried around the Circle of Willis and perfuses the hemisphere contralateral to the side of injection. The amount is small enough for the method to be valid for clinical purposes, but perhaps not to meet the added rigour of the requirements of experimental studies. Finally, the principal distribution of the internal carotid artery does not reach the occipital lobe, the inferior temporal lobe and some other medial aspects of the temporal lobe.

The method is therefore limited to patients who already have abnormal brains, and to crude assessment of cognitive functions. Within these limitations, the data which it can yield is of undoubted value.

Electroconvulsive Therapy

Although electroconvulsive therapy (ECT) has traditionally involved seizure inducement by a pair of bilaterally placed electrodes, it has more recently been administered using unilaterally placed electrodes (Clyma, 1975; d'Élia, 1974), originally with the intention of reducing the confusion and impairment of verbal memory which some patients experienced for a period following each treatment. Providing that the electrodes were placed over the hemisphere nondominant for speech, the unilateral administration was found to reduce the magnitude of these 'side-effects' without lessening the therapeutic power of the treatment significantly (Hesche *et al.*, 1978).

It was subsequently realised that the results of ECT administration could yield data on speech lateralisation in patients, and that the period following administration could be used to study the differential contribution of the two hemispheres to cognitive processes. Recent examples of the way in which this has been done are to be found in Horan *et al.* (1980) and Robertson and Inglis (1978). Geffen *et al.* (1978) also used the results of ECT administration to validate their version of a dichotic listening task for the assessment of speech lateralisation, although Warrington and Pratt (1981) used ECT evidence to argue that dichotic listening does not provide an index of language lateralisation.

The method seems fairly uncontroversial, especially if used merely to establish speech lateralisation. However, how far the after-effects of treatment can be considered to interfere with specifically lateralised processes is uncertain. In addition, as the treatment is only given to clinically depressed patients, and current theories suggest that such patients have a lateral dysfunction of the brain (Gruzelier and Flor-Henry, 1979). The influence of this dysfunction upon the observed results is unclear, but suggests caution in their interpretation.

Psychological Studies with Normal Subjects

Divided Visual Field Presentation

Of the techniques employed with normal intact subjects, this method has been the most profitable, and the most widely employed. Its use to study cerebral lateralisation was stimulated by the split-brain studies in which it was one of the principal methods of investigation, although the technique has a longer history in experimental psychology. An extensive review of the technique and of current findings is to be found in Beaumont (1982c).

The logic of divided visual field presentation is very simple. Because the lateral visual half fields project to the contralateral visual cortex, if stimuli are presented in one lateral visual field then it is certain that the initial reception of such stimuli is by the contralateral hemisphere. Because the information passes through both eyes, and by both crossed and uncrossed fibres (via nasal and temporal hemiretinae) differences in acuity between the eyes and between the crossed and uncrossed pathways should be balanced out, if presentations are arranged for both visual half fields (providing, of course that there is no subtle interaction among these variables). Performance can be observed on some cognitive task relevant to the lateralised stimuli, and referred to the hemisphere in which the stimuli were first received. The methodological problems therefore reduce to ensuring that stimuli can be presented at a given location in one or both visual half fields. Young (1982b) has reviewed and discussed the methodological issues involved.

The first concern is to know just how close to central fixation stimuli may be placed and yet may be safely assumed to be lateralised to the contralateral hemisphere. The concern is difficult to resolve because there is little evidence to inform us about the medial overlap of the visual fields, and much that we have is derived from the study of animals. However, it seems reasonable to assume that there is a central strip with bilateral projections which covers perhaps 1° laterally, and may widen around the fovea. There is a further region of perhaps 3° which has direct cortico-cortical links through the splenium of the corpus callosum. This is probably primarily involved in stereopsis, but whether it is restricted to this function, and therefore not relevant to simple figural or symbolic stimuli, is unclear. See Young (1982b) for a full review of these issues. It seems therefore wise to avoid the central 2° or 3° of vision in divided visual field presentation, although performance asymmetries with more medially placed stimuli have been reported.

The second issue is, given that the eyes are directed at some central fixation point at stimulus onset, how short must stimulus exposure be to obviate the possibility of gaze deviation to the lateral stimulus location? Again, this is difficult to assess from published mean latencies of the various kinds of eye movement which would be likely to be involved, but it would seem that the commonly accepted figure of 150 ms is not unreasonable, and that longer exposure durations, up to perhaps 200 ms may be permissible (Young, 1982b). Longer exposure durations than 200 ms must certainly be suspect without well validated fixation monitoring.

This leads to the third methodological concern, that of fixation monitoring. It now appears that the rather lax approach which has been adopted to this problem may have been a mistake. The assumption is common that to merely instruct adult subjects to fixate, and then present stimuli at one lateral location, randomly to right or left (thereby discouraging anticipatory guessing), is sufficient as a control for fixation. Certainly, most adults appear to be able to fixate with remarkable reliability, but given the very small and subtle nature of the lateral differences in performance observed, together with the known tendency for certain types of task or material to elicit lateral eye movements (see below), perhaps failure of fixation on only a small proportion of trials, with a bias in one lateral direction, could be sufficient to artifactually produce the lateral differences observed.

Various manipulations have been attempted to introduce fixation control. Centrally placed stimuli to be reported before the lateral stimuli have been introduced on each trial (McKeever and Huling, 1971). It is uncertain however whether the introduction of the 'task irrelevant' central item influences subsequent task processing, and the method is not suited to reaction time studies. An alternative strategy is to introduce trials with the stimuli at central fixation and demand that performance of these trials be superior to lateral trials before accepting any subject's data, but this method is cumbersome and its validity uncertain. Other approaches have been to utilise the Haidinger's Brush phenomenon (Gibson *et al.*, 1972), although this is no more than an aid to the subject.

Undoubtedly the best method of fixation monitoring is direct, rather than the above indirect methods, by video monitoring (Geffen et al., 1972; Young et al., 1980) or by electrooculographic recording (Dimond and Beaumont, 1972). The method described by Young et al. is probably the easiest to use in conjunction with tachistoscopic studies, and deserves more widespread adoption.

While unilateral stimulus presentation has been favoured because of the problems of fixation control, bilateral presentation has also been employed, and has been claimed by some to yield lateral asymmetries of larger magnitude. Given that fixation is adequately monitored, then there appears no objection to bilateral presentation, if attention is also paid to the control of report order from left and right visual fields. It is interesting that, given the fierce debate between proponents of unilateral and bilateral presentation, a general review of the research data reveals little conflict between findings obtained with the two forms of presentation (Beaumont, 1982d).

Although most studies have employed the tachistoscope, other forms of apparatus have been employed, including a back-projection system allowing greater stimulus eccentricities and a wider range of stimuli (Dimond and Beaumont, 1974). Apparatus has also been devised to allow continuous presentation of stimulus material. Dimond and Beaumont (1971) used an arrangement with corneal reflection which allowed the suspension of presentation with deviation of fixation, to study vigilance, and methods based upon half occluded contact lenses have been described by Dimond et al. (1975) and, in conjunction with a collimator, by Zaidel (1975). These methods, while promising, are not well validated and cumbersome to employ.

To some extent the findings with divided visual field presentation appear robust and to be not seriously affected by slight artifactual contamination of the technique. Nevertheless the relative ease with which the technique may be employed has meant that many published studies are characterised by less than a fully acceptable degree of methodological control. Some care should therefore be exercised in evaluating evidence from studies using this technique.

Dichotic Listening

The dichotic listening technique, first employed in a neuropsychological context by Kimura (1961), is a direct parallel to divided visual field presentation, but in the auditory modality. There is one important difference, however, in that the auditory pathways do not have a simple contralateral projection to the cortex. From each ear there is both an ipsilateral and a contralateral pathway. From clinical evidence it has been considered that the crossed pathway was the dominant of the two, and this was supported by evidence from commissurotomy patients (Sparks and Geschwind, 1968; Springer and Gazzaniga, 1975; Gordon, 1980) that under conditions of competition, the contralateral crossed pathway suppresses input carried by the ipsilateral uncrossed pathway. This has been questioned more recently by studies on these patients which have shown that the suppression effect only operates for dichotic speech stimuli and not for pure tones (Efron *et al.*, 1977), and that the apparent suppression of left ear material may be a function of the spectral-temporal overlap between competing stimuli (Springer *et al.*, 1978). This means that the dominance of the crossed pathway has not been so clearly validated as was once thought. Interestingly, there are also lateral differences in the size of the tracts of the auditory pathway (Ferraro and Minckler, 1977a,b).

Given that the dominance of the crossed pathway is accepted, and that the logic of lateralised stimulus presentation is upheld, there has been debate about whether competing dichotic stimuli must be presented, or whether single unilateral stimuli may also produce a lateral ear advantage. The question implied by this debate is whether competition between left and right ear stimuli is necessary to produce the ear superiority effect. The answer to this empirical question is to be found in reviews of the literature (Berlin, 1977; Berlin and Cullen, 1977; Blumstein, 1974; Krashen, 1976; Springer, 1979; and with especial reference to music, Damásio and Damásio, 1977; Wyke, 1977; and for a bibliography of monaural studies, Henry, 1979), but the general conclusion seems to be that monaural stimuli may produce an ear superiority under certain conditions, but that the effect is much weaker and less stable than under conditions of dichotic competition.

An important methodological aspect of the technique is the careful construction of the dichotic stimulus tapes, matched with respect to channel characteristics (although all experiments should also balance the assignment of channels to ears across trials or subjects) and carefully aligned for stimulus onset and, perhaps, duration. Technical advice is to be found in Knight and Kantowitz (1973), McDonnell and Perusse (1978), Rubino (1972), and Vincent and Bradshaw (1975). An alternative approach to aligning the left and right ear stimuli, by reference to 'P-centres' has been described by Morton *et al.* (1976).

The form of response demanded, whether for both of the members of a dichotic pair, for the one preferentially perceived, or the one from a channel to be attended, has varied between experiments. There is little study of the effect of selecting one of these response modes, although the study of Millay *et al.* (1977) suggests no main effect of the modes they studied. Out of a particular experimental context, it is not always possible to recommend one of the possible modes, although to control the response mode is preferable to merely allowing free report.

Rather more attention has been devoted to the problems of deriving a laterality index from the left and right ear accuracy scores. This turns out to be less simple than might at first appear, if the effects of overall accuracy, and of guessing in certain forced choice response modes, are to be taken into account. Kuhn (1973) suggested a solution by the use of phi coefficients, but Levy (1977) has shown that these are not entirely independent of accuracy. Alternative solutions have been found by Harshman and Krashen (1972), Birkett (1977), and by Marshall *et al* (1975), refined by Repp (1977). The result, the 'e$_g$' and 'e' coefficients, seem the best solution to date and their use is to be encouraged. Repp also recommends, for statistical reasons, that experimenters should demand a single response for each dichotic stimulus pair. A further discussion of the problems of measuring laterality is to be found in Richardson (1976) and Colbourn (1978).

The reliability of estimates of lateralisation in dichotic listening has been studied by Blumstein *et al*. (1975) and by Pizzamiglio *et al*. (1974), and found to be moderate rather than high. Geffen and co-workers (Geffen *et al*., 1978; Geffen and Caudrey, 1981) describe a particular form of a dichotic listening test which they consider both reliable and valid, and Sidtis (1981) a complex tone test based upon a pitch recognition task.

Finally, there are some methods of lesser importance which are allied to dichotic listening and which deserve mention. Lateralisation of auditory feedback was employed by Greenstadt *et al*. (1978), although their results were not supported by Suter (1980). Tsunoda's method (Tsunoda, 1966; Tsunoda and Oka, 1971), which involves the disruptive effects of lateralised delayed auditory feedback has been used, although recent reports of it have been rather critical (O'Malley, 1978). Elias *et al*. (1977) and Roberts and Gregory (1973) have also used methods based upon delayed auditory feedback. The perception of simultaneity and temporal order has received quite a degree of attention, an example of a recent study being that of Mills and Rollman (1980). Voice onset time has also been a variable in the manipulation of ear superiority effects (Repp, 1978), and shadowing has, of course, also been used in laterality experiments in the auditory modality (Murray and Richards, 1978).

Tactile Presentation

Rather less attention has been paid to presentation in the somesthetic modality (and even less to olfaction: see Hines, 1977). Because the lateralisation of tactual or haptic information would seem to provide opportunities for the simple lateralisation of stimuli, more than the handful of studies which have been performed might have been expected. Although this is probably not the reason for the paucity of studies, tactile information is not as neatly lateralised as is often stated in popular texts. Tactile presentation is, however, particularly important in the present context, as it often leads to findings of right hemisphere superiorities.

In the upward projection of somatosensory information, it would seem that joint and position senses are clearly and absolutely lateralised in the expected contralateral relationship. Passive touch, however, shows a degree of bilateral representation, as is true of stereognostic and tactile localisation abilities, although here, as in audition, the crossed pathway may be dominant. Complete bilateral representation seems to be present for temperature and pain sensations. Much of this information is derived from the commissurotomy patients, and a discussion of the relevant aspects of these studies appears in Gazzaniga and LeDoux (1978).

Some caution must therefore be exercised with respect to studies which have used tactile presentation. Also, it must be admitted, the range of tactile acuity is rather limited, and studies using tactile presentation often preclude response latency measurement. Nevertheless, a number of studies have used such presentation, prompted in part by the work of Nebes (1971) with the split-brain patients. A variety of stimuli have been employed, including lines for bisection (Bowers and Heilman, 1980) and for the judgement of orientation (Zoccolotti *et al.*, 1979), Braille dots (Harriman and Castell, 1979) and raised dots for enumeration (Young and Ellis, 1979). A trail of tactile pulses has also been presented for enumeration (Lechelt and Tanne, 1976) and temporal discrimination (Hammond, 1981), and the tactile perception of direction studied (Benton *et al.*, 1978; Honda, 1977). Lateral vibrotactile sensitivity has been studied by Rhodes and Schwartz (1981).

The most common stimulus material, however, has been nonsense shapes for identification or matching, as a variant of a task originally developed by Witelson (1974) for use with children. A feature of this 'dichhaptic' task is the simultaneous presentation of pairs of stimuli to the left and right hands. Identification of the stimuli, by selection from a response array, can be post-cued by a lateralised light stimulus or some other method. Some recent variations on this technique have been reported by Beaumont (1981b), Gardner and Ward (1979), Hannay and Smith (1979), Nilsson *et al.* (1980) and Schmuller and Goodman (1979). A further variation involving rotation was employed by Yamamoto and Hatta (1980). Some doubts on the validity of the Witelson task have, however, been raised by Cranney and Ashton (1980).

It need hardly be said that many of the methodological problems which apply to studies of divided visual field presentation and of dichotic listening, insofar as they are not strictly related to stimulus presentation, also apply to tactile presentation. The problems of controlling attention, report strategies and other report biasses are equally acute, as is the problem of deriving a measure of the degree of lateralisation. Care must be taken with the careful matching and balancing of all lateral elements in the trial and response sequence, and there is the suspicion that lateral stimulus-response compatibility factors may play a particularly important role in tactile studies which include the demand for a motor response. It will not be clear how serious some of these problems are until there are studies designed to assess the validity of this method of studying hemisphere function.

It is perhaps also worth noting that in studies of the hemisphere specialisation of psychiatric patients, there has been notable use of tactile stimuli (Carr, 1980; Dimond *et al.*, 1980; Green, 1978). A method of assessment suitable for use with quite young children has also been reported by Galin *et al.* (1979).

Lateral Eye Movements

It has been observed that when presented with mental problems subjects tend to divert their gaze to the left or to the right. It has further been reported that problems of a verbal nature induce rightward eye movements, while those of a spatial nature induce leftward movements (Kinsbourne, 1972, 1974; Kocel *et al.*, 1972). This observation has been integrated into theories of hemisphere function by suggesting that activation of one of the hemispheres induces gaze deviation in a contralateral direction.

There are two aspects to this hypothesis. The first is whether the phenomenon is to be reliably observed, and the second whether it can be validly linked to hemisphere specialisation. On a methodological level there has been some study of the effects of the location of the questioner, and whether the questioner actually confronts the subject (Gur, 1975; Gur *et al.*, 1975; Hiscock, 1977). The sequence of the questions and the sex of the questioner have also been reported to affect the deviations observed (Weitan and Etaugh, 1974), and the pattern of initial movements has been generally found to be more variable than first suggested, and to include vertical as well as lateral components. Nevertheless, the review of Ehrlichman and Weinberger (1978) suggests that, given attention to these variables, relatively reliable lateral eye movements are to be observed. Their review concludes, however, that as only about half of the studies reviewed found the predicted relationship between rightward eye movement and problems expected to engage the left hemisphere, the link with hemisphere lateralisation has not been clearly established. The papers which have appeared since their review, taken together, would not radically change this conclusion.

One interesting extension of the lateral eye movement technique has been the study of affective processes (Ahern and Schwartz, 1979). An attempt has also been made to employ the technique in reverse, by taking gaze direction as the independent variable and observing the effect upon responses in a word matching task (Gross *et al.*, 1978; La Torre and La Torre, 1981).

Perceptual Asymmetries in Free Vision

Some lateral asymmetries in free vision have been reported, and although insufficient studies have been conducted to allow evaluation of the validity of the results, the search for such asymmetries constitutes a distinct methodological approach.

Probably the most important of these asymmetries is the reported lateral asymmetry for judgements of aesthetic merit in picture composition. Although the effect had been earlier reported (Swartz *et al.*, 1974) the connection with hemisphere specialisation has been most clearly proposed by Levy (1976), although her hypothesis of how this is mediated, but not her results, has been disputed (Beaumont, in prep). A related effect in the composition of advertisements has been reported by Ellis and Miller (1981). Asymmetries in lateral spatial orientation and judgement have also been reported, and investigated by various strategies (Beaumont, 1979; Cunningham, 1977; Maki *et al.*, 1977).

There are two other phenomena which may be perceptual asymmetries or may be performance asymmetries. It has been reported that the left cheek is more commonly represented in portrait studies (McManus and Humphrey, 1973), although this does not seem to extend to modern photographs (LaBar, 1973) and may be influenced by cultural conventions (Bolton, 1977). Secondly it has been observed that the left side of the face is judged as more emotionally intense than the right (Borod and Caron, 1980; Sackeim and Gur, 1978; Sackeim *et al.*, 1978). Whether this, in particular, is a result of more expression being executed on the left side of the face, or of the lateral perceptual bias of the observer, is still unclear. Some evidence would support the motor view (Schwartz *et al.*, 1979; Sirota and Schwartz, 1982), but some the perceptual view (Campbell, 1982; Moscovitch and Olds, 1982). It remains an interesting phenomenon deserving further investigation.

Lateral Performance Asymmetries

There is of course an enormous literature on the subject of lateral manual preference and associated differences in manual performance. It is only possible to refer the reader to recent reviews (Annett, 1982; Beaumont, 1974; Hardyck, 1977; Hardyck and Petrinovich, 1977; Herron, 1980) to give some idea of the variety of experimental strategies which have been employed in the study of handedness. Handedness, in that it is believed to reflect fundamental differences in cerebral organisation, has also been used as an independent variable to index such inferred patterns of organisation. As a research strategy, this can only be considered unsound. The available evidence has not as yet enabled a clear model of the relationship between cerebral organisation and manual asymmetries to be constructed, and estimates of hemisphere specialisation based upon handedness can be shown to be of insufficient validity (Satz, 1977). It is not reasonable, therefore, to select groups which differ in handedness, and to attribute differences between the performance of these groups to differences in cerebral organisation inferred from what we know about the neuropsychological basis of handedness.

The suggestion by Levy and Reid (Levy, 1982; Levy and Reid, 1976, 1978) that forms of writing posture are related to lateralisation for speech has been treated in a similar fashion. They proposed that an inverted or 'hooked' posture, with either hand, indicated speech representation ipsilateral to the writing hand, while the normal posture indicated contralateral representation. There have been numerous reports which have included measurement of this variable with, as one might expect, rather confused results (Fudin and Lembessis, 1982; Weber and Bradshaw, 1981). It is clear (e.g. Moscovitch and Smith, 1979) that any relationship with cerebral organisation is limited to visual processes, and the theory has been extended to account for this by McKeever and Hoff (1979). Whatever the true relationship, it is not sufficiently well established for writing posture to serve as an index of cerebral organisation.

There are various other performance asymmetries which have been studied. Manual activity during speaking (Dalby *et al.*, 1980; Kimura and Humphrys, 1981) and tapping performance (Ibbotson and Morton, 1981; Peters 1980, 1981; Todor and Kyprie, 1980), may serve as examples. Also the strategy of observing lateral performance during additional tasks which are expected to engage the hemispheres, or conversely engaging one hemisphere by a lateral performance task and then observing the effects on some central cognitive task, has been used. This strategy, of 'dual task performance', is not without considerable methodological difficulties, particularly the problem of predicting whether competition between processes will result in interference or activation (enhancement). Studies in this area have not always avoided rather weak *post hoc* interpretation. Kinsbourne and Hicks (1978) provide a good review of some of the difficulties of this research.

Finally, the Torque Test of Blau (1977) in which the direction of circle-drawing is observed, may be mentioned. Despite some doubts as to the validity of the procedure (Demarest and Demarest, 1980; Jarmen and Nelson, 1980; Tolor, 1981) results have been found to be consistent with other measures in college students (Woods and Oppenheimer, 1980).

The relation of manual asymmetry to lateral preferences in the use of eye, ear and foot has been recently reviewed by Porac and Coren (1981).

Cognitive Style and Neurosociology

Although these ideas are becoming further removed from the actual observation of data which can be linked to lateral cerebral differences, it has been suggested that individuals may differ in the extent to which their thinking or 'cognitive style' represents dominant left or right hemisphere activity. Questionnaires have been designed to enable individuals to be characterised as showing left or right 'hemisphericity'. Probably the most widely known of these is the SOLAT (Style of Learning and Thinking) Questionnaire (Reynolds and Torrance, 1978; Torrance and Mourad, 1978), but other related questionnaires have been described (Bracken *et al.*, 1979; Zenhausern, 1978). There is only the most indirect and tenuous evidence for the validity of any of these instruments, and the inferences to cerebral lateralisation are so distant as to cast grave doubt on whether they bear any relationship to hemisphere function. This is not to say that the hypothesised relationship has been refuted, nor that research using these questionnaires may not be fruitful, but much clearer evidence of their validity is required before they can be accepted as furnishing evidence of hemisphere specialisation (Beaumont *et al.*, in prep.).

Finally, there is the emergent field of neurosociology in which social institutions, linguistic parameters and general cultural phenomena are interpreted in the light of cognitive style or the evolution of lateralised mechanisms. In so far as studies in this field are based upon empirical data, usually of an anthropological nature, they can be seen as a method of studying hemisphere differences. Much of the work stems from the paper of Bogen *et al.* (1972), with more recent discussions being exemplified by Dawson (1977), Levy (1980) and Tenhouten and Kaplan (1977). An illustration of the kind of study which has been devised is that of Martindale (1978) who studied the intelligence pattern of Jews in contrast to Catholic and Protestant subjects. The kind of methodological criticism to which such studies are generally open is well represented by the comment on Martindale's paper by Levinson (1980). As with cognitive style, the inferences from cerebral organisation are distant, and interpretations of sociological phenomena in terms of hemisphere lateralisation should be viewed with scepticism.

Physiological and Anatomical Studies in Normal Subjects

Regional Cerebral Blood Flow

The study of regional cerebral blood flow (rCBF) has been developed at a number of centres, although the number of laboratories in which it can be performed is limited by the demands and expense of the technique. The method is in principle quite simple. Some radioactively labelled material, generally in the form of an inhaled gas, is taken into the body and absorbed into the blood. As the radioactive elements are carried through the head in the bloodstream their passage can be tracked by a bank of detectors placed alongside the head. The most common gas employed is Xenon (Xe-133), but a hydrogen clearance method has also been used. A good relatively non-technical introduction to the technique is to be found in Stump and Williams (1980), and more advanced discussion of the technique in Wood (1980) and Risberg (1980). Indeed, the best introduction to the technique and to current findings with its application is the special issue of *Brain and Language* (vol. **9**, part 1, 1980) in which these papers appear.

The principal result is a demonstration that with engagement in cognitive tasks, and the related activation of cerebral regions, increased blood flow through those regions can be demonstrated. The principal difficulties are that there is a physical limit to the density of the detector array which can be placed alongside the head, and that the temporal resolution is extremely coarse. On a more purely methodological level, to avoid using two detector arrays, measurements from the left and right of the head are often taken in separate recording periods, which is less satisfactory than simultaneous bilateral recording. It is also difficult to control satisfactorily the non-cognitive components of task performance. If task engagement is to be monitored and performance assessed, then great care must be taken that response related artifacts, and more general non-task-related activities, do not introduce confounding into the results.

It may be noted that an indirect measure of blood flow may be obtained from eardrum temperature (Meiners and Dabbs, 1977), but has been little used.

Psychophysiological Measures

Traditional psychophysiological variables have been studied for evidence of lateral asymmetries related to hemisphere engagement on cognitive tasks. The measures have included electrodermal activity (Dawson and Schell, 1982; Gruzelier et al., 1981; Smith et al., 1981) and also muscle tension and finger pulse volume (Diekhof et al., 1978). The results have been interesting but not entirely clear. There is a problem in that not all workers have appreciated the ipsilateral efferent projection of the autonomic nervous system. It is also difficult to predict the direction of change on autonomic variables, and most accounts have employed post hoc explanations of any task-dependent lateral asymmetries observed. Beyond this difficulty, and the general methodological problems of autonomic recording, there is a further problem in the general use of unvalidated cognitive tasks which are expected, on no very clear grounds, to engage either the left or right hemisphere.

Electrophysiological Variables

There has recently been a surge of interest in the lateral asymmetry of electro-physiological variables contingent upon psychological tasks. This is not surprising, as these methods may allow, for the first time, direct observation in real-time of the parallel occurence of psychological and physiological cognitive events. The studies can be broadly divided into studies of the on-going EEG and studies of average evoked responses (AERs).

The studies of on-going EEG are both exciting and frustrating. Exciting, because of the potential value of the data to be extracted, but frustrating because of the methodological difficulties which characterise most, if not all, of the

studies in this field. These difficulties have been extensively reviewed by
Beaumont (1983c), Donchin *et al.* (1977a,b), Galin (1978) and Gevins (1981).
These difficulties centre around the electrode montages to be used, particularly
with regard to the choice of reference electrode placement, recording
parameters, data analysis (including the inappropriate use of ratio scores), and
the nature of the cognitive task employed. There are numerous sources of
potential artifacts which must be carefully controlled, and no study has yet
fulfilled the most stringent requirements which may be demanded. An
additional, fundamental, and as yet insoluble problem is that of anatomical
asymmetries (see below). This means that electrodes placed at homologous
points on the scalp may not be above homologous points on the cortex. This
problem is worse in some regions than in others, but seriously invalidates the
strategy of many investigations.

Studies of AERs suffer from many of the same difficulties as those of on-going
EEG. There are methodological questions, many a matter of debate, about
reference electrode sites, artifact rejection, the control of cognitive set, and the
assumptions which underlie the averaging process. Although there are many
recent collections of research data which present lateralisation studies of AERs,
methodological discussions are to be found particularly in Begleiter (1979),
Desmedt (1977a,b), Lehmann and Callaway (1979) and Rugg (1982). The
general conclusion again is that because of the inadequacy of both the cognitive
models employed and our understanding of the electrophysiological phenomena,
it is rarely possible to make crucial predictions which can be rigorously tested.
Few really well conducted studies have been carried out, and while the method
has great potential, that potential has yet to be realised.

Other Physiological and Anatomical Investigations

Recent studies have revealed a surprising degree of asymmetry in the surface
topography of the left and right hemisphere cortices, which was unsuspected
little over a decade ago. Recent reviews of the latest evidence on such findings
are to be found in Galaburda (1978), LeMay (1976) and LeMay and Geschwind
(1978). Differences in the distribution of the white and grey matter in the body
of the neocortical hemispheres have also been reported (Gur *et al.*, 1980). The
techniques involved in this research are generally outside the competence of
most workers in the field of cerebral lateralisation, but the findings seem now to
be generally accepted by those competent to judge them. There is little doubt
that the advent of relatively accessible computerised axial tomography will
enable more studies correlating gross cerebral anatomy and performance
variables in normals, as well as dramatically improving the data available for
clinical cases. The contribution yet to be made by positron emission
tomography, and NMR scanners, both of which may prove excessively

expensive for all but rare research enterprises, yet which offer greatly increased spatial and temporal resolution, is as yet unknown.

Palaeontological discussions of cerebral evolution have also become relevant to the discussion of hemisphere specialisation (Harnad et al., 1976; Marshack, 1976). There is in addition evidence that, despite some earlier negative reports, there may be lateralisation of neurochemical systems at a subcortical level which in turn affect the operation of the neocortical hemispheres (Knapp and Mandell, 1980; Oke et al., 1978). However, these studies are again beyond the competence of most neuropsychologists, and their results seem less generally accepted.

Two recent reports have described the use of the Hoffmann reflex as an index of lateralised processes (Goode et al., 1980), and the frequency of induced optokinetic nystagmus to the left or right (Rosenberg, 1980). Differential eyelid conditioning has also been employed, but the results using this technique are far from clear (Benish and Grant, 1980), as have studies using hypnotic induction (Sackeim, 1982). We must wait to see if these develop into useful techniques for the study of lateralised cerebral processes.

General Issues

The foregoing has attempted to present an overview of the methods which have been used to investigate hemisphere specialisation, and some of the advantages and disadvantages which attach to each. It seems appropriate to return to some general issues which apply across most of the methods before drawing some final conclusions.

Status of the Concept of Lateralisation

It cannot be emphasied too strongly that neuropsychological investigations of lateralisation proceed by a chain of inference which associates regions of the cerebrum (identified either by the localisation of focal injury, or by the logic of lateralised stimulus presentation) with observed changes in cognitive performance. With the possible exception of the electrophysiological and rCBF studies, the observation of this correlation is never direct. Data are collected under certain conditions of our independent variables, and the conclusions rely upon reasoned inference from the research strategy and a failure to identify methodological artifacts which might account for the results. Such a general research strategy is not unacceptable, but must be operated with care, while greater efforts are made to independently establish the validity of the techniques employed, especially those employed with normal subjects.

More attention might also be paid to the variables used to index cerebral lateralisation. The reliability of these measures has been little studied, as has the interrelationship between them. The study of Fennell *et al.* (1977) has been much quoted as demonstrating reliability and stability within and between divided visual field and dichotic listening measures. The recent critical review of this study by Berenbaum and Harshman (1980), however, casts great doubt on the value of the study. The paper of Hines and Satz (1974) examining divided visual field scores and dichotic listening, and those of Lefevre *et al.* (1977) and Nielsen and Sorensen (1976) associating dichotic listening and lateral eye movements, all suggest that the relationship between these variables may be complex, especially if groups other than consistent dextrals are examined. This may imply that a unitary concept of cerebral lateralisation is unacceptable, and while few would dispute this conclusion, models of hemisphere lateralisation rarely allow for this added dimension.

Cognitive Models

There seems to be a general failure in neuropsychology to take advantage of current models in cognitive psychology. Whatever the quality of these models, and the conceptual status of some is not entirely sound (Lachman *et al.*, 1979), it is patently foolhardy to ignore the very real advances being made by cognitive psychologists. An example might be the treatment of serial and parallel processing. While there are now good methodologies available for the identification of such processes (Das *et al.*, 1979), the terms are used loosely in neuropsychology, as vague conceptual principles, which neither add to the explanation being generated nor yield useful testable hypotheses.

The Design of Experimental Tasks

An associated failure in the design of studies has been in the selection of experimental tasks. The failing has been an unwillingness to employ tasks which are understood in cognitive terms and which have been independently validated as representing some particular process or function. Content to work from one of the loosely conceptualised dichotomies often considered to represent hemisphere differences, such as verbal-nonverbal, serial-parallel, verbal-spatial, analytical-holistic among others, tasks are constructed as expected to engage functions characterising one pole of the selected dichotomy. This is clearly unsatisfactory and accounts for much of the current confusion in the literature. It also permits the unacceptable kind of *post hoc* interpretation of observed asymmetries which has also been all too common in published studies.

The performance tasks which are presented to subjects should be selected to represent some clearly defined process or function, as independently validated from other cognitive research, and where comparisons are to be made between tasks, all other cognitive and performance variables must be carefully controlled.

Particularly where two sets of tasks are taken to engage left and right hemisphere function differentially, they must be carefully matched in all respects other than the single variable which is being investigated for its association with lateral asymmetry. Parametric manipulation of this variable should be the goal of methodological development. Such tasks must at least be matched for difficulty, for aspects of the stimulus presentation and for response factors. This has rarely been attempted, and yet seems methodologically imperative.

I am only too aware of how difficult it is to find or construct such experimental tasks, but the study of hemisphere specialisation has moved beyond the time when pioneering, prospecting studies were acceptable, and the field will not make significant further progress until more attention is paid to the tasks given to subjects.

Subject Variables

While attention has been paid to some subject variables, particularly sex and handedness, other aspects have been neglected. There is at least an increasing acknowledgement of the potential role of subject strategies (Bryden, 1978), although there has been little systematic study of this variable. The way in which strategies of task performance may interact with attentional variables may be of particular importance, as may the way in which such strategies modify the associated cognitive subprocesses which are involved in task performance.

There has also been concern in this context (e.g. Colbourn, 1978) that the practice of reporting group statistics may mask the genuine and relevant variability among subjects. It may well be that it is important to find out why some individuals show clear lateral asymmetries while others only show insignificant differences. There is a need to develop statistical techniques, and valid indices, which will enable within-subject assessment of lateral asymmetry. The trend towards reporting the number of individual subjects who exhibit a particular effect is also to be encouraged. There is probably also a case for more intensive study of individual cases across a wide range of variables and methods, as well as the reporting of correlations between measures when more than one is used in any particular study.

Response Mechanisms

Lastly, there is a general confounding of response mechanisms with more central cognitive processes in many studies. Although many investigators control for hand of response, or balance lateral aspects of response conditions in other ways, there is often an assumption, which may not be warranted, that the involvement of response mechanisms does not account for hemisphere differences. There are certainly studies which can be presented to support such a view, but it may have led to too cavalier a disregard for the importance of the mechanisms which select and control response output. These should be much more explicitly controlled by studies of cerebral lateralisation.

Conclusions

The variety of techniques which have been used to study hemisphere specialisation have been briefly reviewed, although the number of methods listed should not mask the fact that most of the evidence has been derived from only two techniques: observation of the effects of focal lesions in clinical patients and divided visual field studies of normal subjects. The data obtained from commissurotomy patients is also of considerable importance, although it has perhaps been accorded rather more attention than its value merits, and dichotic listening has also had a significant part to play. Hemispherectomy patients and studies using tactile presentation have also contributed to our understanding. By comparison with these methods, if only because of the number of studies which have employed them, all other methods are at present of minor importance.

There are both general and specific methodological problems which attach to each method, besides the general conceptual problems which beset this area of research. It is reasonable to conclude, however, that no method escapes relatively serious methodological problems, although these are perhaps better understood for the divided visual field technique than for other methods. At least there is an increasing recognition of the methodological issues which are of importance, although there are as yet few systematic attempts to study their nature or to find solutions. It must be admitted that, while the evidence accumulates in favour of hemisphere specialisation, the use of almost any method must be regarded with some caution. While increasingly unlikely, it is still possible that alternative explanations not so directly based upon cerebral anatomy may yet be found for many of the performance asymmetries thought to indicate hemisphere specialisation. It would be absurd to discount all the research evidence, often of considerable quality, which has been gathered, but it is not unreasonable to counsel continuing caution in its interpretation. The confusion which has come to be typical of this literature has at last created a mood of reappraisal and re-evaluation, and the result may well be an extensive re-assessment of the part played by cerebral specialisation in observed performance asymmetries.

Finally, it is important not to lose sight of the inferential and correlational nature of most of the research methods which have been discussed above, and not to neglect the important fact that most neuropsychologists are not measuring the brain, but measuring human performance, and hoping that it tells them something about the brain. The degree to which it can is highly dependent upon the quality of both the theories and concepts expressed and the methodology employed. Neuropsychologists neglect careful consideration of either at their peril.

References

AHERN, G. L. and SCHWARTZ, G. E. (1979). Differential lateralisation for positive versus negative emotion. *Neuropsychologia* **17**, 693-698.

ANDREWS, G. and QUINN, P. T. (1972). Stuttering and cerebral dominance. *Journal of Communication Disorders* **5**, 212.

ANNETT, M. (1982). Handedness. In *Divided Visual Field Studies of Cerebral Organisation* (J. G. Beaumont, ed.), pp.195-215. Academic Press, London and New York.

BEAUMONT, J. G. (1974). Hemisphere function and handedness. In *Hemisphere Function in the Human Brain* (S. J. Dimond and J. G. Beaumont, eds), pp.89-120. Elek Science London.

BEAUMONT, J. G. (1979). Lateral asymmetry of orientation to track control in extra-personal space. *Acta Psychologica* **43**, 85-101.

BEAUMONT, J. G. (1981a). Split-brain studies and the duality of consciousness. In *Aspects of Consciousness*, Vol. II (G. Underwood and R. G. Stephens, eds), pp.189-213. Academic Press, London and New York.

BEAUMONT, J. G. (1981b). Activation and interference in tactile perception. *Neuropsychologia* **19**, 151-154.

BEAUMONT, J. G. (1982a). Developmental aspects. In *Divided Visual Field Studies of Cerebral Organisation* (J. G. Beaumont, ed.), pp.113-128. Academic Press, London and New York.

BEAUMONT, J. G. (1982b). The split-brain studies. In *Divided Visual Field Studies of Cerebral Organisation* (J. Beaumont, ed.), pp.217-232. Academic Press, London and New York.

BEAUMONT, J. G. (ed.) (1982c). *Divided Visual Field Studies of Cerebral Organisation.* Academic Press, London and New York.

BEAUMONT, J. G. (1982d). Studies with verbal stimuli. In *Divided Visual Field Studies of Cerebral Organisation* (J. G. Beaumont, ed.), pp.57-86. Academic Press, London and New York.

BEAUMONT, J. G. (1983a). Neuropsychology and the organisation of behaviour. In *Physiological Correlates of Human Behaviour* (A. Gale and J. Edwards, eds). Academic Press, London and New York.

BEAUMONT, J. G. (1983b). *Introduction to Neuropsychology.* Blackwell Scientific Publications, Oxford.

BEAUMONT, J. G. (1983c). The EEG and task performance: a tutorial review. In *Tutorials in ERP Research: Endogenous Components* (A. W. K. Gaillard and W. Ritter, eds), pp.385-406. Elsevier/North Holland, Amsterdam.

BEAUMONT, J. G. (in prep.). Aesthetic preference and lateral dominance: the importance of peripheral visual asymmetries.

BEAUMONT, J. G., MCMANUS, I. C. and YOUNG, A. W. (in prep.). The concept of hemisphericity: a critical review.

BEGLEITER, H. (ed.) (1979). *Evoked Brain Potentials and Behaviour.* Plenum Press, New York.

BENISH, W. A. and GRANT, D. A. (1980). Hemispheric processing in differential classical eyelid conditioning. *Bulletin of the Psychonomic Society* **15**, 433-434.

BENTON, A. L., VARNEY, N. R. and HAMSHER, K. de S. (1978). Lateral differences in tactile directional perception. *Neuropsychologia* **16**, 109-114.

BERENBAUM, S. A. and HARSHMAN, R. A. (1980). On testing group differences in cognition resulting from differences in lateral specialisation: reply to Fennell *et al*. *Brain and Language* **11**, 209-220.

BERLIN, C. I. (1977). Hemispheric asymmetry in auditory tasks. In *Lateralization in the Nervous System* (S. Harnad, R. W. Doty, L. Goldstein, J. Jaynes and G. Krauthamer, eds), pp.303-323. Academic Press, New York and London.

BERLIN, C. I. and CULLEN, J. K. Jr. (1977). Acoustic problems in dichotic listening tasks. In *Language Development and Neurological Theory* (S. J. Segalowitz and F. A. Gruber, eds), pp.75-88. Academic Press, New York and London.

BIRKETT, P. (1977). Measures of laterality and theories of hemispheric processes. *Neuropsychologia* **15**, 693-696.

BLAU, T. H. (1977). The Torque Test: a measurement of cerebral dominance. *Catalog of Selected Documents in Psychology* **7**, 16-17.

BLUME, W. T., GRABOW, J. D., DARLEY, F. L. and ARONSON, A. E. (1973). Intracarotid amobarbital test of language and memory before temporal lobectomy for seizure control. *Neurology* **23**, 812-819.

BLUMSTEIN, S. E. (1974). The use of theoretical implications of the dichotic technique for investigating distinctive features. *Brain and Language* **1**, 337-350.

BLUMSTEIN, S., GOODGLASS, H. and TARTTER, V. (1975). The reliability of ear advantage in dichotic listening. *Brain and Language* **2**, 226-236.

BOGEN, J. E. and BOGEN, G. M. (1976). Wernicke's region—where is it? *Annals of the New York Academy of Sciences* **280**, 834-843.

BOGEN, J. E., DeZURE, R., TENHOUTEN, W. D. and MARSH, J. F. (1972). The other side of the brain IV: the A/P ratio. *Bulletin of the Los Angeles Neurological Societies* **37**, 49-61.

BOLTON, R. (1977). Directionality in Qolla Indian drawings. *Perceptual and Motor Skills* **45**, 419-420.

BOROD, J. C. and CARON, H. S. (1980). Facedness and emotion related to lateral dominance, sex and expression type. *Neuropsychologia* **18**, 237-241.

BOWERS, D. and HEILMAN, K. M. (1980). Pseudoneglect: effects of hemispace on a tactile line bisection task. *Neuropsychologia* **18**, 491-498.

BRACKEN, B. A., LEDFORD, T. L. and McCALLUM, R. S. (1979). Effects of cerebral dominance on college-level achievement. *Perceptual and Motor Skills* **49**, 445-446.

BRANCH, C., MILNER, B. and RASMUSSEN, T. (1964). Intracarotid sodium amytal for the lateralisation of cerebral speech dominance. *Journal of Neurosurgery* **21**, 399-405.

BRYDEN, M. P. (1978). Strategy effects in the assessment of hemispheric asymmetry. In *Strategies of Information Processing* (G. Underwood, ed.), pp.117-149. Academic Press, London and New York.

CAMPBELL, R. (1982). Asymmetries in moving faces. *British Journal of Psychology* **73**, 95-103.

CARR, S. A. (1980). Interhemispheric transfer of stereognostic information in chronic schizophrenics. *British Journal of Psychiatry* **136**, 53-58.

CHIARELLO, C. (1980). A house divided? Cognitive functioning with callosal agenesis. *Brain and Language* **11**, 128-158.

CLYMA, E. A. (1975). Unilateral ECT: how to detect which hemisphere is dominant. *British Journal of Psychiatry* **126**, 372-379.

COLBOURN, C. J. (1978). Can laterality be measured? *Neuropsychologia* **16**, 283-289.

CORBALLIS, M. C. and MORGAN, M. J. (1978). On the biological basis of human laterality. *The Behavioural and Brain Sciences* **1**, 261-366.

CRANNEY, J. and ASHTON, R. (1980). Witelson's dichhaptic task as a measure of hemispheric asymmetry in deaf and hearing populations. *Neuropsychologia* **18**, 95-98.

CUNNINGHAM, M. R. (1977). Notes on the psychological basis of environmental design: the right-left dimension in apartment floor plans. *Environment and Behaviour* **9**, 125-135.

DAMÁSIO, A. R. and DAMÁSIO, H. (1977). Musical faculty and cerebral dominance. In *Music and the Brain* (M. Critchley and R. A. Henson, eds), pp.141-155. Heinemann Medical Books, London.

DALBY, J. T., GIBSON, D., GROSSI, V. and SCHNEIDER, R. D. (1980). Lateralized hand gesture during speech. *Journal of Motor Behavior* **12**, 292-297.

DAS, J. P., KIRBY, J. R. and JARMAN, R. F. (1979). *Simultaneous and Successive Cognitive Processes*. Academic Press, New York and London.

DAWSON, J. L. M. B. (1977). An anthropological perspective on the evolution and lateralisation of the brain. *Annals of the New York Academy of Sciences* **299**, 424-447.

DAWSON, M. E. and SCHELL, A. M. (1982). Electrodermal responses to attended and nonattended significant stimuli during dichotic listening. *Journal of Experimental Psychology: Human Perception and Performance* **8**, 315-324.

d'ÉLIA, G. (1974). Unilateral convulsive therapy. In *Psychobiology of Convulsive Therapy* (M. Fink, S. Kety, J. McGaugh and T. A. Williams, eds), pp.21-34. V. H. Winston & Sons, Washington, D.C.

DEMAREST, J. and DEMAREST, L. (1980). Does the 'Torque Test' measure cerebral dominance in adults? *Perceptual and Motor Skills* **50**, 155-158.

DESMEDT, J. E. (ed.) (1977a). *Progress in Clinical Neurophysiology*. Vol. 1: *Attention, Voluntary Contraction and Event-related Cerebral Potentials*. S. Karger, Basel.

DESMEDT, J. E. (ed.) (1977b). *Progress in Clinical Neurophysiology*. Vol. 3: *Language and Hemispheric Specialisation in Man: Cerebral Event-Related Potentials*. S. Karger, Basel.

DIEKHOF, G. M., GARLAND, J., DANSEREAU, D. F. and WALKER, C. A. (1978). Muscle tension, skin conductance and finger pulse volume — asymmetries as a function of cognitive demands. *Acta Psychologica* **42**, 83-93.

DIMOND, S. J. (1972). *The Double Brain*. Churchill-Livingstone, Edinburgh.

DIMOND, S. J. (1980). *Neuropsychology*. Butterworths, Sevenoaks, Kent.

DIMOND, S. J. and BEAUMONT, J. G. (1971). Hemisphere function and vigilance. *Quarterly Journal of Experimental Psychology* **23**, 443-448.

DIMOND, S. J. and BEAUMONT, J. G. (1972). On the nature of the interhemispheric effects of fatigue. *Acta Psychologica* **36**, 443-449.

DIMOND, S. J. and BEAUMONT, J. G. (eds) (1974). *Hemisphere Function in the Human Brain*. Elek Science, London.

DIMOND, S. J., BUREŠ, J., FARRINGTON, L. J. and BROUWERS, E. Y. M. (1975). The use of contact lenses for the lateralisation of visual input in man. *Acta Psychologica* **39**, 341-350.

DIMOND, S. J., SCAMMELL, R., PRYCE, I. J., HUWS, D. and GRAY, C. (1980). Some failures of intermanual and cross-lateral transfer in chronic schizophrenia. *Journal of Abnormal Psychology* **89**, 505-509.

DONCHIN, E., KUTAS, M. and MCCARTHY, G. (1977a). Electrocortical indices of hemispheric utilisation. In *Lateralization in the Nervous System* (S. Harnad, R. W. Doty, L. Goldstein, J. Jaynes and G. Krauthamer, eds), pp.339-384. Academic Press, New York and London.

DONCHIN, E., MCCARTHY, G. and KUTAS, M. (1977b). Electroencephalographic investigation of hemispheric specialisation. In *Progress in Clinical Neurophysiology*. Vol. 3: *Language and Hemisphere Specialisation in Man: Cerebral Event-Related Potentials* (J. E. Desmedt, ed.), pp.212-242. S. Karger, Basel.

EFRON, R., BOGEN, J. E. and YUND, E. W. (1977). Perception of dichotic chords by normal and commissurotomised human subjects. *Cortex* **13**, 137-149.

EHRLICHMAN, H. and WEINBERGER, A. (1978). Lateral eye movements and hemispheric asymmetry: a critical review. *Psychological Bulletin* **85**, 1080-1101.

ELIAS, J. W., YAIRI, E., WRIGHT, L., ADAMS, L. A. and VILLESCAS, R. (1977). The use of delayed auditory feedback in the identification of the left cerebral hemisphere as a temporal/duration processor. *Journal of Auditory Research* **17**, 155-160.

ELLIS, A. W. and MILLER, D. (1981). Left and wrong in adverts: neuropsychological correlates of aesthetic preference. *British Journal of Psychology* **72**, 225-230.

FENNELL, E. B., BOWERS, D. and SATZ, P. (1977). Within-modal and cross-modal reliabilities of two laterality tests. *Brain and Language* **4**, 63-69.

FERRARO, J. A. and MINCKLER, J. (1977a). The brachium of the inferior colliculus: the human auditory pathways: a quantitative study. *Brain and Language* **4**, 156-164.

FERRARO, J. A. and MINCKLER, J. (1977b). The human lateral lemniscus and its nuclei: the human auditory pathways: a quantitative study. *Brain and Language* **4**, 277-294.

FINGER, S. (ed.) (1978). *Recovery from Brain Damage.* Plenum Press, New York.

FUDIN, R. and LEMBESSIS, E. (1982). Note on criteria for writing posture used to test Levy and Reid's cerebral organisation hypothesis. *Perceptual and Motor Skills* **54**, 551-556.

GALABURDA, A. M., LeMAY, M., KEMPER, T. L. and GESCHWIND, N. (1978). Right-left asymmetries in the brain. *Science* **199**, 852-856.

GALIN, D. (1978). Methodological problems and opportunities in EEG studies of lateral specialisation. In *Symposium on Neurological Bases of Language Disorders in Children.* National Institute of Neurological and Communicative Disorders and Stroke, U.S.A.

GALIN, D., JOHNSTONE, J., NAKELL, L. and HERRON, J. (1979). Development of the capacity for tactile information transfer between hemispheres in normal children. *Science* **204**, 1330-1332.

GARDNER, E. B. and WARD, A. W. (1979). Spatial compatibility in tactile-visual discrimination. *Neuropsychologia* **17**, 421-425.

GAZZANIGA, M. S. (1970). *The Bisected Brain.* Appleton-Century-Crofts, New York.

GAZZANIGA, M. S. (1975a). Beyond lateralisation. In *Les Syndromes de Disconnexion Calleuse chez l'Homme* (F. Michel and B. Schott, eds). Hôpital Neurologique, Lyon.

GAZZANIGA, M. S. (1975b). Partial commissurotomy and cerebral localisation of function. In *Cerebral Localisation* (K. J. Zülch, O. Creutzfeldt and G. C. Galbraith, eds), pp.133-143. Springer-Verlag, Berlin.

GAZZANIGA, M. S. and HILLYARD, S. A. (1971). Language and speech capacity of the right hemisphere. *Neuropsychologia* **9**, 273-280.

GAZZANIGA, M. S. and LeDOUX, J. E. (1978). *The Integrated Mind.* Plenum Press, New York.

GEFFEN, G. and CAUDREY, D. (1981). Reliability and validity of the dichotic monitoring test for language laterality. *Neuropsychologia* **19**, 413-423.

GEFFEN, G., BRADSHAW, J. L. and NETTLETON, N. C. (1972). Hemispheric asymmetry: verbal and spatial encoding of visual stimuli. *Journal of Experimental Psychology* **95**, 25-31.

GEFFEN, G., TRAUB, E. and STIERMAN, I. (1978). Language laterality assessed by unilateral ECT and dichotic monitoring *Journal of Neurology, Neurosurgery and Psychiatry* **41**, 354-360.

GEVINS, A. S. (1981). The use of brain electrical potentials (BEP) to study localization of human brain function. *International Journal of Neuroscience* **13**, 27-41.

GIBSON, A. R., DIMOND, S. J. and GAZZANIGA, M. S. (1972). Left field superiority for word matching. *Neuropsychologia* **10**, 463-466.

GILBERT, J. H. V. and PRATT, L. R. (1977). Cross-modal matching and association under sodium amytal. *Brain and Language* **4**, 558-571.

GOODE, D. J., GLENN, S., MANNING, A. A. and MIDDLETON, J. F. (1980). Lateral asymmetry of the Hoffmann reflex: relation to cortical laterality. *Journal of Neurology, Neurosurgery and Psychiatry* **43**, 831-835.

GORDON, H. W. (1980). Right hemisphere comprehension of verbs in patients with complete forebrain commissurotomy: use of the dichotic method and manual performance. *Brain and Language* **11**, 76-86.

GREEN, P. (1978). Defective interhemispheric transfer in schizophrenia. *Journal of Abnormal Psychology* **87**, 472-480.

GREENSTADT, L., SCHUMAN, M. and SHAPIRO, D. (1978). Differential effects of left versus right monaural biofeedback for heart rate increase. *Psychophysiology* **15**, 233-238.

GROSS, Y., FRANKO, R. and LEWIN, I. (1978). Effects of voluntary eye movements on hemispheric activity and choice of cognitive mode. *Neuropsychologia* **16**, 653-657.

GRUZELIER, J. and FLOR-HENRY, P. eds. (1979). *Hemisphere Asymmetries of Function in Psychopathology*. Elsevier/North Holland, Amsterdam.

GRUZELIER, J., EVES, F. and CONNOLLY, J. (1981). Reciprocal hemispheric influences on response habituation in the electrodermal system. *Physiological Psychology* **9**, 313-317.

GUR, R. C., PACKER, I. K., HUNGERBUHLER, J. P., REIVICH, M., OBRIST, W. D., AMARNEK, W. S. and SACKEIM, H. A. (1980). Differences in the distribution of gray and white matter in human cerebral hemispheres. *Science* **207**, 1226-1228.

GUR, R. E. (1975). Conjugate lateral eye movements as an index of hemispheric activation. *Journal of Personality and Social Psychology* **31**, 751-757.

GUR, R. E., GUR, R. C. and HARRIS, L. J. (1975). Cerebral activation as measured by subjects' lateral eye movements is influenced by experimenter location. *Neuropsychologia* **13**, 35-44.

HAMMOND, G. R. (1981). Finer temporal acuity for stimuli applied to the preferred hand. *Neuropsychologia* **19**, 325-329.

HANNAY, H. J. and SMITH, A. C. (1979). Dichhaptic perception of forms by normal adults. *Perceptual and Motor Skills* **49**, 991-1000.

HARDYCK, C. (1977). A model of individual differences in hemispheric functioning. In *Studies in Neurolinguistics*, Vol. 3 (H. Whitaker and H. A. Whitaker, eds), pp.223-256. Academic Press, London and New York.

HARDYCK, C. and PETRINOVICH, L. F. (1977). Left-handedness. *Psychological Bulletin* **84**, 385-404.

HARNAD, S. R., STEKLIS, H. D. and LANCASTER, J. (eds) (1976). Origins and Evolution of Language and Speech. *Annals of the New York Academy of Science* **280**.

HARRIMAN, J. and CASTELL, L. (1979). Manual asymmetry for tactile discrimination. *Perceptual and Motor Skills* **48**, 290.

HARSHMAN, R. A. and KRASHEN, S. D. (1972). An 'unbiased' procedure for comparing degree of lateralisation of dichotically presented stimuli. *University of California Working Papers in Phonetics* **23**, 3-12.

HÉCAEN, H. and ALBERT, M. L. (1978). *Human Neuropsychology*. Wiley-Interscience, New York.

HEILMAN, K. M. and VALENSTEIN, E. (eds) (1979). *Clinical Neuropsychology*. Oxford University Press, New York.

HENRY, R. G. (1979). Monaural studies eliciting an hemispheric asymmetry: a bibliography. *Perceptual and Motor Skills* **48**, 335-338.

HERRON, J. (ed.) (1980). *Neuropsychology of Left-Handedness.* Academic Press, New York and London.
HESCHE, J., RODER, E. and THEILGAARD, A. (1978). Unilateral and bilateral ECT: a psychiatric and psychological study of therapeutic effect and side effects. *Acta Psychiatrica Scandinavica* (Suppl.) **275**
HINES, D. E. (1977). Olfaction and the right hemisphere. *Journal of Abnormal States of Consciousness* **3**, 47-59.
HINES, D. E. and SATZ, P. (1974). Cross-modal asymmetries in perception related to asymmetry in cerebral function. *Neuropsychologia* **12**, 239-247.
HISCOCK, M. (1977). Effects of examiner's location and subject's anxiety on gaze laterality. *Neuropsychologia* **15**, 409-416.
HONDA, H. (1977). Hemispheric laterality effects on tactile perception of direction in normal subjects. *Tohoku Psychologica Folia* **36**, 68-74.
HORAN, M., ASHTON, R. and MINTO, J. (1980). Using ECT to study hemispheric specialisation for sequential processes. *British Journal of Psychiatry* **137**, 119-125.
IBBOTSON, N. R. and MORTON, J. (1981). Rhythm and dominance. *Cognition* **9**, 125-138.
JARMEN, R. F. and NELSON, J. G. (1980). Torque and cognitive ability: some contradictions to Blau's proposals. *Journal of Clinical Psychology* **36**, 458-464.
KETTERER, M. W. and SMITH, B. D. (1977). Bilateral electrodermal activity, lateralised cerebral processes and sex. *Psychophysiology* **14**, 513-516.
KIMURA, D. (1961). Cerebral dominance and the perception of verbal stimuli. *Canadian Journal of Psychology* **15**, 166-171.
KIMURA, D. and HUMPHRYS, C. A. (1981). A comparison of left- and right-arm movements during speaking. *Neuropsychologia* **19**, 807-812.
KINSBOURNE, M. (1971). Cognitive deficit: experimental analysis. In *Psychobiology* (J. L. McGaugh, ed.), pp.285-348. Academic Press, New York and London.
KINSBOURNE, M. (1972). Eye and head turning indicates cerebral lateralization. *Science* **176**, 539-541.
KINSBOURNE, M. (1974). Direction of gaze and distribution of cerebral thought processes. *Neuropsychologia* **12**, 279-282.
KINSBOURNE, M. (1976). The neuropsychological analysis of cognitive deficits. In *Biological Foundations of Psychiatry*, Vol. I (R. G. Grenell and S. Gabay, eds), pp.527-589. Raven Press, New York.
KINSBOURNE, M. (ed.) (1978). *Asymmetrical Function of the Brain.* Cambridge University Press, Cambridge.
KINSBOURNE, M. and HICKS, R. E. (1978). Functional cerebral space: a model for overflow, transfer and interference effects in human performance: a tutorial review. In *Attention and Performance VII* (J. Requin, ed), pp.345-362. Laurence Erlbaum Associates, Hillsdale, New Jersey.
KINSBOURNE, M. and SMITH, W. L. (eds.) (1974). *Hemispheric Disconnection and Cerebral Function.* Charles C. Thomas, Springfield, Illinois.
KNAPP, S. and MANDELL, A. J. (1980). Lithium and Chlorimipramine differentially alter bilateral asymmetry in mesostriatal serotonin metabolites and kinetic conformations of midbrain tryptophan hydroxylase with respect to tetrahydrobiopterin cofactor. *Neuropharmacology* **19**, 1-7.
KNIGHT, J. L. and KANTOWITZ, B. H. (1973). A minicomputer method for generating dichotic word pairs. *Behavior Research Methods and Instrumentation* **5**, 231-234.
KOCEL, K., GALIN, D., ORNSTEIN, R. and MERVIN, E. L. (1972). Lateral eye movement and cognitive mode. *Psychonomic Science* **27**, 223-224.
KRASHEN, S. D. (1976). Cerebral asymmetry. In *Studies in Neurolinguistics*, Vol. 2

(H. Whitaker and H. A. Whitaker, eds), pp.157-192. Academic Press, New York and London.

KUHN, G. M. (1973). The phi coefficient as an index of ear differences in dichotic listening. *Cortex* **9**, 450-457.

LACHMAN, R., LACHMAN, J. L. and BUTTERFIELD, E. C. (1979). *Cognitive Psychology and Information Processing.* Lawrence Erlbaum Associates, Hillsdale, New Jersey.

LABAR, M. (1973). Turning the left cheek examined using modern photography. *Nature, Lond.* **245**, 338.

LACROIX, J. M. and COMPER, P. (1979). Lateralisation in the electrodermal system as a function of cognitive/hemispheric manipulations. *Psychophysiology* **16**, 116-129.

LATORRE, R. A. and LATORRE, A.-M. (1981). Effect of lateral eye fixation on cognitive processes. *Perceptual and Motor Skills* **52**, 487-490.

LECHELT, E. C. and TANNE, G. (1976). Laterality in the perception of successive tactile pulses. *Bulletin of the Psychonomic Society* **7**, 452-454.

LEFEVRE, E., STARCK, R., LAMBERT, W. E. and GENESIS, F. (1977). Lateral eye movements during verbal and nonverbal dichotic listening. *Perceptual and Motor Skills* **44**, 1115-1122.

LEHMANN, D. and CALLAWAY, E. (eds.) (1979). *Human Evoked Potentials: Applications and Problems.* Plenum Press, New York.

LEMAY, M. (1976). Morphological cerebral asymmetries of modern man, fossil man and nonhuman primate. *Annals of the New York Academy of Sciences* **280**, 349-366.

LEMAY, M. and GESCHWIND, N. (1978). Asymmetries of the human cerebral hemispheres. In *Language Acquisition and Language Breakdown: Parallels and Divergencies* (A. Caramazza and E. B. Zurif, eds), pp.311-328. Johns Hopkins University Press, Baltimore, Maryland.

LEVINSON, B. M. (1980). Comment on Martindale's "Hemispheric asymmetry and Jewish intelligence test patterns". *Journal of Consulting and Clinical Psychology* **48**, 258-260.

LEVY, J. (1976). Lateral dominance and aesthetic preference. *Neuropsychologia* **14**, 431-445.

LEVY, J. (1977). The correlation of the phi function of the difference score with performance and its relevance to laterality experiments. *Cortex* **13**, 458-464.

LEVY, J. (1980). Cerebral asymmetry and the psychology of man. In *The Brain and Psychology* (M. C. Wittrock, ed.), pp.245-321. Academic Press, New York and London.

LEVY, J. (1982). Handwriting posture and cerebral organization: how are they related? *Psychological Bulletin* **91**, 589-608.

LEVY, J. and REID, M. (1976). Variations in writing posture and cerebral organisation. *Science* **194**, 337-339.

LEVY, J. and REID, M. (1978). Variations in cerebral organisation as a function of handedness, hand posture in writing, and sex. *Journal of Experimental Psychology: General* **107**, 119-144.

LEZAK, M. D. (1976). *Neuropsychological Assessment.* Oxford University Press, New York.

LUSSENHOP, A. J., BOGGS, J. S., LABORWIT, L. J. and WALLE, E. L. (1973). Cerebral dominance in stutterers determined by Wada testing. *Neurology* **23**, 1190-1192.

MAKI, R. H., MAKI, W. S. Jr. and MARSH, L. G. (1977). Processing locational and orientational information. *Memory and Cognition* **5**, 602-612.

MARSHACK, A. (1976). Implications of the paleolithic symbolic evidence for the origin of language. *American Scientist* **64**, 136-145.

MARSHALL, J. C., CAPLAN, D. and HOLMES, J. M. (1975). The measure of laterality. *Neuropsychologia* **13**, 315-322.

MARTINDALE, C. (1978). Hemispheric asymmetry and Jewish intelligence test patterns. *Journal of Consulting and Clinical Psychology* **46**, 1299-1301.

McDONNELL, P. M. and PERUSSE, S. (1978). A method for the preparation of audio tapes for dichotic listening research. *Behavior Research Methods and Instrumentation* **10**, 15-17.

McKEEVER, W. F. and HOFF, A. L. (1979). Evidence of a possible isolation of left hemisphere visual and motor areas in sinistrals employing an inverted handwriting posture. *Neuropsychologia* **17**, 445-455.

McKEEVER, W. F. and HULING, M. D. (1971). Lateral dominance in tachistoscopic word recognition performance obtained with simultaneous bilateral input. *Neuropsychologia* **9**, 15-20.

McMANUS, I. C. and HUMPHREY, N. K. (1973). Turning the left cheek. *Nature, Lond.* **243**, 271-272.

MEINERS, M. L. and DABBS, J. M. Jr. (1977). Ear temperature and brain blood flow: laterality effects. *Bulletin of the Psychonomic Society* **10**, 194-196.

MILLAY, K. K., ROESER, R. J. and GODFREY, J. S. (1977). Reliability of performance for dichotic listening using two response modes. *Journal of Speech and Hearing Research* **20**, 510-518.

MILLS, L. and ROLLMAN, G. B. (1980). Hemispheric asymmetry for auditory perception of temporal order. *Neuropsychologia* **18**, 41-47.

MILNER, A. D. and JEEVES, M. A. (1979). A review of behavioural studies of agenesis of the corpus callosum: In *Structure and Function of Cerebral Commissures* (I. Steele Russell, M. W. Van Hoff and G. Berlucchi, eds), pp.428-448. Macmillan, London.

MILNER, B. and TEUBER, H.-L. (1968). Alterations of perception and memory in man: reflections on methods. In *Analysis of Behavioural Change* (L. Weiskrantz, ed.), pp.268-375. Harper and Row, New York.

MORTON, J., MARCUS, S. and FRANKISH, C. (1976). Perceptual centres (P-centres). *Psychological Review* **83**, 405-408.

MOSCOVITCH, M. and OLDS, J. (1982). Asymmetries in spontaneous facial expressions and their possible relation to hemispheric specialisation. *Neuropsychologia* **20**, 71-81.

MOSCOVITCH, M. and SMITH, L. C. (1979). Differences in neural organisation between individuals with inverted and noninverted handwriting postures. *Science* **205**, 710-713.

MURRAY, M. R. and RICHARDS, S. J. (1978). A right-ear advantage in monotic shadowing. *Acta Psychologica* **42**, 495-504.

NEBES, R. D. (1971). Superiority of the minor hemisphere in commissurotomised man for the perception of part-whole relations. *Cortex* **7**, 333-349.

NEBES, R. D. (1974). Hemispheric specialisation in commissurotomised man. *Psychological Bulletin* **81**, 1-14.

NIELSEN, H. and SORENSEN, J. H. (1976). Hemispheric dominance, dichotic listening and lateral eye movement behaviour. *Scandinavian Journal of Psychology* **17**, 129-132.

NILSSON, J., GLENCROSS, D. and GEFFEN, G. (1980). The effect of familial sinistrality and preferred hand on dichaptic and dichotic tasks. *Brain and Language* **10**, 390-404.

OJEMANN, G. A. (1979). Individual variability in cortical localisation of language. *Journal of Neurosurgery* **50**, 164-169.

OJEMANN, G. A. and WHITAKER, H. A. (1978). Language localisation and variability. *Brain and Language* **6**, 239-260.

OKE, A., KELLER, R., MEFFORD, I. and ADAMS, R. N. (1978). Lateralisation of norepinephrine in human thalamus. *Science* **200**, 1411-1413.

O'MALLEY, H. (1978). Assumptions underlying the delayed auditory feedback task in the study of ear advantage. *Brain and Language* **5**, 127-135.

PETERS, M. (1980). Why the preferred hand taps more quickly than the non-preferred hand: three experiments on handedness. *Canadian Journal of Psychology* **34**, 62-71.

PETERS, M. (1981). Attentional asymmetries during concurrent bimanual performance. *Quarterly Journal of Experimental Psychology* **33A**, 95-103.

PIZZAMIGLIO, L., PASCALIS, C. de and VIGNATI, A. (1974). Stability of dichotic listening test. *Cortex* **10**, 203-205.

PORAC, C. and COREN, S. (1981). *Lateral Preferences and Human Behavior*. Springer-Verlag, New York.

RASMUSSEN, T. and MILNER, B. (1975). Clinical and surgical studies of the cerebral speech areas in man. In *Cerebral Localization* (K. J. Zülch, O. Creutzfeldt and G. C. Galbraith, eds), pp.238-257. Springer-Verlag, Berlin.

REPP, B. H. (1977). Measuring laterality effects in dichotic listening. *Journal of the Acoustic Society of America* **62**, 720-737.

REPP, B. H. (1978). Stimulus dominance and ear dominance in the perception of dichotic voicing contrasts. *Brain and Language* **5**, 310-330.

REYNOLDS, C. R. and TORRANCE, E. P. (1978). Perceived changes in styles of learning and thinking (hemisphericity) through direct and indirect training. *Journal of Creative Behaviour* **12**, 247-252.

RHODES, D. L. and SCHWARTZ, G. E. (1981). Lateralized sensitivity to vibrotactile stimulation: individual differences revealed by interaction of threshold and signal detection tasks. *Neuropsychologia* **19**, 831-835.

RICHARDSON, J. T. E. (1976). How to measure laterality. *Neuropsychologia* **14**, 135-136.

RISBERG, J. (1980). Regional cerebral blood flow measurement by ^{133}Xe-inhalation: methodology and applications in neuropsychology and psychiatry. *Brain and Language* **9**, 9-34.

RISSE, G. L. and GAZZANIGA, M. S. (1978). Well-kept secrets of the right hemisphere: a carotid amytal study of restricted memory transfer. *Neurology* **28**, 950-953.

ROBERTS, L. D. and GREGORY, A. H. (1973). Ear differences and delayed auditory feedback. *Journal of Experimental Psychology* **101**, 269-272.

ROBERTSON, A. D. and INGLIS, J. (1978). Memory deficits after electro-convulsive therapy: cerebral asymmetry and dual encoding. *Neuropsychologia* **16**, 179-187.

ROSENBERG, B. A. (1980). Mental-task instructions and optokinetic nystagmus to the left and right. *Journal of Experimental Psychology: Human Perception and Performance* **6**, 459-472.

RUBINO, C. A. (1972). A simple procedure for constructing dichotic listening tapes. *Cortex* **8**, 335-338.

RUGG, M. D. (1982). Electrophysiological studies of divided visual field stimulation. In *Divided Visual Field Studies of Cerebral Organisation* (J. G. Beaumont, ed.), pp.129-146. Academic Press, London and New York.

SACKEIM, H. A. (1982). Lateral asymmetry in bodily response to hypnotic suggestions. *Biological Psychiatry* **17**, 437-448.

SACKEIM, H. A. and GUR, R. C. (1978). Lateral asymmetry in intensity of emotional expression. *Neuropsychologia* **16**, 473-481.

SACKEIM, H. A., GUR, R. C. and SAUCY, M. C. (1978). Emotions are expressed more intensely on the left side of the face. *Science* **202**, 434-436.

SATZ, P. (1977). Laterality tests: an inferential problem. *Cortex* **13**, 208-212.

SCHMULLER, J. and GOODMAN, R. (1979). Bilateral tachistoscopic perception, handedness and laterality. *Brain and Language* **8**, 81-91.

SCHWARTZ, G. E., AHERN, G. L. and BROWN, S.-L. (1979). Lateralised facial muscle response to positive and negative emotional stimuli. *Psychophysiology* **16**, 561-571.

SEARLEMAN, A. (1977). A review of right hemisphere linguistic capabilities. *Psychological Bulletin* **84**, 503-528.

SIDTIS, J. J. (1981). The complex tone test: implications for the assessment of auditory laterality effects. *Neuropsychologia* **19**, 103-112.

SIROTA, A. D. and SCHWARTZ, G. E. (1982). Facial muscle patterning and lateralisation during elation and depressive imagery. *Journal of Abnormal Psychology* **91**, 25-34.

SMITH, B. D., KETTERER, M. W. and CONCANNON, M. (1981). Bilateral electrodermal activity as a function of hemisphere-specific stimulation, hand preference, sex and familial handedness. *Biological Psychology* **12**, 1-11.

SPARKS, R. and GESCHWIND, N. (1968). Dichotic listening in man after section of neocortical commissures. *Cortex* **4**, 3-16.

SPRINGER, S. P. (1979). Speech perception and the biology of language. In *Handbook of Behavioral Neurobiology*. Vol. 2: *Neuropsychology* (M. S. Gazzaniga, ed.), pp.153-177. Plenum Press, New York.

SPRINGER, S. P. and GAZZANIGA, M. S. (1975). Dichotic testing of partial and complete split-brain subjects. *Neuropsychologia* **13**, 341-346.

SPRINGER, S. P., SIDTIS, J., WILSON, D. and GAZZANIGA, M. S. (1978). Left ear performance in dichotic listening following commissurotomy. *Neuropsychologia* **16**, 305-312.

STUMP, D. A. and WILLIAMS, R. (1980). The noninvasive measurement of regional cerebral circulation. *Brain and Language* **9**, 35-46.

SUTER, S. (1980). Left versus right monaural biofeedback for finger temperature changes. *Perceptual and Motor Skills* **50**, 70.

SWARTZ, P., SWARTZ, S. and DICARLO, D. (1974). Lateral organisation in pictures and aesthetic preference: III. *Perceptual and Motor Skills* **38**, 867-874.

TENHOUTEN, W. D. and KAPLAN, C. D. (1977). More on split-brain research and anthropology. *Current Anthropology* **18**, 344-350.

TEUBER, H.-L. (1975). Recovery of function after brain injury in man. In *Outcome of Severe Damage to the CNS*. CIBA Foundation Symposium 34 (new series), pp.159-190. Elsevier, Amsterdam.

TODOR, J. I. and KYPRIE, P. M. (1980). Hand differences in the rate and variability of rapid tapping. *Journal of Motor Behavior* **12**, 57-62.

TOLOR, A. (1981). Torque behaviour in schizophrenics, elderly persons and other special groups. *Journal of Nervous and Mental Disease* **169**, 357-363.

TORRANCE, E. P. and MOURAD, S. (1978). Some creativity and style of learning and thinking correlates of Guglielmino's Self-directed Readiness Scale. *Psychological Reports* **43**, 1167-1171.

TREVARTHEN, C. (1975). Psychological activities after forebrain commissurotomy in man: concepts, and methodological hurdles in testing. In *Les Syndromes de Disconnexion Calleuse chez l'Homme* (F. Michel and B. Schott, eds), pp.181-210. Hôpital Neurologique, Lyon.

TSUNODA, T. (1966). Tsunoda's method: a new objective testing method available for the orientation of the dominant cerebral hemisphere towards various sounds and its clinical use. *Indian Journal of Otology* **18**, 78-88.

TSUNODA, T. and OKA, M. (1971). Cerebral hemispheric dominance test and localisation of speech. *Journal of Auditory Research* **11**, 117-189.

VINCENT, T. and BRADSHAW, J. (1975). A simple device for the preparation of exactly aligned dichotic tapes. *Behavior Research Methods and Instrumentation* **7**, 534-538.

WADA, J. (1949). A new method for determination of the side of cerebral speech dominance: a preliminary report on the intracarotid injection of sodium amytal in man. *Medical Biology (Tokyo)* **14**, 221-222.

WALSH, K. W. (1978). *Neuropsychology: A Clinical Approach.* Churchill-Livingstone, Edinburgh.

WARRINGTON, E. K. and PRATT, R. T. C. (1981). The significance of laterality effects. *Journal of Neurology, Neurosurgery and Psychiatry* **44**, 193-196.

WEBER, A. M. and BRADSHAW, J. L. (1981). Levy and Reid's neurological model in relation to writing hand/posture: an evaluation. *Psychological Bulletin* **90**, 74-88.

WEISKRANTZ, L. (ed.) (1968). *Analysis of Behavioural Change.* Harper and Row, New York.

WEISKRANTZ, L. (1973). Problems and progress in physiological psychology. *British Journal of Psychology* **64**, 511-520.

WEITAN, W. and ETAUGH, C. (1974). Lateral eye-movement as a function of cognitive mode, question sequence, and sex of subject. *Perceptual and Motor Skills* **38**, 439-444.

WHITAKER, H. A. and OJEMANN, G. A. (1977). Lateralisation of higher cortical functioning: a critique. *Annals of the New York Academy of Sciences* **299**, 459-473.

WHITAKER, H. A. and SELNES, O. A. (1976). Anatomic variations in the cortex: individual differences and the problem of the localisation of language functions. *Annals of the New York Academy of Sciences* **280**, 844-854.

WITELSON, S. F. (1974). Hemispheric specialisation for linguistic and nonlinguistic tactual perception using a dichotomous stimulation technique. *Cortex* **10**, 3-17.

WITELSON, S. F. (1977). Early hemisphere specialisation and interhemispheric plasticity: an empirical and theoretical review. In *Language Development and Neurological Theory* (S. J. Segalowitz and F. A. Gruber, eds), pp.213-287. Academic Press, New York and London.

WOOD, F. (1980). Theoretical, methodological and statistical implications of the inhalation rCBF technique for the study of brain-behaviour relationships. *Brain and Language* **9**, 1-8.

WOODS, D. J. and OPPENHEIMER, K. C. (1980). Torque, hemispheric dominance and psychosocial adjustment. *Journal of Abnormal Psychology* **89**, 567-572.

WYKE, M. (1977). Musical ability: a neuropsychological interpretation. In *Music and the Brain* (M. Critchley and R. A. Henson, eds), pp.156-173. Heinemann Medical Books, London.

YAMAMOTO, M. and HATTA, T. (1980). Hemispheric asymmetries in a tactile thought task for normal subjects. *Perceptual and Motor Skills* **50**, 467-471.

YOUNG, A. W. (1982a). Asymmetry of cerebral hemispheric function during development. In *Brain and Behavioural Development* (J. Dickerson and H. McGurk, eds), pp.168-202. Blackie, Glasgow.

YOUNG, A. W. (1982b). Methodological and theoretical bases of visual hemifield studies. In *Divided Visual Field Studies of Cerebral Organisation*, (J. G. Beaumont, ed.), pp.11-27. Academic Press, London and New York.

YOUNG, A. W. and ELLIS, A. W. (1979). Perception of numerical stimuli felt by fingers of the left and right hands. *Quarterly Journal of Experimental Psychology* **31**, 263-272.

YOUNG, A. W., BION, P. J. and ELLIS, A. W. (1980). Studies toward a model of laterality effects for picture and word naming. *Brain and Language* **11**, 54-65.

ZAIDEL, E. (1975). A technique for presenting lateralised visual input with prolonged exposure. *Vision Research* **15**, 283-289.

ZAIDEL, E. (1978). Auditory language comprehension in the right hemisphere following cerebral commissurotomy and hemispherectomy: a comparison with child language and aphasia. In *Language Acquisition and Language Breakdown: Parallels and Divergencies* (A. Caramazza and E. B. Zurif, eds), pp.229-276. Johns Hopkins University Press, Baltimore, Maryland.

ZENHAUSERN, R. (1978). Imagery, cerebral dominance and style of thinking: a unified field model. *Bulletin of the Psychonomic Society* **12**, 381-384.

ZOCCOLOTTI, P., PASSAFIUME, D. and PIZZAMIGLIO, L. (1979). Hemispheric superiorities on a unilateral tactile test: relationship to cognitive dimensions. *Perceptual and Motor Skills* **49**, 735-742.

6

THE DEVELOPMENT OF RIGHT HEMISPHERE ABILITIES

Andrew W. Young

Introduction

ALTHOUGH MUCH attention has been recently given to questions concerning the abilities of the right cerebral hemisphere, comparatively few studies have been directly addressed to the topic of the development, during infancy and childhood, of these abilities. This is in marked contrast to the relatively large number of studies of the ontogeny of left hemisphere abilities. In reviewing our knowledge of the development of right hemisphere abilities it is, therefore, necessary to consider a wide range of studies whose bearing on the topic is sometimes quite indirect.

Despite the lack of a really extensive body of directly relevant studies, ambitious theoretical statements have been attempted by a number of authors. These may well be useful in both guiding and stimulating interest in the area, but they also make it necessary to consider to what extent they are supported by the available findings, and to what extent they are capable of being supported or falsified by any conceivable set of data gathered under the limitations of existing research methods.

In order to orientate the reader I will now give a plan of how I have structured the material at my disposal. This introductory section is followed by a brief discussion of questions of research method, and then an introduction to ideas and evidence concerning lateralisation and plasticity of cerebral hemisphere function during infancy and childhood. These sections are followed by

FUNCTIONS OF THE RIGHT CEREBRAL HEMISPHERE
0-12-773250-0
Copyright © 1983 by Academic Press, London.
All rights of reproduction in any form reserved.

comparatively detailed consideration of the evidence relating to the development of the right hemisphere's visuospatial abilities, face recognition abilities, auditory and musical abilities, and language abilities. A short conclusions section completes the chapter.

In all cases the term 'right hemisphere abilities' is used to refer to the abilities shown by the right cerebral hemisphere in the majority of right-handed people. Thus, for instance, right hemisphere language abilities refers to the language abilities of the right hemispheres of people with what is regarded as left cerebral dominance for language functions, and should not be confused with the separate point that a minority of people have right cerebral dominance for language. Questions relating to such topics as individual differences in right hemisphere abilities, and the extent of right hemisphere language dominance, will not be directly discussed.

Questions of Research Method

The available methods are reviewed by Beaumont in Chapter 5 of this book, so it is only necessary here to provide a brief introduction to each of the methods employed. However, there are a number of special problems involved in their application to developmental studies which do need to be explained. Only points that apply generally to studies using each method will be discussed here, with specific points relating to particular studies discussed together with those studies in later sections.

The simplest way of classifying the methods for present purposes is into those that have been used primarily for studies of development in normal children and those based on clinical subject populations. The methods used with normal children have involved the lateralised presentation of visual, tactile and auditory stimuli, or the use of electrophysiological measures. Studies based on clinical subject populations have generally concerned themselves with effects of, and recovery from, unilateral cerebral injuries and hemispherectomy.

The majority of studies of normal children have involved the use of lateralised stimulus presentations. An excellent introduction to these methods is provided by Cohen (1977), and their application to developmental studies has been discussed in Witelson (1977a) and Young (1982a). They depend on the predominance of contralateral projections in the nervous system, which connect the left visual hemifield (LVF) to the right cerebral hemisphere, the right visual hemifield (RVF) to the left hemisphere, the left hand to the right hemisphere, the right hand to the left hemisphere, the left ear to the right hemisphere, and the right ear to the left hemisphere. Although substantial ipsilateral tactile and auditory projections are known to exist connecting the left hand to the left cerebral hemisphere, the right hand to the right hemisphere, the left ear to the left hemisphere, and the right ear to the right hemisphere, their functions and efficiency are generally considered to be subservient to those of the contralateral projections. This is thought to be particularly the case when active exploration of tactile stimuli (Gibson, 1962; Wall, 1975), relatively fine motor movements (Brinkman and Kuypers, 1973) and simultaneous bilateral (dichotic) stimulation of the ears are involved (Kimura, 1967).

It is possible, then, to take advantage of the arrangement of the nervous system in order to present stimuli to the left or right cerebral hemispheres, though it must be remembered that this can only determine the initial projection of stimuli, and that the subsequent interhemispheric coordination and integration of information by the cerebral commissures is but poorly understood. Nonetheless, the attractions of the possibility of studying the development of cerebral hemisphere function in the normal, intact brain are obvious. There are, however, a number of problems involved in such developmental studies.

Most of these problems can be summed up in the statement that it is difficult to ensure that children of different ages (and also different children of the same age) are doing the same thing.

It is important, for instance, that any changes across age in obtained laterality effects do not simply reflect age-related changes in subject strategies, since this possibility would preclude conclusions concerning the ontogeny of cerebral asymmetry (Young and Ellis, 1981; Young, 1982a). It is particularly tricky to avoid quite marked age differences in task difficulty, which may again influence obtained laterality effects. In addition, it is possible for spurious developmental differences in laterality effects to arise if some components of experimental tasks are disproportionately difficult to particular age groups (Porter and Berlin, 1975).

Such difficulties of interpretation led Colbourn (1978) to argue that between-group comparisons in laterality research, of which comparisons across age can be seen as a particular kind of example, should be based on conservative measures. Beaumont (1982), in reviewing the developmental studies using visual stimulus presentations, went even further by implying that it may not be possible to arrive at definite conclusions concerning cerebral organisation from studies of this type. This latter position is, however, excessively pessimistic. There are a number of experimental procedures that can be used to minimise these difficulties of method (Young and Ellis, 1981; Young, 1982a), and it is clear that the findings of studies that have employed such procedures exhibit a remarkable degree of agreement (Beaumont, 1982; De Renzi, 1982; Witelson, 1977a; Young, 1982a). Moreover, there are several good grounds for believing that these procedures do tap cerebral asymmetries in adult subjects, such as differences in obtained asymmetries between left and right handers, and differences in obtained asymmetries with different stimuli and experimental tasks. Thus it would seem that valid across age comparisons of cerebral asymmetries can be made under appropriate conditions. In particular, as Young and Bion (1980a) have pointed out, when the same asymmetries are found at different ages there are good grounds for concluding that cerebral asymmetry for the processes investigated does not change across age. It is when across age differences in laterality effects are found that it is difficult to mount a convincing argument that they reflect changes in cerebral asymmetry, since there are so many more prosaic alternative explanations that must be ruled out. It should be noted that this point of interpretation applies not only to developmental studies of cerebral asymmetry, but is simply a particular example of a general point applicable to all across age comparisons (Bryant, 1974). Whenever the same findings can be made for both younger and older subjects it can be inferred that young people possess the abilities investigated; when differences across age are found it is always difficult to establish convincingly that young people lack some quality present in those who are older.

A special problem that arises in studies using visual stimulus presentation concerns fixation control. There is no purpose in presenting stimuli left or right of a central fixation spot if subjects are not looking at that spot, and the problem of establishing fixation is especially pressing in developmental studies. Fortunately a number of simple techniques of fixation control have been developed whose use has been reviewed by Beaumont (1982) and Young (1982b). Studies that have tried to present LVF and RVF stimuli to children without fixation control will not be discussed in this review.

The other research strategy that has been adopted in studies of normal children involves the use of electrophysiological measures. These are particularly useful in studies of infants, but they are often made difficult to interpret by our lack of understanding of what is being measured, and the fact that the symmetric placement of electrodes on the scalp does not guarantee placement over corresponding locations in the left and right cerebral hemispheres. These, and other points, concerning electrophysiological measures are explained by Beaumont in Chapter 5.

Most of the studies of clinical subject populations have looked at the effect of age on the immediate symptoms and the extent of recovery following unilateral cerebral injuries. Such studies face a number of serious difficulties of method and interpretation, which have been discussed by Kinsbourne (1976), Witelson (1977a) and St. James-Roberts (1979). These include the need to establish that types of injury do not differ across age, that the injuries are genuinely unilateral, and that different biases in the selection and reporting of cases do not operate at different ages. A further difficulty is to establish the relative contributions to observed symptoms and recovery made by the injured hemisphere itself, and by the uninjured hemisphere. At first sight this latter problem is avoided in studies of hemispherectomy, where the cortex of one of the cerebral hemispheres has been surgically removed, and such cases have received considerable attention.

However, there remains the problem of the contribution of subcortical structures after hemispherectomy, and the further problem that the neurological status of the remaining cerebral hemisphere is often particularly difficult to assess (St. James-Roberts, 1979, 1981).

It is clear, then, that there is no available way of studying cerebral organisation in children that is not beset with considerable problems of method. However, it is equally clear that researchers have become well aware of such difficulties, and that several can be adequately dealt with by careful and ingenious experimental design. The long list of problems is thus reason for caution in interpreting findings, not despair. Moreover, the characteristic problems of each of the types of study are mostly quite different, so that it is possible to have considerable confidence in findings that have been confirmed by different methods. It is mainly when particular results are out of line with those arising from other studies or other methods that they need to be especially carefully examined.

Lateralisation and Plasticity

As already stated, existing research activity has been largely directed toward understanding the development of left hemisphere abilities. The findings from such studies provide a useful context for studies of right hemisphere abilities. This context will now be outlined, together with the theoretical concepts of lateralisation and plasticity that have dominated so much of the research into the ontogeny of both left and right hemisphere abilities.

Lenneberg (1967) proposed that cerebral asymmetry develops gradually throughout childhood from an initial symmetric organisation of functions. Thus a particular set of skills, such as language, would at first be acquired by both cerebral hemispheres, and then normally become gradually lateralised to one of the cerebral hemispheres — in this case, the left. This process of lateralisation would be completed around the age of puberty. In the event of injury to one of the cerebral hemispheres, the degree to which the intact hemisphere could assume the other's functions would depend on the extent to which lateralisation had already occurred, with a much greater degree of takeover (i.e. plasticity) being possible at younger ages. In the case of the hypothesised bilaterally symmetric organisation during the first two years of life, perfect equipotentiality was thought to obtain, with the right hemisphere potentially as capable of supporting language acquisition, should it prove necessary, as the left.

This view of the ontogeny of cerebral hemisphere function was not entirely new but Lenneberg (1967) did give it its most eloquent and thoroughly documented expression. Three aspects of his views need to be particularly carefully noted. Firstly, the idea that lateralisation of function proceeds in a regular and progressive manner during childhood. Secondly, the idea that the initial organisation of functions is bilaterally symmetric. Thirdly, the idea that lateralisation and plasticity are intimately and inversely related, with increasing lateralisation being inevitably linked to decreasing plasticity.

More recent theoretical statements can be divided into those that continue to accept the idea of progressive lateralisation, and those that have questioned or rejected it. Amongst those who accept the idea of lateralisation, two kinds of disagreement have arisen. The first concerns the age at which lateralisation is held to be complete. Lenneberg (1967) set this at puberty, whereas Krashen (1973) wanted to lower it to age 5 years. Brown and Jaffe (1975), on the other hand, have argued that it should be raised, and that lateralisation continues even into old age. The second disagreement between the proponents of progressive lateralisation concerns whether or not the abilities of the two hemispheres lateralise concurrently, as it has been suggested that the abilities of the left hemisphere lateralise earlier than those of the right (Corballis and Morgan, 1978; Carey and Diamond, 1977).

A number of recent reviews have, however, expressed dissatisfaction with the idea of progressive lateralisation (Kinsbourne, 1976; Kinsbourne and Hiscock, 1977; De Renzi, 1982; Young, 1982a). There are several empirical reasons for this dissatisfaction, of which the most important will be briefly examined here.

One of the reasons was the demonstration of neuroanatomical asymmetries in adult, infant, newborn and foetal human brains (Geschwind and Levitsky, 1968; Teszner *et al.*, 1972; Witelson and Pallie, 1973; Wada *et al.*, 1975; Chi *et al.*, 1977). Although it was possible to argue that these asymmetries simply represent the neuroanatomical substrate of later developing functional specialisations, their existence made it difficult not to suspect that Lenneberg's ideas of perfect equipotentiality and bilaterally symmetric organisation in infancy might well prove false. This was soon found to be the case. Detailed studies of hemispherectomy patients showed that perfect equipotentiality does not obtain even in infancy (Dennis and Kohn, 1975; Dennis and Whitaker, 1976, 1977). At the same time, studies of normal infants (reviewed by Molfese, 1977, and De Renzi, 1982) revealed the presence of extensive functional asymmetries. These demonstrations of infant asymmetries were in turn consistent with a considerable body of evidence from studies of performance asymmetries in normal children indicating that such asymmetries are typically quite stable across age, and do not change in the manner that the concept of progressive lateralisation would imply (Kinsbourne, 1976; Witelson, 1977a; De Renzi, 1982; Young, 1982a).

It is clear, then, that the ideas of perfect equipotentiality and bilaterally symmetric organisation of cerebral functions in infancy are false. The cerebral hemispheres of the infant's brain are both structurally and functionally asymmetric. Moreover, positive evidence of the gradual lateralisation of abilities has not been found, though some theorists have continued to find the idea attractive.

In order to reconcile their view of cerebral asymmetry as a relatively fixed and structural characteristic of the human brain at all ages with the evidence from clinical studies, Kinsbourne (1976), De Renzi (1982) and Young (1982a) all drew attention both to the difficulties in interpreting the clinical developmental data and to the point that the available data are often more relevant to the question of plasticity than to that of lateralisation. This latter point denies the link Lenneberg (1967) saw between plasticity and lateralisation, and maintains that these are quite separate issues. Although sceptical as to the occurrence of progressive lateralisation, Kinsbourne (1976), De Renzi (1982) and Young (1982a) all thought that the clinical data indicated the existence of a relatively marked degree of plasticity in infancy. However, this view has also come under critical scrutiny, and St. James-Roberts (1979, 1981) and Parker (1982) have argued convincingly that both the degree of plasticity itself, and the size of age differences in plasticity, may well have been overestimated.

Having looked at the methods and theoretical positions that have been adopted, the evidence deriving from studies that have examined the development of right hemisphere abilities can now be considered. This will be done under the headings visuospatial abilities, face recognition, auditory and musical abilities, and language abilities (corresponding to Chapters 1 to 4 of this book).

Visuospatial Abilities

Most of the studies of normal children that have been carried out would fall under the headings 'form recognition' and 'recognition and enumeration of stimulus configurations' used in Chapter 1.

Considering firstly form recognition (but excluding verbal forms, which are discussed under language abilities, and faces), investigators have tended to follow Witelson's (1974) dichhaptic procedure, in which different tactile stimuli are simultaneously explored by the two hands. With this type of procedure, left hand superiorities for the identification of tactually perceived nonsense shapes have been reported by Witelson (1974, 1977b), Cioffi and Kandel (1979), Flanery and Balling (1979), and Klein and Rosenfield (1980). These left hand superiorities were stable across age down to 6 years, the youngest age tested, but inconsistent sex differences have been observed.

Turning to studies of recognition and enumeration of stimulus configurations, a similar pattern emerges of right hemisphere superiorities and somewhat inconsistent sex differences at all ages tested. Hermelin and O'Connor (1971) found that blind children aged 8-10 years were, like adults, better at reading braille with the left than the right hand. Rudel et al. (1974a, 1977) found that sighted children aged over 10 years were better able to learn tactile configurations felt with the left hand. These authors did not, however, find left hand superiorities in children below age 10, but for reasons explained by De Renzi (1982) and Young (1982a) it is difficult to interpret this latter result, as changes in subject strategies may have occurred. Young and Bion (1979) found LVF superiorities for dot enumeration in children of 5 years and above, with the suggestion of a sex difference in subject strategies, as shown by apparent differences in speed–accuracy tradeoffs.

There are also a number of other studies of visuospatial information processing in children, using an assortment of procedures. Witelson (1977b) found a LVF superiority for matching simultaneously presented pairs of human figures in boys aged 6–14 years. Kershner *et al.* (1977) and Carter and Kinsbourne (1979) reported LVF superiorities in children that were apparently a consequence of an induced spatial mental set. Grant (1980, 1981) found LVF superiorities in children for colour naming. Ingram (1975) showed that 3–5-year-old children were better at copying hand postures and finger spacings with their left than with their right hands. A study of infants by Davis and Wada (1977) revealed a greater amplitude of evoked potentials to flashes recorded from the occipital lobe of the right hemisphere.

These studies of visuospatial abilities in normal infants and children have thus demonstrated right hemisphere superiorities at all of the ages it has proved possible to work with. These right hemisphere superiorities occur under the same conditions as the right hemisphere superiorities for visuospatial information processing found in adults (see Chapter 1), and there is no evidence of any age-related change in the degree of cerebral hemisphere asymmetry. There have, however, been some findings consistent with age and sex differences in subject strategies, and this factor needs to be carefully controlled whenever possible.

In discussing studies of tactile information processing in normal children, the findings reported by Galin *et al.* (1979) should also be mentioned. Galin *et al.* (1979) asked 3-year-old and 5-year-old children to compare fabric samples presented either to the same hand or to different hands. Their finding of a relatively greater proportion of errors made by the younger children when the comparisons were across different hands suggests some degree of difficulty in interhemispheric communication of information in the younger children. Such a conclusion would be consistent with anatomical evidence of comparatively late development of the cerebral commissures (Yakovlev and LeCours, 1967). The result is of clear theoretical significance and is badly in need of replication and extension.

A few studies have looked at the recovery of visuospatial functions following right hemisphere injuries sustained during childhood, and these have been well reviewed by De Renzi (1982). The studies have tended to confirm the conclusion deriving from studies of normal children, that right hemisphere superiorites for visuospatial information processing are present at all ages of postnatal development, since a number of visuospatial abilities have been found to be more impaired following unilateral injuries or hemispherectomy of the right hemisphere at any age (Fedio and Mirsky, 1969; Kohn and Dennis, 1974a, 1974b; Rudel and Denckla, 1974; Rudel et al., 1974). It has been suggested (e.g. Kohn and Dennis, 1974a,b) that it is the later developing spatial abilities that are particularly susceptible to disruption following right hemisphere injuries, but the confounding effect of task difficulty, with the later developing abilities tending to be associated with more difficult tasks, needs to be more fully explored before this interesting idea can be accepted.

Face Recognition

Two approaches have been used in studying the development of the right hemisphere's ability to recognise faces. One involves the presentation of pictures of faces briefly presented in the left and right visual hemifields, and the other involves an attempt to infer maturational status from performance with faces seen under comparatively free viewing conditions.

The original series of visual hemifield studies all employed photographs of upright faces as stimuli, and were able to demonstrate LVF superiorities down to age 5 years (Marcel and Rajan, 1975; Young and Ellis, 1976; Broman, 1978). A slightly discrepant result was recorded by Leehey (unpub.), who found LVF superiorities down to age 8 years (the youngest age she tested) for familiar faces, but only down to age 10 for unfamiliar faces. This may, however, have been due to her failure to control children's order of reporting her bilaterally presented stimuli (Young and Bion, 1980a). Reynolds and Jeeves (1978) also found no visual hemifield difference in a group of 7-8-year-old girls. Although Reynolds and Jeeves (1978) only employed a fixation control on one of their blocks of trials, the most likely explanation of their result is, as Beaumont (1982) pointed out, that LVF superiority has been masked by the excessive variance of the reaction times recorded from this subject group.

The general finding, then, has been one of LVF superiorities for upright faces presented to children. However, it was not certain whether these LVF superiorities reflected right hemisphere involvement in the processing of faces per se, or a more general right hemisphere superiority for processing complex visual stimuli. This problem is exacerbated by the fact that all of the studies so far mentioned required subjects to recognise the same photographs of the same faces, a task that can be solved using either face recognition or stimulus recognition strategies (Hay and Young, 1982). As an example of a stimulus recognition strategy, subjects might remember the presence of a strikingly dark spot in one of the pictures.

Fortunately, a suitable way of disentangling these possibilities was offered by

Leehey *et al.* (1978). Leehey *et al.* (1978) were able to demonstrate that the LVF superiority for face recognition by adult subjects was reduced by inversion of the stimulus faces. A face is an equally complex visual stimulus whether upright or inverted, but it will often fail to look 'face-like' as a consequence of inversion. Thus Leehey *et al.* (1978) argued that inverted faces can provide an adequate assessment of any visual hemifield differences introduced by cerebral hemisphere differences for processing complex visual stimuli, whereas the greater LVF superiority for upright faces can be seen as arising from a right hemisphere superiority for the processing of faces as such. A previous finding of an equal degree of LVF superiority for upright and inverted faces (Ellis and Shepherd, 1975) was argued by Leehey *et al.* (1978) to have involved such brief presentations that subjects were unable to encode presented stimuli as faces (but see Chapter 2 for a different line of reasoning).

Using Leehey *et al.*'s (1978) general procedure of presenting both upright and inverted faces at relatively long exposures within the acceptable range Young and Bion (1980a, Experiment 1) demonstrated a LVF superiority for recognising a small set of upright faces in children aged 7 years and above. The degree of visual hemifield asymmetry was unrelated to age, and there was no visual hemifield difference for inverted faces. With a larger set of faces, LVF superiorities for upright faces unrelated to age were again found by Young and Bion (1980a, Experiment 2), but for boys only. The fact that a LVF superiority had been demonstrated in girls with a small set of stimulus faces (Young and Bion, 1980a, Experiment 1) shows that the sex difference does not simply reflect any lesser degree of lateralisation in the female brain.

The study of Young and Bion (1980a) thus demonstrates a right hemisphere superiority for face (as opposed to stimulus) recognition which did not change in the age range studied. The faces used were all those of people not known personally by the children involved. Essentially similar findings were made by Young and Bion (1981a) in a study of the recognition of faces of people already known personally to the subjects (photographs of classmates and colleagues). LVF superiorities for upright known faces, and no visual hemifield differences for inverted faces, were found to be unrelated to age in the age range 7 years to adult. This study was again able to demonstrate that the right hemisphere superiorities involved were face recognition superiorities because of the absence of visual hemifield differences to inverted faces.

The results of studies using brief lateral presentations of faces, then, have demonstrated the existence of right hemisphere superiorities across a wide range of ages, with no changes in the degree of cerebral asymmetry. The second approach used in studies of children has been much less direct, involving attempts to infer the maturational status of the right hemisphere from performance with faces seen under comparatively free viewing conditions.

Carey and Diamond (1977) proposed that faces can be represented in the brain in terms of both piecemeal information concerning specific facial features (large lips, scar on cheek, etc.) and configurational information specifying the spatial relations of individual features. The piecemeal representations are seen as operating equally effectively for upright or inverted faces, whereas the configurational representations are claimed to be sensitive to orientation, and adversely affected by inversion. Carey and Diamond (1977), Diamond and Carey (1977) and Carey (1978) maintain that between the ages of 6 and 10 years children shift from relying predominantly on piecemeal to relying on configurational encoding of faces, and that maturational changes in the right cerebral hemisphere are responsible for this shift. These two claims are logically distinct and will be considered separately.

The claim for a shift from piecemeal to configurational representation of faces depends largely on data presented by Carey and Diamond (1977) and Diamond and Carey (1977), and is not really convincing. Carey and Diamond (1977) found that 6-year-old children recognised upright and inverted faces equally well, whereas 10-year-olds were better with upright faces. They argue that ability to use the orientation-sensitive configurational face representations develops between ages 6 and 10. However, the subsequent studies of Young and Bion (1980a; 1981a) indicate that Carey and Diamond's (1977) finding of an interaction of face orientation and age only arises when a sizeable set of unfamiliar faces is used (as in Carey and Diamond, 1977, and Young and Bion, 1980a, Experiment 2). When sets of known faces (Young and Bion, 1981a, Experiment 1), or a small set of initially unfamiliar faces (Young and Bion, 1980a, Experiment 1), were used as stimuli, 7-year-olds were as much affected by inversion as were older children. It is thus clear that young children do use configurational methods to represent known faces, and to make unknown faces familiar if given an adequate opportunity. When dealing with tasks with a relatively demanding memory component, however, the encoding or retrieval processes used by young children do not manage to attain higher levels of performance with upright than with inverted faces.

Carey and Diamond (1977) and Diamond and Carey (1977) also tried to show a shift from piecemeal to configurational encoding by showing that 6-year-old children were misled by changes in clothing when trying to recognise unfamiliar people. The use of clothing as a cue certainly can be seen as involving piecemeal encoding, though it is hardly piecemeal face encoding. The task concerned was very difficult, with the unfamiliar people being quite similar in appearance. Even adults I have asked to do this task in fact report that they also rely on piecemeal strategies; one of the unfamiliar people, for instance, has bushy eyebrows, and the photographs of one of the others look under-exposed. Thus the difference between older and younger people is not in the use of piecemeal or configurational encoding, since both use piecemeal encoding in this case. Moreover, both groups are also willing to resort to the use of nonfacial cues. The difference is that the piecemeal cues selected by adults are valid for identifying the people concerned, whereas the experiment is designed in such a way that the piecemeal cues used by 6-year-olds happen to be invalid. The results would seem to be telling us nothing about face encoding under everyday conditions, and in fact when Diamond and Carey (1977) gave children a comparable but easier task, with photographs of people known personally to them used as stimuli, even 6-year-old children were not misled by changes in clothing. This latter experiment again demonstrates the point that young children can use configurational representations under appropriate conditions; that they do not do this under inappropriate conditions is unsurprising.

Although the evidence adduced to support Carey and Diamond's (1977) claim for a shift from piecemeal to configurational representations of faces thus remains open to simpler explanations that do not involve such a change, this need not affect their second claim, that developmental differences in face recognition ability reflect underlying maturational changes in the right cerebral hemisphere.

Carey (1978) found that ability to recognise upright unfamiliar faces improved between ages 6 and 10 years, but then declined after age 10, with a recovery to the 10-year-old level of performance occurring between ages 14 and 16. The recognition of inverted faces, in contrast, remained at a relatively constant level of performance across this age range. Comparable results for recognising upright unfamiliar faces were reported by Flin (1980). Carey (1978) suggested that this unusual pattern of development, with a dip in the level of performance, may arise through an effect on right hemisphere abilities of the maturational changes associated with puberty.

A more immediately appealing explanation of the findings of Carey (1978) and Flin (1980) would be that the observed developmental differences are associated with changes in the strategies used to perform the task. Such strategy changes might arise for a variety of non-maturational reasons, such as the need to learn large numbers of new faces when moving to secondary schooling. Blaney and Winograd (1978), for instance, have shown that the performance of 6-10-year-old children on face recognition tasks is affected by strategies that they are asked to use. However, a study reported by Carey et al. (1980) simultaneously demonstrated both that strategies do affect performance at all ages and that the pattern of results found by Carey (1978) and Flin (1980) holds even when people are all using the same strategy. It should be noted that the presence of a main effect of strategy at all ages implies that Carey et al.'s (1980) instructions to use particular strategies were not simply disregarded. Thus, although such a study cannot entirely rule out the possibility of strategy changes across age being responsible for Carey's (1978) and Flin's (1980) findings, as it remains possible that Carey et al. (1980) examined the wrong strategies, the burden of proof has shifted such that anyone propsing a strategy change explanation would need to make clear what the different strategies actually are. Moreover, a study of age differences in ability to recognise voices by Mann et al. (1979) produced results that are remarkably comparable to Carey's (1978) and Flin's (1980) findings for recognition of upright faces. Although I know of no direct evidence to indicate that voice recognition is a right hemisphere ability, this does not detract from the parallel with the findings for upright face recognition. A maturational explanation would at present seem more readily able to account for this result.

There is, then, evidence consistent with the idea of maturational changes in some right hemisphere abilities. However, a number of reservations must be expressed. The evidence is at present very indirect, and it has to be said that it is hard to see why maturational changes in these particular skills should be expected to occur across such a prolonged period. Both face and voice recognition are well established in early infancy, and it is likely that there are innate mechanisms that make even neonates especially responsive to such stimuli (Schaffer, 1971; Mills and Melhuish, 1974; Goren et al., 1975). In addition, the findings of the visual hemifield studies already reviewed show that any maturational changes in right hemisphere abilities do not take the form of increases or decreases in lateralisation proposed by Carey (1978) and Carey et al. (1980).

In summary, then, the findings of studies of ability to recognise faces have shown that right hemisphere superiority is present from at least age 5 years, and that the degree of superiority does not change across age. The possibility that changes in overall performance levels for upright face recognition are associated with maturational changes of a form other than increasing or decreasing lateralisation, although based on indirect evidence, remains open and intriguing. It is a matter for considerable regret that studies of right hemisphere involvement in processing faces in infancy and in developmental clinical subject populations have not been reported.

Auditory and Musical Abilities

Only a few studies have looked at the development of the auditory and musical abilities that have been found to be associated with right hemisphere superiorities in adults. Environmental sounds were found to be associated with left ear (and hence right hemisphere) superiorities when dichotically presented to 3-5-year-old children by Knox and Kimura (1970). Auditory evoked responses to a C major piano chord and a burst of noise composed of frequencies between 250 Hz and 4 Hz were found to be larger in amplitude when recorded from the right hemispheres of infants, children and adults by Molfese et al. (1975). This asymmetry was most marked in the infants, a finding that Molfese et al. (1975) thought might reflect the lack of myelinisation of the interhemispheric

' the infant's brain. As was mentioned in the section of this
~~ned~~ with visuospatial abilities, there are both anatomical
~~L~~eCours, 1967) and functional (Galin *et al.*, 1979) findings to
~~support an argument~~ of this type. Gardiner and Walter (1977) also found greater
changes in right than left hemisphere EEG when infants were presented with
musical stimuli, and Glanville *et al.* (1977) demonstrated a greater degree of
habituation for music stimuli presented to infants' left ears.

Language Abilities

Although cases of right hemisphere language dominance are not being discussed
here, so that there are no instances of any right hemisphere superiority for
language abilities, it is none the less clear that the right hemisphere is not
entirely lacking in language abilities (reviewed by Searleman, 1977, and
Chapter 4 in this book; Coltheart, 1980). This raises the interesting question as
to how these somewhat limited language abilities are acquired. In discussing this
question it is necessary to distinguish language comprehension from language
production, and spoken from written language. There is considerable evidence
indicating that the right hemisphere is much better at comprehending than
producing language (Searleman, 1977), and Zaidel's (1976, 1978, 1979) studies
have suggested that its comprehension of spoken language may be greater than
its comprehension of written language.

An obvious hypothesis would be that the right hemisphere acquires its
language abilities during the early years of childhood. This might occur either
because lateralisation is not complete in early childhood, or because greater
plasticity of cerebral organisation in early childhood allows the acquisition of
some limited language ability despite the presence of left hemisphere language
dominance. Given the very substantial evidence against the idea of progressive
lateralisation of abilities already discussed the latter version of the hypothesis,
in terms of plasticity, might be thought more appealing. However, this too runs
into considerable difficulties when faced with the available evidence.

Zaidel's (1976, 1978, 1979) studies of commissurotomy and hemispherectomy
patients have shown that their right hemisphere language abilities do not map
easily onto the patterns of abilities found in children of different ages. The
difference between left and right hemisphere language abilities in these patients
seems to be qualitative in nature, rather than a reflection of an arrested or slowed
right hemisphere language development. The same conclusion emerges from
studies of normal adults by Ellis and Young (1977), Young and Bion (1980b),
Young and Ellis (1980) and Young *et al.* (1982). These have shown that ear
and visual hemifield asymmetries are not affected by the age of spoken or reading
acquisition of stimulus words, thus providing no grounds for the views that

words in the right hemisphere's auditory or visual comprehension vocabularies are those learnt early in life.

This view of the acquisition of right hemisphere language abilities is also supported by studies of normal children. Young and Bion (1981b) and Ellis and Young (1981) looked at visual hemifield differences for pictures, three-letter imageable nouns, and three-letter verbs, all of which should be within the right hemisphere's visual comprehension ability (see Searleman, Chapter 4). No changes across age in the nature or degree of visual hemifield asymmetries for these stimuli were observed by Young and Bion (1981b) and Ellis and Young (1981), which again implies that the differences between right and left hemisphere language abilities do not change during childhood.

At first sight, these findings from studies of right hemisphere language abilities in commissurotomy and hemispherectomy patients, and adults and children acting as normal subjects, would seem to conflict with the view deriving from studies of cerebral injuries in childhood, that the right hemisphere is involved in the early stages of language acquisition. However, this view has recently had to be reconsidered, for reasons which must be explained.

The proportion of children over 5 years of age who experience language difficulties following left as opposed to right hemisphere injuries is known to be comparable to the proportion found in adults (Krashen, 1973; Hécaen, 1976). For children aged under 5 years, however, language difficulties following right hemisphere injuries were originally thought to be relatively frequent. Witelson (1977a) arrived at a rough figure of 30%, but both she and Kinsbourne (1976) drew attention to a number of difficulties in taking such a figure at its face value. The most important of these is the possibility that many of the presumed right hemisphere injuries were so extensive as to also involve parts of the left hemisphere. This suggestion would find support in Annett's (1973) study of childhood hemiplegia, where a test of manual dexterity indicated the likelihood of additional injury to the supposedly healthy hemispheres in a number of cases. Woods and Teuber (1978) also noted that more recent reports do not find such a marked frequency of language disturbances following right hemisphere injury in childhood. They pointed out that many of the early reports are of cases where hemiplegias and language disturbances were complications of infectious illnesses, and that they precede the introduction of antibiotics.

It would appear, then, that right hemisphere language abilities are acquired throughout childhood, and that the differences between left and right hemisphere language abilities reflect structural factors. This answer is not fully satisfactory, however, because it is clear that the extent of the language abilities that the right hemisphere is capable of supporting in response to left hemisphere injury is much greater than the language abilities it shows in the absence of left hemisphere injury. Cleary, the way in which 'structural factors' operate to limit language acquisition in the right hemisphere of the normal brain whilst permitting an extensive degree of right hemisphere language in response to left hemisphere injury needs to be clarified. The relevant evidence derives entirely from clinical studies, and has to be interpreted with caution.

It is possible to think up a number of factors that might underly recovery from unilateral cerebral injuries. These would include recovery of the injured cortical areas themselves, acquisition of functions by corresponding areas of the intact cerebral hemisphere, and (in theory at least) acquisition of functions by uncommitted areas of cortex of the injured hemisphere. It is clear, however, that acquisition of functions by the intact cerebral hemisphere can occur. For instance, cases are known where patients have regained some degree of speech following left hemisphere injury only to lose their recovered speech after injury to the corresponding part of the right hemisphere (Nielsen, 1946). The Wada test, which involves the temporary anaesthesis of one of the cerebral hemispheres, has also been used to establish that the right hemisphere can be the source of speech after left hemisphere injury (Kinsbourne, 1971; Rasmussen and Milner, 1977). The proportion of cases of right hemisphere language acquisition following left hemisphere injuries in right-handers identified by Rasmussen and Milner (1977) was, though, rather low and it seems likely that considerable intrahemispheric recovery also occurs.

In hemispherectomy cases, however, intrahemispheric recovery is not possible, though the influence of remaining subcortical structures should not be neglected. Studies of the consequences of left hemispherectomy have again shown that a considerable degree of recovery of language functions can occur (Smith and Sugar, 1975). None the less, it is now known that despite the remarkable degree of recovery that can sometimes be achieved, the right hemisphere is not able to support language abilities as well as the left (Dennis and Kohn, 1975; Dennis and Whitaker, 1976; Dennis and Whitaker, 1977). In other words, equipotentiality of the cerebral hemispheres for language acquisition does not obtain.

The right hemisphere, then, can show considerable ability to support language in the face of left hemisphere injury, but it does not attain the same level of linguistic competence as an uninjured left hemisphere. It is no longer certain, though, to what extent the degree to which the right hemisphere can support language varies with age. It has often been thought that recovery from unilateral injuries sustained early in childhood is better than recovery from unilateral injuries sustained comparatively late in childhood or in adulthood (e.g. Hécaen and Albert, 1978; De Renzi, 1982; Young, 1982a). However, there are several reasons why the degree of age differences in plasticity may have been overestimated (St. James-Roberts, 1979, 1981; Parker, 1982). These include age differences in the aetiology of symptoms, and the tendency only to consider the subsection of adult cases in which substantial recovery does not occur.

Thus the reasons why the right hemisphere can be capable of a considerable degree of language acquisition under some circumstances, yet does not normally do so, remain to be established. The idea that an intact left hemisphere will actually inhibit activity in language areas of the right hemisphere has been advanced by some authors (see Moscovitch, 1976, and Searleman's discussion in Chapter 4), but others have seen this idea both as lacking substantial supporting evidence and as creating as many problems as it solves (Selnes, 1974, 1976). We simply do not know at present.

Conclusions

Studies of the development of right hemisphere abilities are, in comparison with studies of the development of left hemisphere abilities, scant and diverse. None the less, a consistent pattern of findings emerges. Studies that have examined the development of visuospatial abilities, face recognition, and auditory abilities, have revealed right hemisphere superiorities at all of the ages studied. Such studies, and those of right hemisphere language abilities, have produced no evidence of any progressive lateralisation of function. This conclusion holds regardless of whether these abilities have been studied early or late in life, and at ages close to or distant from those at which they are first acquired. Although it is possible to question the conclusions that may properly be drawn from some of the methods employed, and caution often needs to be exercised in interpreting particular results, this pattern of findings has emerged from studies employing methods that are themselves very varied. It is difficult to believe that such a consistent pattern could arise from an accumulation of the very different potential artifacts and pitfalls of each type of study. Rather, it would seem to be the case that the theory of progressive lateralisation of abilities during development is wrong.

The fact that the brain functions asymmetrically at all ages during infancy, childhood and adulthood demands a change in research strategies (Young, 1982a). The dominant type of study arising from the idea of progressive lateralisation has consisted of a search for gradual changes in the cerebral organisation of well established abilities across quite wide range of ages. Whilst this strategy may well continue to be of limited use, it now needs to be supplemented by investigations directed to the question as to how newly acquired abilities are integrated with existing abilities that are already asymmetrically (or symmetrically) organised. Such investigations will differ from the previous strategy in that they involve comparatively detailed studies of particular skills whilst they are being acquired, and hence often across rather narrow age ranges.

Given the existing evidence of asymmetries of cerebral hemispheric function at all ages of postnatal development, and for the existence of neuroanatomical asymmetries in foetal brains, it is most likely that differences between left and right hemisphere abilities arise for structural reasons. This is rather disappointing, as it is probably the least interesting of the possible conclusions, both for developmental researchers themselves and for the potential importance of developmental studies in understanding hemisphere function in the adult brain. Progressive lateralisation might have been wrong, but it was exciting. However, the details of the 'structural difference' hypothesis remain to be properly worked out, and from this many interesting new findings and lines of enquiry may well arise. The importance of studying laterality effects whilst skills are being acquired has already been mentioned. Much more needs to be known, too, about the various forms of plasticity, and the extent to which these may themselves be age dependent. The possible role of maturational factors in the development of right hemisphere abilities has also been noted. Such open questions continue to offer satisfying challenges to the ingenuity of researchers investigating the development of right hemisphere abilities.

Acknowledgements

The assistance provided by SSRC Grant HR6876 is gratefully acknowledged.

References

ANNETT, M. (1973). Laterality of childhood hemiplegia and the growth of speech and intelligence. *Cortex* **9**, 4-33.
BEAUMONT, J. G. (1982). Developmental aspects. In *Divided Visual Field Studies of Cerebral Organisation* (J. G. Beaumont, ed.), pp.113-128. Academic Press, London and New York.
BLANEY, R. L. and WINOGRAD, E. (1978). Developmental differences in children's recognition memory for faces. *Developmental Psychology* **14**, 441-442.
BRINKMAN, J. and KUYPERS, H. G. J. M. (1973). Cerebral control of contralateral and ipsilateral arm, hand and finger movements in the splitbrain rhesus monkey. *Brain* **96**, 653-674.
BROMAN, M. (1978). Reaction-time differences between the left and right hemispheres for face and letter discrimination in children and adults. *Cortex* **14**, 578-591.
BROWN, J. W. and JAFFE, J. (1975). Hypothesis on cerebral dominance. *Neuropsychologia* **13**, 107-110.
BRYANT, P. E. (1974). *Perception and Understanding in Young Children*. Methuen, London.
CAREY, S. (1978). A case study: face recognition. In *Explorations in the Biology of Language*. (E. Walker, ed.), pp.175-201. Bradford Books, Vermont.
CAREY, S. and DIAMOND, R. (1977). From piecemeal to configurational representation of faces. *Science* **195**, 312-314.
CAREY, S., DIAMOND, R. and WOODS, B. (1980). Development of face recognition—a maturational component? *Developmental Psychology* **16**, 257-269.

CARTER, G. L. and KINSBOURNE, M. (1979). The ontogeny of right cerebral lateralization of spatial mental set. *Developmental Psychology* **15**, 241-245.

CHI, J. G., DOOLING, E. C. and GILLES, F. H. (1977). Left-right asymmetries of the temporal speech areas of the human fetus. *Archives of Neurology* **34**, 346-348.

CIOFFI, J. and KANDEL, G. L. (1979). Laterality of stereognostic accuracy of children for words, shapes, and bigrams: a sex difference for bigrams. *Science* **204**, 1432-1434.

COHEN, G. (1977). *The Psychology of Cognition.* Academic Press, New York and London.

COLBOURN, C. J. (1978). Can laterality be measured? *Neuropsychologia* **16**, 283-289.

COLTHEART, M. (1980). Deep dyslexia: a right hemisphere hypothesis. In *Deep Dyslexia* (M. Coltheart, K. Patterson and J. C. Marshall, eds), pp.326-380. Routledge and Kegan Paul, London.

CORBALLIS, M. C. and MORGAN, M. J. (1978). On the biological basis of human laterality. I. Evidence for a maturational left-right gradient. *Behavioral and Brain Sciences* **1**, 261-269.

DAVIS, A. E. and WADA, J. A. (1977). Hemispheric asymmetries in human infants: spectral analysis of flash and click evoked potentials. *Brain and Language* **4**, 23-31.

DE RENZI, E. (1982). *Disorders of Space Exploration and Cognition.* Wiley, Chichester.

DENNIS, M. and KOHN, B. (1975). Comprehension of syntax in infantile hemiplegics after cerebral hemidecortication: left-hemisphere superiority. *Brain and Language* **2**, 472-482.

DENNIS, M. and WHITAKER, H. A. (1976). Language acquisition following hemidecortication: linguistic superiority of the left over the right hemisphere. *Brain and Language* **3**, 404-433.

DENNIS, M. and WHITAKER, H. A. (1977). Hemispheric equipotentiality and language acquisition. In *Language Development and Neurological Theory* (S. J. Segalowitz and F. A. Gruber, eds), pp.93-106. Academic Press, New York and London.

DIAMOND, R. and CAREY, S. (1977). Developmental changes in the representation of faces. *Journal of Experimental Child Psychology* **23**, 1-22.

ELLIS, A. W. and YOUNG, A. W. (1981). Visual hemifield asymmetry for naming concrete nouns and verbs in children between seven and eleven years of age. *Cortex* **17**, 617-623.

ELLIS, H. D. and SHEPHERD, J. W. (1975). Recognition of upright and inverted faces presented in the left and right visual fields. *Cortex* **11**, 3-7.

ELLIS, H. D. and YOUNG, A. W. (1977). Age-of-acquisition and recognition of nouns presented in the left and right visual fields: a failed hypothesis. *Neuropsychologia* **15**, 825-828.

FEDIO, P. and MIRSKY, A. F. (1969). Selective intellectual deficits in children with temporal lobe or centrencephalic epilepsy. *Neuropsychologia* **7**, 287-300.

FLANERY, R. C. and BALLING, J. D. (1979). Developmental changes in hemispheric specialization for tactile spatial ability. *Developmental Psychology* **15**, 364-372.

FLIN, R. H. (1980). Age effects in children's memory for unfamiliar faces. *Developmental Psychology* **16**, 373-374.

GALIN, D., JOHNSTONE, J., NAKELL, L. and HERRON, J. (1979). Development of the capacity for tactile information transfer between hemispheres in normal children. *Science* **204**, 1330-1332.

GARDINER, M. F. and WALTER, D. O. (1977). Evidence of hemispheric specialization from infant EEG. In *Lateralization in the Nervous System* (S. Harnad, R. W. Doty, L. Goldstein, J. Jaynes and G. Krauthamer, eds), pp.481-502. Academic Press, New York and London.

GESCHWIND, N. and LEVITSKY, W. (1978). Human brain: left-right asymmetries in temporal speech region. *Science* **161**, 186-187.

GIBSON, J. J. (1962). Observations on active touch. *Psychological Review* **69**, 477-491.
GLANVILLE, B., BEST, C. and LEVENSON, R. (1977). A cardiac measure of cerebral asymmetries in infant auditory perception. *Developmental Psychology* **13**, 54-59.
GOREN, C. G., SARTY, M. and WU, P. Y. K. (1975). Visual following and pattern discrimination of face-like stimuli by newborn infants. *Pediatrics* **56**, 544-549.
GRANT, D. W. (1980). Visual asymmetry on a colour-naming task: a developmental perspective. *Perceptual and Motor Skills* **50**, 475-480.
GRANT, D. W. (1981). Visual asymmetry on a colour naming task: a longitudinal study with primary school children. *Child Development* **52**, 370-372.
HAY, D. C. and YOUNG, A. W. (1982). The human face. In *Normality and Pathology in Cognitive Functions* (A. W. Ellis, ed.), pp.173-202. Academic Press, London and New York.
HÉCEAN, H. (1976). Acquired aphasia in children and the ontogenesis of hemispheric functional specialization. *Brain and Language* **3**, 114-134.
HÉCAEN, H. and ALBERT, M. L. (1978). *Human Neuropsychology*. Wiley, New York.
HERMELIN, B. and O'CONNOR, N. (1971). Functional asymmetry in the reading of Braille. *Neuropsychologia* **9**, 431-435.
INGRAM, D. (1975). Motor asymmetries in young children. *Neuropsychologia* **13**, 95-102.
KERSHNER, J., THOMAE, R. and CALLAWAY, R. (1977). Nonverbal fixation control in young children induces a left-field advantage in digit recall. *Neuropsychologia* **15**, 569-576.
KIMURA, D. (1967). Functional asymmetry of the brain in dichotic listening. *Cortex* **3**, 163-178.
KINSBOURNE, M. (1971). The minor hemisphere as a source of aphasic speech. *Transactions of the American Neurological Association* **96**, 141-145.
KINSBOURNE, M. (1976). The ontogeny of cerebral dominance. In *The Neuropsychology of Language* (R. W. Rieber, ed.), pp.181-191. Plenum Press, New York.
KINSBOURNE, M. and HISCOCK, M. (1977). Does cerebral dominance develop? In *Language Development and Neurological Theory* (S. J. Segalowitz and F. A. Gruber, eds), pp.171-191. Academic Press, New York and London.
KLEIN, S. P. and ROSENFIELD, W. D. (1980). Hemispheric specialization for linguistic and non-linguistic tactile stimuli in third grade children. *Cortex* **16**, 205-212.
KNOX, C. and KIMURA, D. (1970). Cerebral processing of nonverbal sounds in boys and girls. *Neuropsychologia* **8**, 227-237.
KOHN, B. and DENNIS, M. (1974a). Selective impairment of visuo-spatial abilities in infantile hemiplegics after right cerebral hemidecortication. *Neuropsychologia* **12**, 505-512.
KOHN, B. and DENNIS, M. (1974b). Patterns of hemispheric specialization after hemidecortication for infantile hemiplegia. In *Hemispheric Disconnection and Cerebral Function* (M. Kinsbourne and W. L. Smith, eds), pp.34-47. Charles C. Thomas, Springfield, Illinois.
KRASHEN, S. (1973). Lateralization, language learning and the critical period: some new evidence. *Language Learning* **23**, 63-74.
LEEHEY, S. C. (unpub.). Face recognition in children. Evidence for the development of right hemisphere specialization. Ph.D. thesis, Massachusetts, Institute of Technology, 1976.
LEEHEY, S. C., CAREY, S., DIAMOND, R. and CAHN, A. (1978). Upright and inverted faces: the right hemisphere knows the difference. *Cortex* **14**, 411-419.
LENNEBERG, E. H. (1967). *Biological Foundations of Language*. Wiley, New York.
MANN, V. A., DIAMOND, R. and CAREY, S. (1979). Development of voice recognition:

parallels with face recognition. *Journal of Experimental Child Psychology* **27**, 153-165.

MARCEL, T. and RAJAN, P. (1975). Lateral specialisation for recognition of words and faces in good and poor readers. *Neuropsychologia* **13**, 489-497.

MILLS, M. and MELHUISH, E. (1974). Recognition of mother's voice in early infancy. *Nature, Lond.* **252**, 123-124.

MOLFESE, D. L. (1977). Infant cerebral asymmetry. In *Language Development and Neurological Theory* (S. J. Segalowitz and F. A. Gruber, eds), pp.21-35. Academic Press New York and London.

MOLFESE, D. L., FREEMAN, R. B., and PALERMO, D. S. (1975). The ontogeny of brain lateralization for speech and nonspeech stimuli. *Brain and Language* **2**, 356-368.

MOSCOVITCH, M. (1976). On the representation of language in the right hemisphere of right-handed people. *Brain and Language* **2**, 47-71.

NIELSEN, J. M. (1946). *Agnosia, Apraxia, Aphasia: Their Value in Cerebral Localization.* Hoeber, New York.

PARKER, D. M. (1982). Determinate and plastic principles in neuropsychological development. In *Brain and Behavioural Development* (J. W. T. Dickerson and H. McGurk, eds), pp.203-232. Blackie, Glasgow.

PORTER, R. J. and BERLIN, C. I. (1975). On interpreting developmental changes in the dichotic right-ear advantage. *Brain and Language* **2**, 186-200.

RASMUSSEN, T. and MILNER, B. (1977). The role of early left brain injury in determining lateralisation of cerebral speech function. In *Evolution and Lateralization of the Brain* (S. J. Dimond and D. A. Blizard, eds). *Annals of the New York Academy of Science* **299**, 355-369.

REYNOLDS, D. McQ. and JEEVES, M. A. (1978). A developmental study of hemisphere specialization for recognition of faces in normal subjects. *Cortex* **14**, 511-520.

RUDEL, R. G. and DENCKLA, M. B. (1974). Relation of forward and backward digit repetition to neurological impairment in children with learning disabilities. *Neuropsychologia* **12**, 109-118.

RUDEL, R. G., DENCKLA, M. B. and SPALTEN, E. (1974a). The functional asymmetry of Braille letter learning in normal, sighted children. *Neurology* **24**, 733-738.

RUDEL, R. G., TEUBER, H.-L. and TWITCHELL, T. E. (1974b). Levels of impairment of sensori-motor functions in children with early brain damage. *Neuropsychologia* **12**, 95-108.

RUDEL, R. G. DENCKLA, M. B. and HIRSCH, S. (1977). The development of left-hand superiority for discriminating Braille configurations. *Neurology* **27**, 160-164.

SCHAFFER, H. R. (1971). *The Growth of Sociability.* Penguin, Harmondsworth.

SEARLEMAN, A. (1977). A review of right hemisphere linguistic capabilities. *Psychological Bulletin* **84**, 503-528.

SELNES, O. A. (1974). The corpus callosum: some anatomical and functional considerations with reference to language. *Brain and Language* **1**, 111-139.

SELNES, O. A. (1976). A note on 'on the representation of language in the right hemisphere of right-handed people'. *Brain and Language* **3**, 583-589.

SMITH, A. and SUGAR, O. (1975). Development of above normal language and intelligence 21 years after left hemispherectomy. *Neurology* **25**, 813-818.

ST. JAMES-ROBERTS, I. (1979). Neurological plasticity, recovery from brain insult, and child development. *Advances in Child Development and Behavior* **14**, 253-319.

ST. JAMES-ROBERTS, I. (1981). A reinterpretation of hemispherectomy data without functional plasticity of the brain. *Brain and Language* **13**, 31-53.

TESZNER, D., TZAVARAS, A., GRUNER, J. and HÉCAEN, H. (1972). L'asymétrie droite-gauche du planum temporale: a propos de l'étude anatomique de 100 cervaux. *Revue Neurologique* **126**, 444-449.

WADA, J. A., CLARK, R. and HAMM, A. (1975). Cerebral hemispheric asymmetry in humans: cortical speech zones in 100 adult and 100 infant brains. *Archives of Neurology* **32**, 239-246.

WALL, P. D. (1975). The somatosensory system. In *Handbook of Psychobiology* (M. S. Gazzaniga and C. Blakemore, eds), Academic Press, New York and London.

WITELSON, S. F. (1974). Hemispheric specialization for linguistic and nonlinguistic tactual perception using a dichotomous stimulation technique. *Cortex* **10**, 3-17.

WITELSON, S. F. (1977a). Early hemisphere specialization and interhemisphere plasticity: an empirical and theoretical review. In *Language Development and Neurological Theory* (S. J. Segalowitz and F. A. Gruber, eds), pp.213-287. Academic Press, New York and London.

WITELSON, S. F. (1977b). Neural and cognitive correlates of developmental dyslexia: age and sex differences. In *Psychopathology and Brain Dysfunction* (C. Shagass, S. Gershon, and A. J. Friedhoff, eds), pp.15-49. Raven Press, New York.

WITELSON, S. F. and PALLIE, W. (1973). Left hemisphere specialization for language in the newborn: neuroanatomical evidence of asymmetry. *Brain* **96**, 641-646.

WOODS, B. T. and TEUBER, H.-L. (1978). Changing patterns of childhood aphasia. *Annals of Neurology* **3**, 273-280.

YAKOVLEV, P. and LECOURS, A. (1967). The myelogenetic cycles of regional maturation of the brain. In *Regional Development of the Brain in Early Life* (A. Minkowski, ed.). Blackwell, Oxford.

YOUNG, A. W. (1982a). Asymmetry of cerebral hemispheric function during development. In *Brain and Behavioural Development* (J. W. T. Dickerson and H. McGurk, eds), pp.168-202. Blackie, Glasgow.

YOUNG, A. W. (1982b). Methodological and theoretical bases of visual hemifield studies. In *Divided Visual Field Studies of Cerebral Organisation* (J. G. Beaumont, ed.), pp.11-27. Academic Press, London and New York.

YOUNG, A. W. and BION, P. J. (1979). Hemispheric laterality effects in the enumeration of visually presented collections of dots by children. *Neuropsychologia* **17**, 99-102.

YOUNG, A. W. and BION, P. J. (1980a). Absence of any developmental trend in right hemisphere superiority for face recognition. *Cortex* **16**, 213-221.

YOUNG, A. W. and BION, P. J. (1980b). Hemifield differences for naming bilaterally presented nouns varying on age of acquisition. *Perceptual and Motor Skills* **50**, 366.

YOUNG, A. W. and BION, P. J. (1981a). Accuracy of naming laterally presented known faces by children and adults. *Cortex* **17**, 97-106.

YOUNG, A. W. and BION, P. J. (1981b). Identification and storage of line drawings presented to the left and right cerebral hemispheres of adults and children. *Cortex* **17**, 459-463.

YOUNG, A. W. and ELLIS, A. W. (1981). Asymmetry of cerebral hemispheric function in normal and poor readers. *Psychological Bulletin* **89**, 183-190.

YOUNG, A. W. and ELLIS, H. D. (1976). An experimental investigation of developmental differences in ability to recognise faces presented to the left and right cerebral hemispheres. *Neuropsychologia* **14**, 495-498.

YOUNG, A. W. and ELLIS, H. D. (1980). Ear asymmetry for the perception of monaurally presented words accompanied by binaural white noise. *Neuropsychologia* **18**, 107-110.

YOUNG, A. W. BION, P. J. and ELLIS, A. W. (1982). Age of reading acquisition does not affect visual hemifield asymmetries for naming imageable nouns. *Cortex* **18**, 477-482.

ZAIDEL, E. (1976). Auditory vocabulary of the right hemisphere following brain bisection or hemidecortication. *Cortex* **12**, 191-211.

ZAIDEL, E. (1978). Lexical organization in the right hemisphere. In *Cerebral Correlates of Conscious Experience* (P. A. Buser and A. Rougeul-Buser, eds), pp.177-197. North Holland Publishing, Amsterdam.

ZAIDEL, E. (1979). Performance on the ITPA following cerebral commissurotomy and hemispherectomy. *Neuropsychologia* 17, 259-280.

7

THE RIGHT HEMISPHERE AND DISORDERS OF READING

Max Coltheart

AFTER DAMAGE to the left cerebral hemisphere has produced a severe aphasia, linguistic abilities may show a gradual and partial recovery over a period of months or years. One can interpret the existence of such partial recovery in two ways. On the one hand, the view can be taken that these abilities reflect some recovery of the use of the left hemisphere mechanisms subserving language. Such recovery might be consequent upon improvements in the neurological condition of the damaged left hemisphere, and the reason why the recovered language is imperfect is because it is being produced by a damaged system.

As Searleman and Young observe in their chapters in this volume, however, an alternative interpretation of partial recovery from aphasia exists, and has been advanced on various occasions throughout the past hundred years. On this interpretation, the limited linguistic ability exhibited by the partially recovered aphasic depends, not upon the use of a damaged linguistic system in the left hemisphere, but upon the use of an intact linguistic system in the right hemisphere. Here the reason why the recovered language is imperfect is because it is being produced by a system whose linguistic capabilities are intrinsically limited, at least in the majority of people.

As a way of thinking about the linguistic capabilities of the partially recovered aphasic, this right hemisphere interpretation is quite widespread and quite influential, especially amongst those concerned with the rehabilitation of aphasia. For example, Lesser (1981) refers to the exploration of right hemisphere functions as a 'significant aspect of aphasia rehabilitation'; Code (1982) describes

FUNCTIONS OF THE RIGHT CEREBRAL HEMISPHERE
0-12-773250-0 *Copyright © 1983 by Academic Press, London.*
All rights of reproduction in any form reserved.

a rehabilitation programme based entirely on attempts to develop the linguistic capabilities of the right hemisphere; and

> in severe cases of aphasia, therapies which purely try to re-establish normal language are fighting an uphill battle because one potential seat of new learning, the left hemisphere, is severely damaged . . . the alternative solution in severe cases is to devise a communication system that the right hemisphere can properly mediate. (Powell, 1980, p.112)

It has almost always been the case that discussions of the role of the right hemisphere in mediating partially recovered aphasic language have considered only spoken language—that is, speech production and speech comprehension. Nevertheless, if it is plausible that the right hemisphere plays a part in aphasic processing of spoken language, it must also be reasonable to consider the possible role of the right hemisphere when the aphasic is attempting to deal with written language—to read, to write or to spell. The aim of this chapter is to discuss what contributions the right hemisphere may be making in cases of disordered reading, writing and spelling.

Reading disorders (dyslexias) arise in two different ways—they can be *acquired* or they can be *developmental*. The term 'acquired dyslexia' refers to the occurrence of a disorder of reading as a consequence of damage to the brain in a previously literate person (adult or child). The term 'developmental dyslexia' refers to a failure ever to reach a normal level of literacy. I will be concerned here mainly with acquired dyslexias, but will also briefly consider developmental dyslexias, because suggestions have been made concerning contributions by the right hemisphere in cases of developmental dyslexia.

In the term 'acquired dyslexias', the plural is used advisedly, because damage to the brain can impair reading in a number of different ways. This has become particularly clear in recent years, as experimental psychologists have begun to investigate reading disorders from an information-processing or psycholinguistic perspective (Coltheart, 1982). This work has led to the definition and description of a variety of acquired dyslexias, including *surface dyslexia* (Marshall and Newcombe, 1973; Coltheart *et al.*, in press), *deep dyslexia* (Marshall and Newcombe, 1973; Coltheart, 1980b), *phonological dyslexia* (Beauvois and Derouesne, 1979; Derouesne and Beauvois, 1979; Patterson, 1982), *attentional dyslexia* (Shallice and Warrington, 1977), *concrete-word dyslexia* (Warrington, 1981), and *letter-by-letter reading* (Patterson and Kay, 1982) also known as *word-form dyslexia* (Warrington and Shallice, 1980) and probably equivalent to the traditional 'pure alexia' or 'alexia without agraphia'. General surveys of this approach to the acquired dyslexias are provided by Coltheart (1981a), Newcombe and Marshall (1981), Patterson (1981) and Shallice (1981).

Since for all six of the acquired dylexias listed above there is usually damage to the left hemisphere, one can raise the question of right hemisphere mediation of impaired reading in relation to each of these dyslexias. However, in this chapter I will be discussing only three of the disorders: deep dyslexia, letter-by-letter reading and concrete-word dyslexia. The reason for this is that no one has yet proposed that there is any contribution from the right hemisphere to the forms of disordered reading seen in surface dyslexia, phonological dyslexia or attentional dyslexia. Hence, at least at present, these three disorders are not relevant to discussions of the role of the right hemisphere in reading.

The other three disorders, however, are all relevant. Deep dyslexia is relevant because of claims (Coltheart, 1980a; Saffran *et al.* 1980) that the right hemisphere is solely responsible for reading in deep dyslexia. Letter-by-letter reading and concrete-word dyslexia are relevant because, as will be discussed below, the properties of each of these disorders raise difficulties for the right hemisphere account of deep dyslexia, and attempts to resolve these difficulties lead to more precise views concerning possible roles played by the right hemisphere in disorders of reading.

Deep Dyslexia

Early reports of this acquired dyslexia include those by Franz (1930) and Low (1931). The first detailed case study was published by Marshall and Newcombe (1966), who subsequently proposed the term 'deep dyslexia' (Marshall and Newcombe, 1973) to describe the condition. A recent book (Coltheart *et al.*, 1980) is entirely devoted to deep dyslexia, and includes a review (Coltheart, 1980b) of 22 cases reported during the period 1930–1979. Since then, several further cases have been described (Shallice and Coughlin, 1980; Patterson, 1981; Nolan and Caramazza, 1982; Friedman and Perlman, in press; Coltheart *et al.*, in prep.).

According to the review by Coltheart (1980b), the characteristics of deep dyslexia are as follows:

1. Semantic errors occur in the reading aloud of single isolated words—for example, *vision* → 'focus', *tram* → 'line', and *great* → 'bigger'. Semantic errors also occur when writing from dictation.

2. Visual errors in reading also occur—for example, *heart* → 'heaven', *weak* → 'wear', and *needed* → 'needle'.

3. There are also derivational errors: *write* → 'writing', *slept* → 'sleeper', and *theft* → 'thief'.

4. Function words are much less likely to be read correctly than content words;

and when a function word is misread, the incorrect response is commonly another (often entirely unrelated) function word—for example, *there* → 'and', *my* → 'is', *ours* → 'on' and *he* → 'in'.

5. Words which are concrete and/or high in imageability are more likely to be read aloud correctly than words which are low in imageability and/or abstract.

6. Reading non-words aloud is impossible, or nearly so, as are tasks requiring silent judgements about phonological properties of non-words.

7. In Japanese cases of deep dyslexia (of which seven have been reported) reading of the ideographic script *kanji* is much better than reading of the syllabic script *kana*; indeed, the reading of *kana* may be entirely abolished (Sasanuma, 1980).

8. Writing, spontaneously or from dictation, is severely impaired.

9. Auditory-verbal short-term memory is impaired.

It was claimed by Coltheart (1980b) that these are the essential characteristics of deep dyslexia in the sense that, if the first symptom is seen in an acquired dyslexic, then every one of the remaining eight symptoms will also be seen.

Deep Dyslexia as Right Hemisphere Reading

It has been proposed (Coltheart, 1980a) that deep dyslexia arises when a left hemisphere lesion prevents access to the left hemisphere linguistic system from printed representations. If this is so, lexical access from print must be achieved by using a right hemisphere lexicon. The input side of reading, therefore, depends (in deep dyslexia) upon the use of the right hemisphere.

What of the ouput side? For example, when words are read aloud by a deep dyslexic, which hemisphere produces the spoken response? It was assumed (Coltheart, 1980a, p.351) that spoken responses are produced from the left hemisphere. It was pointed out, however, that the view that deep dyslexia represents right hemisphere reading is not committed to the assumption that spoken responses are produced by the left hemisphere, and that if one assumed instead that spoken output in deep dyslexia arises from the right hemisphere, this would entail only the modification, not the abandonment, of a right hemisphere interpretation of deep dyslexic reading.

One can attempt to establish *prima facie* plausibility for the right hemisphere hypothesis by attempting to demonstrate parallels between the reading abilities of the right hemisphere (as inferred from, for example, visual hemifield experiments with normal readers) and the reading abilities of the deep dyslexic;

and Coltheart (1980a) proposed that several such parallels exist, some of which will now be discussed.

Derivation of Phonology from Print

Evidence from Klatzky and Atkinson (1971), Moscovitch (1976) and Cohen and Freeman (1979) indicates that in reading tasks which involve the derivation of phonology from print the right hemisphere makes no contribution when normal readers are studied, and this is consistent with the view that, even if the right hemisphere can perform certain kinds of reading tasks, the derivation of phonology from print is not one of these. The split-brain studies of Levy and Trevarthen (1977) and of Zaidel (1978) suggest somewhat more directly that print-to-phonology conversion is not possible for the right hemisphere.

More recently, Zaidel and Peters (1981) have studied the phonological capabilities of two split-brain patients, N.G. and L.B. The disconnected right hemisphere of N.G. could not match pictures on the basis of homophony or rhyme, nor match a word to a picture on the basis of rhyme, nor match printed words or non-words on the basis of rhyme. The same pattern of results was produced by the disconnected right hemisphere of L.B., except that matching pictures by rhyme or homophony yielded above-chance performance by the right hemisphere. These phonological tasks could all be performed easily by the left hemispheres of these patients; and semantic tasks such as picture-word matching can be performed by their right hemispheres (although not very well in the case of N.G.). On the basis of these results, Zaidel and Peters (1981) concluded that

> the ideographic, nonphonetic reading of the disconnected right hemisphere is reminiscent of so-called acquired phonemic, deep or literal alexia, where patients suffering from left hemisphere lesions apparently lack phonetic encoding and can consequently access meaning in the lexicon directly.

Semantic Errors

The results of Gott (1973) might be taken as indicating that a propensity to make semantic errors is an intrinsic characteristic of a right hemisphere reading system. Gott investigated the reading abilities of a girl whose left hemisphere had been removed at the age of ten. This patient's reading, which pre-operatively was poor, was not completely abolished by the hemispherectomy. When she was given 20 short words to read, she attempted nine: five responses were correct and the rest were semantic errors such as *book* → 'poem'. The relevance of such results to a discussion of the properties of the right hemisphere in people whose brain was normal until maturity is often challenged on the ground that the juvenile brain is plastic, so that the right hemisphere can take over linguistic functions when there is damage to the left hemisphere in childhood, but can do so much less or not at all when the damage occurs after the brain has matured. A close examination of the evidence adduced to supported this view reveals that it is not strong (St. James-Roberts, 1981), and it can be argued that the juvenile brain is in fact no more plastic than the adult brain. If so, then there is no reason for dismissing Gott's patient as being irrelevant for explanations of the behaviour of patients whose brain damage occurred in adulthood. It follows that the semantic errors made by Gott's patient in reading aloud provide at least some reason for believing that, if damage to the left hemisphere in adulthood forces a patient to read via the right hemisphere, semantic errors will occur.

Additional evidence for a propensity of the right hemisphere to make semantic errors in reading is provided by Zaidel (1982). His subjects were two split-brain patients, N. G. and L. B., and he carried out various tests of the ability of their right hemispheres to choose, from a set of written words, that which matched a picture or spoken word. The written distractors in the recognition test included items semantically similar, visually similar, or auditorily similar to the target item. When the words were presented to the right hemisphere, the patients sometimes chose the semantically similar distractors. In a similar picture–word matching task, at least one deep dyslexic has been shown to make semantic errors in his choice of a picture to match the printed word (Newcombe and Marshall, 1980). If the tests used with N.G. and L.B. by Zaidel were to be carried out also with some deep dyslexic patients, the results would permit a direct comparison between deep dyslexic reading and right hemisphere reading.

The results of Zaidel and Peters (1981) and Zaidel (1982), in connection with their phonological and semantic-error tests of the disconnected right hemisphere, led them to argue that

> the present findings suggest that [deep dyslexics] may use their intact right hemispheres for ideographic reading (Zaidel and Peters, 1981)

and that

> the right hemisphere is particularly likely to support reading in cases of acquired deep dyslexia (Zaidel, 1982)

Visual Hemifield Differences in Deep Dyslexic Reading

The view that deep dyslexics read with the right hemisphere

> predicts that [deep dyslexics] with good visual fields will show a left visual half-field advantage in recognizing words flashed on the left or right of a central fixation point. (Zaidel and Peters, 1981, p.231)

This prediction was investigated by Saffran *et al.* (1980) with three deep dyslexics who, according to standard perimetry, were free of visual field defects. Two of these patients consistently showed a left visual half-field advantage for lexical decision: the third showed this effect when there was bilateral stimulus presentation. These results were obtained after exposure durations had been adjusted, independently for the two visual half-fields if necessary, until performance was equal in the two half-fields on elementary letter-recognition tasks such as deciding whether all four letters in a row presented to one half-field or the other were identical. Equivalence of the two half-fields on this task rules out explanations of the left half-field lexical decision superiority in terms of elementary visual-field defects or unilateral neglect undetected by perimetry. Thus these results provide reasonable confirmation of the prediction that there should be left visual half-field advantages in tachistoscopic reading by deep dyslexics, and hence provide support for the right hemisphere hypothesis.

Kanji and Kana: Visual Hemifield Differences

Studies reviewed by Coltheart (1980a) report that, with lateralised presentation of single *kanji* or *kana* stimuli to Japanese subjects, a left visual field advantage occurs for the ideographic script *kanji* and a right visual field advantage occurs for the syllabic script *kana* (Hatta, 1977a, 1977b, 1978; Hirata and Osaka, 1967; Sasanuma *et al.*, 1977: in this paper the left-visual-field advantage for *kanji* was not significant). A left visual field advantage for tachistoscopic recognition of single Chinese characters was reported by Tzeng *et al.* (1978). When multiple *kanji* or Chinese characters are used as stimuli, a right visual field advantage has been reported (Hatta, 1978; Tzeng *et al.*, 1978).

Since the review of this work by Coltheart (1980a), a considerable amount of further work on visual hemifield differences for *kanji*, *kana* and Chinese ideographs has appeared. With *kana* stimuli, Shimuzu and Endo (1981) found a RVF superiority in classifying disyllabic non-words. Hatta (1981) presented colour names written in *kana* or *kanji* and coloured either congruently or incongruently, and asked subjects to classify the colour of the stimulus by a button press response. With *kanji* stimuli, Stroop effects were much larger in the LVF than in the RVF. With *kana* stimuli, the two visual hemifields yielded equivalent Stroop effects (a result which, as Hatta observes, conflicts with what one would expect from the remaining literature on tachistoscopic reading of *kana*). Sasanuma *et al.* (1980) found that, when subjects were required to perform a phonological task (deciding whether a pair of *kana* characters rhymed, or whether a pair of *kanji* characters was homophonous), both forms of script yielded a RVF advantage. When a visual task was performed (are these two characters visually identical?), neither script showed any visual hemifield difference.

Elman *et al.* (1981a) asked subjects to classify *kanji* words as nouns or as non-nouns (adjectives or verbs). With *kanji* nouns, reaction time was shorter with LVF presentation; with adjectives or verbs, the two visual hemifields yielded equivalent mean reaction times. As the authors note, the interaction between visual hemifield and word type might not be a syntactic effect: since the nouns were more concrete than the verbs and adjectives, the interaction may really be between concreteness and visual hemifield. Investigations of this interaction between concreteness and visual hemifield will be discussed later in this chapter. Elman *et al.* (1981b) investigated naming latency for concrete and abstract *kanji* nouns: for abstract nouns, latencies were shorter with RVF presentation, whilst with concrete nouns latencies did not differ between the visual hemifields. Besner *et al.* (1982) investigated the verbal report of the numbers 4 through 9 written as *kanji* and presented tachistoscopically followed by a mask: their Japanese subjects showed better performance in the RVF.

With Chinese subjects, and Chinese characters as stimuli, Besner *et al.* (1982) obtained an RVF superiority for tachistoscopic report of numbers; Huang and Jones (1980) found no naming latency differences between the two visual hemifields; and Nguy *et al.* (1980) found that, with verbal report of tachistoscopically presented characters, there was RVF superiority except for those characters they considered to be pictographic, which yielded equivalent performance in the two visual hemifields; as they acknowledge, the characters they classified as pictographic were also much more concrete, so the interaction they observed may have been due to concreteness, not the nature of a character *per se*.

These investigations are relevant to deep dyslexia, and to its interpretation in terms of right hemisphere reading, because of the relative sparing of *kanji* reading in Japanese cases of deep dyslexia. For example, in the case reported by Sasanuma (1980) reading aloud and comprehension of *kana* was impossible, whilst reading aloud and comprehension of *kanji* was fair. In terms of the right hemisphere account of deep dyslexia, this pattern of results could be explained if the right hemisphere is much better at reading *kanji* (and presumably Chinese ideographs) than at reading *kana*. The tachistoscopic studies reviewed by Coltheart (1980a) provided some evidence that this is so, and the subsequent studies have by and large provided further evidence for a right hemisphere competence at the reading of ideographs, at least when these represent concrete words. The only evidence which conflicts with this is the finding by Besner *et al.* (1982) of an RVF superiority for ideographically written numbers (numbers cannot be considered to be abstract, since they receive relatively high ratings in rating studies of imageability or concreteness). However, since this finding does not necessarily mean that the right hemisphere cannot read ideographic numbers — the finding implies only that the left hemisphere is better than the right with this kind of stimulus material — there is no direct challenge to the right hemisphere account of deep dyslexia.

It is sometimes proposed that LVF advantages for the reading of ideographs arise, not because of the necessity of reading via ideographic mechanisms, but because most ideographs are visually complex and the right hemisphere is specialised for the processing of visually complex material. Besner *et al.* (1982), pointing out that the ideographic representations of the number 4 through 9 are visually much simpler than most Chinese or Japanese ideographs, suggest it is because of the visual simplicity of their stimuli that a LVF superiority was not evident in their results. Taking this view, one might expect an LVF advantage to occur in visual matching of complex ideographs, but Sasanuma *et al.* (1980) found that the two visual hemifields did not differ in the accuracy with which visual matching of kanji characters was performed. Furthermore, if the LVF advantage for *kanji* is a purely perceptual effect, it is not clear why it should be larger for concrete than for abstract *kanji* (if indeed this can be conclusively demonstrated).

A body of literature which is now quite substantial thus provides considerable evidence that, in normal readers of Japanese or Chinese, the right hemisphere is competent at reading ideographic characters. From this it would follow that a dyslexic reader of Japanese who was relying upon the right hemisphere would be better at reading *kanji* than *kana*, and hence that the right hemisphere account of deep dyslexia would predict relative sparing of *kanji* reading in Japanese deep dyslexia, as is observed. However, the observation of LVF superiorities in the *kanji* reading of normal subjects does not imply that the left hemisphere is not competent at reading *kanji*; it merely implies that the right hemisphere is superior. Hence one cannot infer from these studies that the right hemisphere actually plays a part in the *normal* reading of Japanese (especially since tachistoscopic studies of the reading of two-character *kanji* stimuli produce RVF superiorities: *see* Hatta, 1978; Elman *et al.*, 1981b).

There is something puzzling about the existence (Sasanuma, 1980) of partial preservation of *kanji* reading accompanied by abolition of *kana* reading. Even if it is the case in normal reading that *kanji* is read ideographically whilst *kana* is read via phonological recoding using the syllable as a unit, why should it be that, if brain damage abolishes the ability to perform phonological recoding, the Japanese dyslexic cannot then read *kana* words by treating them as ideographs? A possible answer is that, even if one is careful to control for word type by presenting the *same words* in the two script forms when carrying out investigations of dyslexic readings, the *kana* form of any word which possesses a *kanji* form will be much less familiar than the *kanji* form (because, of course, the word is normally written in *kanji* and not in *kana*). In these circumstances, the poor performance with *kana* may be an effect of visual unfamiliarity, not script type. This cannot be the correct explanation of Sasanuma's results, however, because the *kana* nouns she used with her deep dyslexic subjects were nouns which *are* normally written in *kana*.

If *kana* reading is entirely abolished in deep dyslexia, this may be because the script is syllabic in nature and is read via intermediate phonological recoding. It is therefore of interest to attempt to discover whether other kinds of syllabic script suffer so severely in deep dyslexia. One widely used syllabic script is Devanagari (used to write several Indian languages, including Nepalese). In an investigation of a Nepalese-English bilingual, biscriptal deep dyslexic, Coltheart *et al.* (in prep.) found that reading comprehension, although impaired, was no worse for Nepalese words than words in the Roman alphabet. It is therefore not true in general that the reading of syllabic scripts is abolished in deep dyslexia: in fact, this may only be true for Japanese.

Imageability/Concreteness

A number of studies reviewed by Coltheart (1980a) investigated differences between the two visual hemifields in the reading of abstract versus concrete words. In several of these studies (Ellis and Shepherd, 1974; Hines, 1976, 1977; Day, 1977; Tzeng *et al.*, 1979; Bradshaw and Gates, 1978), the RVF advantage was larger for abstract words than for concrete words, implying a right hemisphere contribution to the reading of concrete words. In some studies, however, (Hatta, 1977b; Saffran *et al.*, 1980) this result was not obtained; the RVF advantage was equally large for concrete and for abstract words.

More recent work has not, unfortunately, clarified these discrepancies. Some of this work is perhaps less than satisfactory. For example, in the lexical decision study by Shanon (1979) error rates ranged from 32% to 43% (where 50% would be chance), and there were only eight words presented per hemifield/word-type combination. The very small number of correct responses per condition would make this an extremely insensitive experiment (the interaction between visual hemifield and concreteness was not significant). In the study by Bradshaw *et al.* (1981) abstractness/concreteness was blocked, and subjects were informed in advance as to the nature of the block of words they were about to see. In view of suggestions that the hemispheres might differ in their ability to use expectancies (Cohen, 1975), it is unclear what effects should be predicted here. An added complication in this experiment is that concreteness was deliberately confounded with word frequency: the concrete words were all of high frequency, and the abstract words all of low frequency.

Recent studies in which it was found that the RVF superiority was smaller for concrete than for abstract words include those of Elman *et al.* (1981b) using *kanji*, Nguy *et al.* (1980) using Chinese characters, and Day (1979) using English words. In Day's study, the visual field/concreteness interaction was significant for nouns and for adjectives, but not significant for verbs (although for both reaction times and error rates the RVF superiority was smaller for concrete than for abstract words). Graves *et al.* (1981) investigated lexical decision for emotional and non-emotional words presented to one visual field or the other. Since emotionality is presumably correlated with imageability, which is in turn correlated with concreteness, it is to be expected that their emotional words would have been more concrete than their non-emotional words, and indeed for male subjects the RVF advantage was smaller for emotional than non-emotional words; but for female subjects there was no significant interaction between visual hemifield and emotionality. Visual hemifield effects were generally smaller for females than for males, and a substantial number of female subjects showed LVF advantages, a result observed in some other visual hemifield experiments (e.g. Day, 1977; Bradshaw and Gates, 1978).

The words used in the experiment by Graves *et al.* (1981) were given to 22 aphasics to read. Across words, the correlation beteen percent correct reading by the aphasics and percent correct performance in the LVF by normals was +0·56 ($P < 0.003$). In contrast, the correlation between aphasic reading and percent correct performance in the RVF by normals was -0·05 (n.s.), leading Graves *et al.* to conclude:

> whatever processing allows the aphasics to succeed with some words and not others
> also operates on the LVF for normal males . . . it seems likely that this processing
> involves the right hemisphere.

Unfortunately, the authors provide no information about the nature of the dyslexic reading exhibited by the 22 aphasic patients. Their results would count as evidence for the right hemisphere account of deep dyslexia only if the significant correlation they observed arose because of the presence in their aphasic group of a sufficient number of deep dyslexics.

In most of the studies reviewed here, then, it is found that the RVF superiority observed with abstract words is reduced, often eliminated, when concrete words are used. Failures to obtain this interaction, however, have occurred, but at least some of these failures may be due to the use of insensitive methods. It remains reasonable, then, to believe that the right hemisphere can be shown to be superior at dealing with concrete words than at dealing with abstract words. This conclusion allows one to interpret the beneficial effect of concreteness on deep-dyslexic reading within the context of the right-hemisphere account of deep dyslexia.

Two Difficulties for the Right Hemisphere
Account of Deep Dyslexia

Much of the evidence assembled earlier (Coltheart, 1980a) to establish a *prima facie* case for the view that deep dyslexia reflects right hemisphere reading has retained its validity in relation to subsequent experimental results. It is still possible to claim that, independently of studies of deep dyslexia, there is evidence to indicate that the right hemisphere is better at reading concrete than abstract words, is better at reading single *kanji* than *kana*, is prone to semantic error, and cannot derive phonology from print whilst sometimes being able to derive semantics from print. Since these four properties of the right hemisphere are also properties of deep dyslexic reading, a case is made that deep dyslexic reading is right hemisphere reading.

There have been two recent challenges, however, to this account of deep dyslexia. These have emerged from studies of other forms of acquired dyslexia — one from a study of letter-by-letter reading or 'pure alexia' (Patterson and Kay, 1982) and the other from a study of concrete-word dyslexia (Warrington, 1981).

In cases of letter-by-letter reading, the right hemisphere is usually undamaged: this was so for all four cases studied by Patterson and Kay (1982). Consequently, these letter-by-letter readers should have available to them the right hemisphere reading system, and hence should be able, as deep dyslexics are, to comprehend promptly at least some words which they cannot read aloud promptly. Patterson and Kay therefore investigated single-word reading comprehension in their four letter-by-letter readers. Despite the fact that pure alexia was one of the first varieties of acquired dyslexia to be identified, no adequate study of reading comprehension in pure alexia had been carried out until the work of Patterson and Kay. They found that their letter-by-letter readers could not comprehend words until they were able to read them aloud, and so:

> We therefore challenge theorists who maintain that the normal right hemisphere can support rapid comprehension of written words to explain why many letter-by-letter readers fail to demonstrate this ability. (Patterson and Kay, 1982)

In the syndrome of concrete-word dyslexia described by Warrington (1981), the patient is better at reading abstract words than concrete words. In relation to deep dyslexia, an effect of concreteness on reading is explained by assuming that the left hemisphere can read both concrete and abstract words, whilst the right hemisphere can read only concrete words. If this is how the brain is organised, then clearly a large enough lesion in the left hemisphere could produce a dyslexic who could read concrete words better than abstract words; but what kind of lesion could produce a patient who could read abstract words better than concrete words? Thus, as Warrington (1981, p.184) points out,

> This concrete word dyslexic syndrome poses considerable problems for the hypothesis that there is a right hemisphere lexicon which can subserve concrete word reading.

Anyone who still wishes to entertain the right hemisphere hypothesis concerning deep dyslexia must attempt to meet these two challenges. Hence the work of Patterson and Kay and of Warrington will be described in more detail, and the possibilities for reconciliation of their results with the right hemisphere hypothesis will be discussed.

Concrete-Word Dyslexia

This disorder has been described for one patient, C.A.V., (Warrington, 1981), and, as Warrington notes, it is important to keep in mind the chronology of this patient's testing, since all testing was carried out over a brief period, during which his cognitive functions steadily improved. He was admitted to hospital on 21st October, 1978 for investigation of severe headaches, right hemianopia, right sensory loss and mild right hemiparesis. A necrotic glioma of the left posterior hemisphere was diagnosed, and confirmed by biopsy on 27 October. His reading and other cognitive abilities were tested over a period from 5 days after onset of his symptoms to 20 days after onset (i.e. from 26 October to 10 November). During this period his reading improved considerably. The patient's condition deteriorated rapidly from 10 November onwards, and he died on 25 November, 1978.

Apart from his dyslexia, to be discussed shortly, the patient exhibited the following symptoms:

1. Some nominal dysphasia, indicated by word-finding difficulties in otherwise fluent speech, by impaired ability to name from description, and by impaired picture naming. This nominal dysphasia improved hardly at all over the period 31 October to 10 November.

2. Visual object agnosia, as indicated on 31 October by inability to match two visual objects in terms of their functions, with preserved ability to match usual with unusual views of objects. This agnosia is reported to have resolved, though no test results relevant to this are reported.

3. Poor recognition memory both for words and for faces, at an early stage of testing.

4. Marked dysgraphia at an early stage of testing.

5. Some impairment of speech comprehension. On 31 October, when he failed at a test involving matching objects by their function, he achieved a mental age score of 11:9 on the Peabody Picture Vocabulary Test (involving matching of single spoken words to one of four pictures). Matching of printed words to pictures was worse than matching spoken words to pictures on this occasion.

Two days later, his ability to match spoken words to pictures was normal for abstract words but poorer than normal for concrete or emotional words.

The most important aspect of the patient's dyslexia for our present purposes was, of course, the finding that his reading was poorer with concrete words than with abstract words. He was tested on four occasions with a set of 36 concrete words and 36 abstract words. His reading aloud of the concrete words improved steadily from 5/36 (2nd November) to 26/36 (10 November). Reading aloud of the abstract words improved from 15/36 (2nd November) to 29/36 (10 November). Thus the advantage for abstract words, initially marked, was virtually absent by 10 November — and, indeed, since nominal dysphasia was still evident on 9 November (e.g. naming objects from description 60% correct, picture naming 48% correct) all 17 failures to read aloud on 10 November may have been naming difficulties rather than failures of word recognition or comprehension. Indeed, on 9 November the patient was somewhat better at reading picture names (65%) than at naming the corresponding pictures (48%):

This patient's dyslexia was not, however, solely an output difficulty, at least not in its early stages, because on 1 November his matching of printed words to pictures, for those words which he could not read aloud, was at chance; on 31 October picture-word matching was worse with printed words than spoken words; and lexical decision with printed words was at chance. Nearly all of his 260 errors in reading aloud were either visual errors (29·2%) or failures to respond (54·2%).

When 80 words of four syntactic categories were presented for reading aloud on 6 November, no effect of part-of-speech was evident (nouns 10/20, verbs 8/20, adjectives 8/20, function words 9/20). However, since concreteness was not controlled here, and since there is a correlation between concreteness and part of speech (Shallice and Warrington, 1975), and since on the same day a large effect of concreteness on ability to read aloud was observed (concrete words 9/36, abstract words 25/36), it is difficult to interpret the part-of-speech data.

As indicated above, the existence of a patient with an intact right hemisphere whose reading of concrete words is *inferior* to his reading of abstract words conflicts with the view that there is a right hemisphere sysem capable of reading concrete words, a view that is the basis of the right hemisphere account of deep dyslexia.

A defender of the view that the right hemisphere is capable of supporting the reading of concrete words might wish to reconcile this view with the existence of concrete-word dyslexia by proposing that, after left hemisphere damage, the right hemisphere takes some time to display whatever linguistic abilities it has — a time measurable in months or years. This proposal might be supported by pointing out that the role of the right hemisphere in partial recovery of language after left hemisphere damage has been inferred from:

1. the effect on language of subsequent *right* hemisphere damage (Nielsen, 1965; Heilman *et al.*, 1979);

2. the effects of right-sided intracarotid injection of sodium amytal (Kinsbourne, 1971; Czopf, 1979);

3. the development of a left-ear superiority in dichotic listening (Pettit and Noll, 1979); and

4. the occurrence of attenuation of click-evoked potentials in the *right* hemisphere of aphasics performing a verbal encoding task (and in the left hemisphere of controls and non-aphasic patients) (Papanicolaou *et al.*, unpub.).

In all of these cases, the slow recovery of some language, inferred to be due to the right hemisphere, occupied a period of several months. Hence one might argue that C.A.V.'s failure to display the putative reading capacity of the right hemisphere was due to the fact that his reading disorder had largely resolved 3 weeks after the onset of his left hemisphere damage and that in any case investigations of his reading were confined to the 3 weeks immediately following this damage. In direct contrast, there have been no reports of the existence of deep dyslexic reading in the first few months following left hemisphre damage. The deep dyslexic described by Low (1931) may have exhibited deep dyslexic symptoms about 4 months after his left hemisphere damage; in all other published studies of deep dyslexia, the interval between the occurence of left hemisphere damage and the first observations of deep dyslexic symptoms has been at least a year. I do not mean to claim here that there is any evidence to show that deep dyslexia is never evident very soon after left hemisphere damage. I mean instead simply to point out that the absence of any evidence that deep dyslexia can exist shortly after left hemisphere damage allows one to attempt to explain away the apparent absence of right hemisphere reading in C.A.V.

I believe that this line of argument is generally compatible with many ideas about right hemisphere language and its emergence after the onset of aphasia. Nevertheless, as an attempt to reconcile the case of C.A.V. with the view that the right hemisphere has some ability to read, I cannot see that the argument can succeed. The obstacle to its success is that part of the basis for the view that the right hemisphere possesses some ability to read is that, with normal subjects, the results of tachistoscopic studies may be taken as evidence for some right hemisphere contribution to the reading of concrete nouns. Here the right hemisphere is considered to be displaying some linguistic capabilities which are manifested in the reader's behaviour: yet the reader, instead of having had left hemisphere damage months before, has an *intact* left hemisphere. If these intact readers can read concrete nouns with their right hemispheres, why could not C.A.V. do this *immediately* after the occurrence of damage to his left hemisphere?

Exactly the same objection can be made to a rather different attempt to reconcile concrete word dyslexia with the possibility of right hemisphere reading. It might be argued that the right hemisphere possesses some ability to read, but that this is usually suppressed or inhibited by the left hemisphere: this is a familiar account of relationships between the two hemispheres, and is discussed in Searleman's chapter in this volume. On this view, right hemisphere language can be displayed in behaviour only when there is very extensive damage to the left hemisphere, damage sufficiently extensive to abolish the inhibitory capabilities of this hemisphere. One can apply this idea to C.A.V. and deep dyslexia simply by arguing that C.A.V.'s left hemisphere damage was much less extensive than the left hemisphere damage suffered by deep dyslexics (and there is good evidence to support this view of the relative sizes of the lesions: compare Fig. 1 of Warrington, 1981, with Appendix 1 of Coltheart *et al.*, 1980). Thus C.A.V.'s left hemisphere was still suppressing his right, whereas this suppression is abolished in deep dyslexia. If, however, an intact or fairly mildly damaged left hemisphere is believed to prevent the right hemisphere from exerting its capacity to read, it cannot be argued that in normal readers the right hemisphere contributes to the reading of tachistoscopically displayed concrete nouns.

As far as I can see, then, neither of these two attempts to reconcile concrete word dyslexia with the existence of a right hemisphere reading capability (one attempt based on the idea that it requires time after damage for this capacity to be displayed, the other on the idea that it requires sufficiently extensive damage to the inhibitory left hemisphere) can be entertained if one still wishes to use data from tachistocopic studies of normal readers as part of the evidence for the existence of a right hemisphere reading system.

Without wishing to minimise this difficulty, a major one, it is worth pointing out some ways in which the data obtained from C.A.V. are not entirely clear.

Firstly, it is difficult to understand why C.A.V. was not worse at reading nouns (10/20) than function words (9/20), since these nouns were very concrete and the function words were abstract.

More generally, if a patient is believed to exhibit a dyslexia in which there is an inverse relationship between concreteness and probability of correct reading, one would expect that percent correct reading would be lower for concrete words (defined, let us say, as words whose concreteness rating is above the median value for concreteness) than for abstract words (those with concreteness values below the median value). Exactly this is shown for C.A.V. by Table 3 of Warrington (1981). A set of 456 words were drawn from the 650 words of the norms of Brown and Ure (1969) and administered to C.A.V., who read correctly 125 of the 228 words with below-median concreteness and only 81 of the 228 words with above-median concreteness. This difference (54·8% correct versus 35·5% correct) is highly significant ($\chi^2_{(1)} = 17\cdot2, P < 0\cdot001$).

A more detailed analysis of the relationship of concreteness to percent correct, however, could be made by treating concreteness as a somewhat more continuous variable, rather than a dichotomy: for example, by using deciles, to divide concreteness into ten levels rather than just two. For each decile, one can compute percent correct reading responses. Thus, for example, from the set of 456 words given to C.A.V., the 45 or 46 words with the lowest concreteness values would be the words in the first decile, and the percentage of these words read correctly would be the first of 10 points in a plot of percent correct against concreteness. One would expect percentage correct to decline as concreteness increased across the ten concreteness levels.

The result of this analysis for C.A.V.'s reading of the 456 words from the Brown and Ure norms are shown in Fig. 1. It is clear that percent correct does

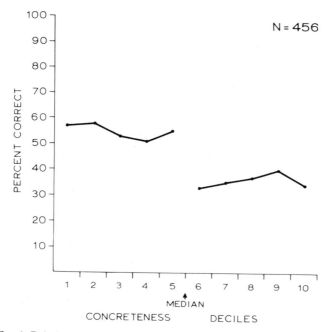

FIG. 1. Relation of concreteness of words to C.A.V.'s ability to read them.

not decline monotonically as concreteness increases. Across the five concreteness levels *below* the median, percent correct does not vary as concreteness increases ($\chi^2_{(4)} = 0.60$, $P > 0.95$); nor does percent correct vary with concreteness across the five levels of concreteness *above* the median ($\chi^2_{(4)} = 0.32$, $P > 0.975$).

An alternative way of investigating this point is to compare the mean concreteness of those words which are read correctly to the mean concreteness of those words which are read wrongly. What one would expect, if there is an inverse relationship between concreteness and probability of correct reading, is that correctly read words will have a lower mean concreteness than wrongly read words. This effect is not shown by C.A.V., at least not when one considers separately abstract words (lower than median concreteness) and concrete words (above median concreteness). One can make the comparison between the concreteness of correctly read words and the concreteness of wrongly read words for 11 sets of words administered to C.A.V., ignoring the testing session whose data are presented in Fig. 1, and the results of these comparisons are shown in Table 1. It is clear that correctly read words show no tendency to be less concrete than wrongly read words in these comparisons.

TABLE 1

Mean Brown-Ure concreteness values (first eight rows) or imageability values (last three rows) of words correctly read and of words wrongly read by C.A.V. Some of the words from Appendices IV and V were not present in the imageability norms (Coltheart, 1981b) and so do not figure in these calculations.

Source	Correct	Wrong	Difference
Appendix II, Concrete words:			
1st presentation	602	620	-18
2nd presentation	634	612	+22
3rd presentation	611	620	-9
4th presentation	619	613	+6
Appendix II, Abstract words:			
1st presentation	332	361	-29
2nd presentation	347	354	-7
3rd presentation	358	331	+27
4th presentation	348	361	-13
Appendix IV (N = 66)	452	446	+6
Appendix V, Set A (N = 35)	600	584	+16
Appendix V, Set B (N = 17)	588	566	+22
MEANS	499	497	+2

These two analyses indicate that it is far from obvious that one can claim that the more concrete a word was the less likely it was that C.A.V. could read it correctly. If one considers separately words above and below the median in concreteness, there is no evidence that concreteness had any influence at all on C.A.V.'s reading. On the other hand, percent correct oral reading was significantly lower for concrete than for abstract words. Given the conflicting

results of the various analyses which may be performed upon the data yielded by
C.A.V., it seems fair to conclude that a clearer demonstration of concrete-word
dyslexia is needed before one need regard the existence of this disorder as a
decisive refutation of the view that the right hemisphere possesses some reading
capability.

Letter-by-Letter Reading

A variety of terms has been used to describe what appears to be a single
syndrome: pure alexia, alexia without agraphia, word-blindness, word-form
dyslexia, verbal alexia, spelling dyslexia and letter-by-letter reading. The first
two terms emphasise the fact that in this syndrome writing and spelling can be
intact whilst reading is severely disordered. The other three terms emphasise
that, when a word cannot be read normally, it is usually identified by a slow
serial identification of its individual letters.

The major features of letter-by-letter reading, as described by Patterson and
Kay (1982), are as follows:

1. In tests of reading aloud of single words, those words which cannot be read
promptly are identified via a process of identifying the individual letters of the
word: this usually takes the form of naming these letters aloud from left to right.
On such occasions, word-reading latency is very long, and is monotonically
related to the number of letters in the word.

2. The naming of individual letters is imperfect in most patients, though not all.

3. Writing to dictation, writing spontaneously, spelling, and the identification of
words which are spelled aloud to the patient may all be intact.

4. A right homonymous hemianopia is almost always present.

5. Speech production and comprehension can be intact.

6. Copying of letters is slow and 'slavish': that is, letters may be copied as if they
were entirely novel visual stimuli. Copying may lead to correct identification of a
letter, and indeed many letter-by-letter readers trace letters with their fingers in
order to identify them.

Under certain conditions—for example, with long words, or with tachistoscopic presentation—the oral reading performance of the letter-by-letter reader
is very much worse than that of the deep dyslexic. Since the letter-by-letter
reader has an intact right hemisphere, why can he not read at least as well as the
deep dyslexic? In considering this point, Coltheart (1980a, p.329) noted that
studies of reading comprehension in letter-by-letter reading had been

perfunctory, and that there were hints from such studies of some comprehension of words which could not be read aloud. Subsequently a rigorous study of reading comprehension in letter-by-letter reading has been carried out by Patterson and Kay (1982). In one task, the patient is shown single words and asked to make an *immediate* spoken semantic judgement about the word (e.g. does it refer to something animate or inanimate?). After this judgement, the patient attempts to read the word aloud. Occasions on which the word is read aloud promptly are not relevant here. The crucial question is: for those words which are not read promptly and which have to be identified letter-by-letter, does the prior semantic judgement reveal any evidence of comprehension? The answer was no; this indicates that in letter-by-letter reading a word cannot be comprehended until after it has been identified. This is in marked contrast to deep dyslexia, where it is common for printed words which are not read aloud correctly to be comprehended. It is this contrast which presents problems for the right hemisphere hypothesis: if the right hemisphere possesses the ability to understand at least some printed words, the letter-by-letter reader should be able to use this ability to make above-chance semantic judgements concerning those words which cannot immediately be read aloud via the left hemisphere. Why does this not happen?

Letter-by-letter readers generally have relatively mild damage to the left hemisphere, and are as a rule only mildly aphasic, sometimes not aphasic at all. If the left hemisphere suppresses right hemisphere linguistic potentialities except when there is very extensive left hemisphere damage, one might offer an explanation of the letter-by-letter reader's behaviour in terms of suppression of the right hemisphere; but, as was discussed in connection with concrete-word dyslexia, this kind of explanation cannot be offered if one at the same time wishes to argue that normal readers (in whom this suppression, of course, ought to be at its strongest) exhibit evidence of right hemisphere contributions to the reading of concrete words.

It is necessary to look elsewhere, therefore, for possible ways to resolve this issue. Consider the nature of the interhemispheric transfer of information required if LVF stimuli are to gain access to the left hemisphere. Let us distinguish between *uncategorised* and *categorised* transfer. I use the term 'uncategorised transfer' to refer to cases where no use has been made of any putative capabilities of the right hemisphere at identifying visual stimuli. The visual input is simply relayed from right hemisphere to left as if it were entirely unfamiliar to the right hemisphere. It must be possible for uncategorised transfer to occur, of course, since stimuli which *are* uncategorised by the right hemisphere (for example, words written in completely unfamiliar scripts) can be described even when they are presented briefly to the LVF.

If the right hemisphere is capable of categorising at least some classes of visual input (for example, is capable of recognising concrete words), then it will be possible for interhemispheric transfer of the *results* of such categorisation to occur. Here the left hemisphere does not receive a comparatively raw and unprocessed representation of the stimulus which needs to be submitted to left hemisphere categorising systems. It receives an already categorised representation of the stimulus. This I refer to as *categorised* transfer.

When the visual stimulus in the LVF is a letter string, more than one form of categorical information is possible. The stimulus might be represented as a set of abstract letter identities (orthographic categorisation) or as a meaning (semantic categorisation). I assume, on the basis of evidence discussed earlier, that phonological categorisation is not possible in the right hemisphere. I assume also that in the right hemisphere semantic categorisation is possible for concrete words to a far greater extent than it is possible for abstract words.

I will also make the assumption that responses to printed words in the LVF are made by the left hemisphere even when the responses are non-verbal — even, indeed, when they are made by the left hand. Specifically, it is assumed that when a printed stimulus is categorised by the right hemisphere, the results of this categorisation are interrogated by the left hemisphere in order for the subject to decide what response should be made (for example, to decide whether or not the semantic representation of the stimulus contains the semantic feature /+animate/ when the task is to classify printed words according to whether they refer to animate or inanimate objects). The only exception to this principle is the split brain patient, in whom such left hemisphere interrogation of representations attained in the right hemisphere is not possible. Apart from this exception, the assumption being made is that even when stimuli are identified by the right hemisphere and the musculature governing the responses required to the stimuli are controlled by the right hemisphere, the decision as to which response to make is taken by the left hemisphere.

These ideas allow one at least to sketch out an account of normal reading, deep dyslexic reading, and letter-by-letter reading, an account which includes some attempt to explain why no use is made of the right hemisphere reading system by the letter-by-letter reader.

The Normal Reader

The LVF inferiority in performance with abstract words, non-words and *kana* occurs because semantic categorisation in the right hemisphere is not possible for these stimuli. Hence the left hemisphere cannot receive from the right a single representation representing the whole visual stimulus. Instead, it receives a sequence of representations, either orthographically categorised (if the items making up the stimulus are letters and hence can each be categorised by the right hemisphere) or even uncategorised (if, for example, the stimulus is a *kana* word and the right hemisphere cannot even categorise *kana* stimuli). If transfer of a set of representations is either slower, or more error-prone, or both, than transfer of the single semantic representation obtained for concrete words, the (usually) observed interaction between word concreteness and visual hemifield will arise.

The Deep Dyslexic

The right hemisphere account of deep dyslexia stems from the proposal that the left hemisphere reading system is now incapable of identifying words from their orthographic representations. Words must therefore be identified by a right hemisphere system. Identification using uncategorised transfer is not possible, of course, because the left hemisphere no longer possesses the ability to identify a word from its orthographic representation by categorising information received by uncategorised transfer. For the same reason, word identification using orthographic categorisation as the basis of transfer is not possible in the left hemisphere. It is only interhemispheric transfer of the results of right hemisphere *semantic* categorisation that provides the left hemisphere with any information about the nature of the printed stimulus: and, of course, the reliance on right hemisphere sematic categorisation will mean that performance will be much better with concrete words than with abstract words.

The Letter-by-Letter Reader

So far it has been suggested that the normal reader can use both uncategorised and categorised transfer, whilst the deep dyslexic can use only categorised transfer; next it is suggested that the letter-by-letter reader can only use uncategorised transfer, at least on many occasions (those occasions when a word cannot be read promptly). On such occasions, a printed letter string is processed as if it consisted of a sequence of entirely unfamiliar visual stimuli. These stimuli can, of course, be categorised by the right hemisphere, but this is not relevant for the task, since the results of such categorisation cannot be communicated to the left hemisphere. The only interhemispheric communication which is possible is the communication of uncategorised representations. It is assumed that the slow, serial, letter-by-letter quality of the reading in this syndrome is a consequence of the need to rely on interhemispheric transfer of an uncategorised representation of each of the letters in the stimulus.

The reason that interhemispheric transfer is needed in the first place is, of course, that there is a disconnection between input from the RVF and those left hemisphere centres needed for making decisions about letter strings or retrieving their phonological representations. This disconnection is, in most cases, due simply to left occipital damage and a resulting right homonymous hemianopia.

The existence of just this disconnection, however, would not force the letter-by-letter reader to rely solely on *uncategorised* transfer. One needs to assume, then, a second disconnection, which impairs left hemisphere receipt of categorised transfer from the right hemisphere. Although it is tempting to attribute this disconnection, at least in most letter-by-letter readers, to damage to the splenium of the corpus callosum (since such damage is present in most letter-by-letter readers) this line of argument conflicts with observations by Sidtis et al. (1981). Their patient had had a complete surgical section of the splenium: yet it would appear that right-to-left interhemispheric transfer of semantic information was possible, since the patient could provide verbal descriptions appropriate to the meaning of words presented in the LVF, even when he could not identify a word precisely.

Varieties of Developmental Dyslexia

Although the possibility that there are distinguishable varieties of developmental dyslexia has often been mentioned in the past, it is only fairly recently that serious attempts have been made to investigate the characteristics of putative varieties of this disorder. Some of these attempts have been of a neurological or broadly neuropsychological orientation (e.g. Mattis et al., 1975; Petrauskas and Rourke, 1979) and are not useful here since this kind of work does not involve psycholinguistic differentiation between various patterns of reading error. Such differentiation is the *sine qua non* of the approach to *acquired* dyslexia adopted in most of the work referred to in this chapter.

However, there has been one attempt at distinguishing varieties of developmental dyslexia on a psycholinguistic basis—that of Boder (1973). In particular, she distinguishes between *dysphonetic* dyslexia and *dyseidetic* dyslexia.

The child who is a *dysphonetic dyslexic*, as characterised by Boder, exhbits the following symptoms:

1. Semantic errors in reading aloud (examples given by Boder include *laugh* → 'funny', *duck* → 'chicken', *cattle* → 'animals').

2. Visual errors (e.g. an incorrect response sharing only the first and last letters with the stimulus).

3. Non-words cannot be read aloud.

4. Spelling is poor, and spelling errors are usually not even phonologically plausible representations of the correct word.

There is an obvious resemblance between this syndrome and deep dyslexia, and indeed one can argue that dysphonetic dyslexia is the developmental form of deep dyslexia. For this argument to rest on sufficiently secure foundations, one would first of all need to be sure that the semantic errors mentioned by Boder occur in the reading of isolated words. Such errors in the reading of text could simply reflect guessing from context. Boder did not specify what kind of material was being read when semantic errors occurred. What is also needed is much more detailed information about dysphonetic dyslexia, information in the form of extensive single case studies. Boder (1973) did not provide any information of this kind, but it is needed if one is to be confident that a developmental form of deep dyslexia does exist.

The child who is a *dyseidetic* dyslexic, as characterised by Boder, exhibits these symptoms:

1. Words which are irregularly spelled are especially difficult to read, and may be misread in ways suggesting the use of elementary letter-to-sound rules.

2. Irregularly spelled words are also especially likely to be mis-spelled in writing.

3. Spelling errors are frequently phonologically plausible, such as spelling 'listen' as *lisn* or 'business' as *bisnis*.

This form of developmental dyslexia resembles a particular form of acquired dyslexia, namely, surface dyslexia. Detailed single case studies of developmentally dyslexic children exhibiting this form of developmental dyslexia have been carried out (Holmes, unpub.; Coltheart *et al.*, in press) and it now seems quite clear that surface dyslexia exists, in exactly the same form, as an acquired dyslexia and as a developmental dyslexia (Coltheart, 1982).

If it is plausible that in acquired deep dyslexia the reading of the dyslexic depends upon a right hemisphere reading system, and if deep dyslexia exists in a developmental form, then the possibility that *developmental* deep dyslexics rely upon right hemisphere reading obviously deserves consideration. There has been a large amount of work on language lateralisation in dyslexic children. In a brief review of this work, Keefe and Swinney (1978) list a number of studies suggesting that language tends to be lateralised in the right hemisphere in dyslexic children, a number of studies suggesting that in dyslexic chidren there is bilateral representation of language, and a number of studies suggesting that dyslexic children have normal left hemisphere language lateralisation. They suggest that this chaos has resulted from pooling dyslexic children and treating developmental dyslexia as a single, homogeneous condition.

In their two experiments—one involving dichotic listening and the other tachistoscopic report of trigram pairs, with one trigram presented in each visual hemifield—a group of developmentally dyslexic children and a control group were used. In the first experiment, the dyslexics and the normals showed right ear advantages. In the second experiment, the dyslexics and the normals showed RVF advantages. However, when a laterality quotient (LQ) was calculated for each subject, reflecting the magnitude of the right-ear or RVF advantage, the distribution of these quotients was unimodal for normal readers but bimodal for dyslexics, in both experiments. Keefe and Swinney therefore suggested that

> . . . there appear to be at least two categories of dyslexic children with respect to hemispheric lateralisation of linguistic material. One type demonstrates what might be labeled, at least in comparison to the normal controls, a Left-Hemisphere Deficit, and the other demonstrates, again by comparison, a Right-Hemisphere Deficit.

Unfortunately, the evidence for bimodality of the dyslexics' LQs in Keefe and Swinney's experiment does not provide very strong support for this suggestion. Positive LQs in their paper represent left-hemisphere superiority. Now, if their suggestion were correct, one would expect that there would be more dyslexic children than normal children having LQs greater than the modal LQ for normal children: these dyslexics would be the Right Hemisphere Deficit group. One would also expect that there would be more dyslexic children than normal children having LQs *smaller* than the modal LQ for normal children: these dyslexics would be the Left Hemisphere group. This is not the pattern Keefe and Swinney observed. In their *dichotic* study, there was no suggestion of the existence of a subgroup of dyslexics with higher-than-normal LQs. In their *tachistoscopic* study, there was no suggestion of the existence of a sub-group of dyslexics with lower-than-normal LQs. Although both studies yielded bimodal LQ distributions for the dyslexics, then, neither provided evidence supporting Keefe and Swinney's interpretation of this bimodality.

If it really is the case, however, that there is a subset of dyslexic children (the 'Left-Hemisphere Deficit' children) who exhibit LVF and left-ear advantages (or even abnormally small though still positive LQs), and if it is also the case that there is a subset of dyslexic children (the 'dysphonetic dyslexic') who exhibit a form of developmental dyslexia which corresponds to deep dyslexia, then clearly one would like to know whether the two subsets are coextensive. There have been four investigations of this question (Omenn and Weber, 1978; Obrzut, 1979; Dalby and Gibson, 1981; Fried *et al.*, 1981). These four attempts to relate type of developmental dyslexia to lateralisation pattern have yielded inconclusive and inconsistent results. There are hints that the dysphonetic dyslexic child might show greater right hemisphere involvement in language, but these are merely hints, and in any case the results of Obrzut (1979) do not show this pattern. It is unfortunate that none of these studies has attacked the problem in the most direct way, which is to look at visual hemifield differences in dysphonetic and dyseidetic children. There are methodological difficulties for such studies (Young and Ellis, 1981) but these can be avoided (though they rarely are). Furthermore, the methods used to identify dysphonetic dyslexics (the putative 'developmental deep dyslexics') are less than ideal, since they do not require the occurrence of semantic errors in single-word reading as a prerequisite for the diagnosis: this limits the degree to which these investigations are comparable to studies of acquired deep dyslexia. For example, the methods used to identify dysphonetic dyslexics would not distinguish between phonological dyslexia and deep dyslexia if applied to cases of acquired dyslexia. Hence the dysphonetic dyslexics tested in these studies may still be a heterogeneous group.

Until studies meeting these objections are carried out it would seem premature to claim that:

> the pattern of ideographic reading in the disconnected right hemisphere bears resemblance to the reading of the so-called congenital "dysphonetic dyslexics" . . . this group of congenital dyslexics may rely on their right hemisphere for reading. (Zaidel and Peters, 1981)

Concluding Comments

Quotations given at the beginning of this chapter provided illustrations of the popularity of the view than the right hemisphere is capable of displaying considerable linguistic abilities. This view has been taken not only in connection with the perception and production of spoken language, but also in connection with reading. Zaidel and Peters (1981), Zaidel (1982) and Graves *et al.* (1981) are amongst those who have explicitly proposed an explanation of experimental results in terms of right hemisphere reading capacities, and many other recent examples could be cited—for instance, Landis *et al.* (1981) argue, in connection with results obtained with a letter-by-letter reader, that

> . . . it is likely that within the unimpaired right hemisphere the written name was associated with the object image and that this iconic reading strategy enabled him to point correctly to the corresponding object.

The characteristics of deep dyslexic reading have also been interpreted by Coltheart (1980a) and by Saffran *et al.* (1980) as evidence for the existence of some reading ability in the right hemisphere.

The properties of concrete-word dyslexia and of letter-by-letter reading, however, directly challenge the view that the right hemisphere possesses some ability to read. I have attempted to outline some of the ways in which one might attempt to meet these challenges and hence to defend the claim that right hemisphere reading does occur. I would not wish to claim, however, that the attempts to meet these challenges are yet fully satisfactory. One cannot meet the challenge of concrete-word dyslexia by arguments based on the slowness with which right hemisphere reading emerges after left hemisphere damage, nor by arguments based on left hemisphere suppression of right hemisphere language, since both types of argument conflict with the use made of data from normal subjects to provide evidence for right hemisphere reading of concrete words. Analyses of the data provided by Warrington (1981), analyses showing a less than uniform effect of concreteness on reading in concrete-word dyslexia, do not completely meet the challenge posed by this syndrome, since other analyses do show significantly worse performance with concrete than with abstract words.

The challenge of letter-by-letter reading was met by constructing an elaborate argument, *ad hoc* in several places, concerning the nature of the interhemispheric transfer of information derived from printed words and the impairments of this transfer in deep dyslexia and in letter-by-letter reading. Of course, although the argument is both elaborate and *ad hoc*, the claims made are not necessarily false; and at least they represent an advance, in terms of specificity, over previous rather general accounts of the role of the right hemisphere in reading.

Contributions from the right hemisphere have also been proposed in discussions of developmental dyslexia, but it is clear that at present there is no satisfactory evidence in support of the view that some cases of developmental dyslexia represent an abnormal reliance upon the right hemisphere during reading. It is unlikely that such evidence will emerge unless some progress is first made in identifying distinguishable varieties of developmental dyslexia and in describing the forms of abnormal reading associated with each variety.

Acknowledgements

I thank K. Patterson and A. Young for many helpful criticisms and suggestions.

References

BEAUVOIS, M. F., and DEROUESNE, J. (1979). Phonological alexia: three dissociations. *Journal of Neurology, Neurosurgery and Psychiatry* 42, 1115-1124.

BESNER, D., DANIELS, S. and SLADE, C. (1982). Ideogram reading and right hemisphere language. *British Journal of Psychology* 73, 21-28.

BODER, E. (1973). Developmental dyslexia: a diagnostic approach based on three atypical reading-spelling patterns. *Developmental Medicine and Child Neurology* 15, 663-687.

BRADSHAW, J. L. and GATES, A. (1978). Visual field differences in verbal tasks: effects of task familiarity and sex of subject. *Brain and Language* 5, 166-187.

BRADSHAW, J. L., NETTLETON, N. C. and TAYLOR, M. J. (1981). Right hemisphere language and cognitive deficit in sinistrals. *Neuropsychologia* 19, 113-132.

BROWN, W. P. and URE, D. M. J. (1969). Five rated characteristics of 650 word association stimuli. *British Journal of Psychology* 60, 233-249.

CODE, C. (1982). Hemispheric specialisation retraining in aphasia: possibilities and problems. In *Aphasia Therapy* (C. Code and D. Müller, eds). Edward Arnold, London.

COHEN, G. L. (1975). Hemispheric differences in the effects of cueing. *Journal of Experimental Psychology: Human Perception and Performance* 1, 366-373.

COHEN, G. and FREEMAN, R. (1979). Individual differences in reading strategies in relation to handedness and cerebral asymmetry. In *Attention and Performance VII* (J. Requin, ed.). Erlbaum, Hillsdale, New Jersey.

COLTHEART, M. (1980a). Deep dyslexia: a right hemisphere hypothesis. In *Deep Dyslexia* (M. Coltheart, K. Patterson and J. C. Marshall, eds). Routledge and Kegan Paul, London.

COLTHEART, M. (1980b). Deep dyslexia: a review of the syndrome. In *Deep Dyslexia* (M. Coltheart, K. Patterson and J. C. Marshall, eds). Routledge and Kegan Paul, London.

COLTHEART, M. (1981a). Disorders of reading and their implications for models of normal reading. *Visible Language* **XV**(2), 245-286.

COLTHEART, M. (1981b). The MRC Psycholinguistic Database. *Quarterly Journal of Experimental Psychology* **33A**, 497-508.

COLTHEART, M. (1982). The psycholinguistic analysis of acquired dyslexia: some illustrations. *Philosophical Transactions of the Royal Society of London* **B298**, 151-164.

COLTHEART, M., PATTERSON, K. E. and MARSHALL, J. C. (eds) (1980). *Deep Dyslexia.* Routledge and Kegan Paul, London.

COLTHEART, M., BYNG, S., MASTERSON, J., PRIOR, M. and RIDDOCH, J. (in prep.). Bilingual biscriptal deep dyslexia. (Submitted for publication.)

COLTHEART, M., MASTERSON, J., BYNG, S., PRIOR, M. and RIDDOCH, J. (in press). Surface dyslexia. *Quarterly Journal of Experimental Psychology.*

CZOPF, C. (1979). The role of the non-dominant hemisphere in speech recovery in aphasia. *Aphasia, Apraxia, Agnosia* **1**, 27-33.

DALBY, J. T. and GIBSON, D. (1981). Functional cerebral lateralization in subtypes of disabled readers. *Brain and Language* **14**, 34-48.

DAY, J. (1977). Right-hemisphere language processing in normal right-handers. *Journal of Experimental Psychology: Human Perception and Performance* **3**, 518-528.

DAY, J. (1979). Visual half-field word recognition as a function of syntactic class and imageability. *Neuropsychologia* **17**, 515-519.

DEROUESNE, J. and BEAUVOIS, M. F. (1979). Phonological processing in reading: data from alexia. *Journal of Neurology, Neurosurgery and Psychiatry* **42**, 1125-1132.

ELLIS, H. D. and SHEPHERD, J. W. (1974). Recognition of abstract and concrete words presented in left and right visual fields. *Journal of Experimental Psychology* **103**, 1035-1036.

ELMAN, J. L., TAKAHASHI, K. and TOHSAKU, Y. (1981a). Asymmetries for the categorization of kanji nouns, adjectives and verbs presented to the left and right visual fields. *Brain and Language* **13**, 290-300.

ELMAN, J. L., TAKAHASHI, K. and TOHSAKU, Y. (1981b). Lateral asymmetries for the identification of concrete and abstract kanji. *Neuropsychologia* **19**, 407-412.

FRANZ, S. J. (1930). The relations of aphasia. *Journal of General Psychology* **3**, 401-411.

FRIED, I., TANGUAY, P. E., BODER, E., DOUBLEDAY, C. and GREENSITE, M. (1981). Development dyslexia: electrophysiological evidence of clinical subgroups. *Brain and Language* **12**, 14-22.

FRIEDMAN, R. and PERLMAN, M. (in press). On the underlying causes of semantic paralexias in a patient with deep dyslexia. *Neuropsychologia.*

GOTT, P. S. (1973). Language after dominant hemipherectomy. *Journal of Neurology, Neurosurgery and Psychiatry* **36**, 1082-1088.

GRAVES, R., LANDIS, T. and GOODGLASS, H. (1981). Laterality and sex differences for visual recognition of emotional and non-emotional words. *Neuropsychologia* **19**, 95-102.

HATTA, T. (1977a). Recognition of Japanese kanji in the left and right visual fields. *Neuropsychologia* **15**, 685-688.

HATTA, T. (1977b). Lateral recognition of abstract and concrete kanji in Japanese. *Perceptual and Motor Skills* **45**, 731-734.

HATTA, T. (1978). Recognition of Japanese kanji and hirakana in the left and right visual fields. *Japanese Psychological Research* **20**, 51-59.

HATTA, T. (1981). Differential processing of kanji and kana stimuli in Japanese people: some implications from Stroop-test results. *Neuropsychologia* **19**, 87-93.

HEILMAN, K. M., ROTHI, L., CAMPANELLA, D. and WOLFSON, S. (1979). Wernicke's global aphasia without alexia. *Archives of Neurology* **36**, 129-133.

HINES, D. (1976). Recognition of verbs, abstract nouns and concrete nouns from the left and right visual half fields. *Neuropsychologia* **14**, 211-216.

HINES, D. (1977). Differences in tachistoscopic recognition between abstract and concrete words as a function of visual half-field and frequency. *Cortex* **13**, 66-73.

HIRATA, K. and OSAKA, R. (1967). Tachistoscopic recognition of Japanese letter materials in left and right visual fields. *Psychologia* **10**, 7-18.

HOLMES, J. M. (unpub.). Dyslexia: a neurolinguistic study of traumatic and developmental disorders of reading. Ph.D. thesis, University of Edinburgh, 1973.

HUANG, Y. and JONES, B. (1980). Naming and discrimination of Chinese ideograms presented in the right and left visual fields. *Neuropsychologia* **18**, 703-706.

KEEFE, B. and SWINNEY, D. (1979). On the relationship of hemispheric specialisation and developmental dyslexia. *Cortex* **15**, 471-481.

KINSBOURNE, M. (1971). The minor cerebral hemisphere as a source of aphasic speech. *Archives of Neurology* **25**, 302-306.

KLATZKY, R. L. and ATKINSON, R. C. (1971). Specialisation of the cerebral hemispheres in scanning for information in short-term memory. *Perception and Psychophysics* **10**, 335-338.

LANDIS, T., REGARD, M. and SERRAT, A. (1981). Iconic reading in a case of alexia without agraphia caused by a brain tumour: a tachistoscopic study. *Brain and Language* **11**, 45-53

LESSER, R. (1981). Book review. *British Journal of Disorders of Communication* **16**, 213-217.

LEVY, J. and TREVARTHEN, C. (1977). Perceptual, semantic and phonetic aspects of elementary language processes in split-brain patients. *Brain* **100**, 105-118.

LOW, A. A. (1931). A case of agrammatism in the English language. *Archives of Neurology and Psychiatry* **25**, 556-597.

MARSHALL, J. C. and NEWCOMBE, F. (1966). Syntactic and semantic errors in paralexia. *Neuropsychologia* **4**, 169-176.

MARSHALL, J. C. and NEWCOMBE, F. (1973). Patterns of paralexia: a psycholinguistic approach. *Journal of Psycholinguistic Research* **2**, 175-199.

MATTIS, S., FRENCH, J. H. and RAPIN, L. (1975). Dyslexia in children and young adults: three independent neurological syndromes. *Developmental Medicine and Child Neurology* **17**, 150-163.

MOSCOVITCH, M. (1976). On the representation of language in the right hemisphere of right-handed people. *Brain and Language* **3**, 47-71.

NIELSEN, J. M. (1965). *Agnosia, Apraxia, Aphasia*. Hoeber, New York.

NEWCOMBE, F. and MARSHALL, J. C. (1980). Response monitoring and response blocking in deep dyslexia. In *Deep Dyslexia* (M. Coltheart, K. Patterson, and J. C. Marshall, eds). Routledge and Kegan Paul, London.

NEWCOMBE, F. and MARSHALL, J. C. (1981). On psycholinguistic classifications of the acquired dyslexias. *Bulletin of the Orton Society* **31**, 29-46.

NGUY, T. V., ALLARD, F. and BRYDEN, M. P. (1980). Laterality effects for Chinese characters: differences between pictorial and nonpictorial characters. *Canadian Journal of Psychology* **34**, 270-273.

NOLAN, K. A. and CARAMAZZA, A. (1982). Modality-independent impairments in word processing in a deep dyslexic patient. *Brain and Language* **16**, 237-264.

OBRZUT, J. E. (1979). Dichotic listening and bisensory memory skills in qualitatively diverse dyslexic readers. *Journal of Learning Disabilities* **12**, 304-314.

OMENN, G. S. and WEBER, B. A. (1978). Dyslexia: search for phenotypic and genetic heterogeneity. *American Journal of Medical Genetics* **1**, 333-342.

PAPANICOLAOU, A. C., LEVIN, H. S. and EISENBERG, H. M. (unpub.). Evoked potential correlates of hemsipheric dominance shifts in recovered aphasics. Paper presented at Academy of Aphasia, 1981.

PATTERSON, K. E. (1981). Neuropsychological approaches to the study of reading. *British Journal of Psychology* **72**, 151-174.

PATTERSON, K. E. (1982). The relation between reading and phonological coding: further neuropsychological observations. In *Normality and Pathology in Cognitive Function* (A. W. Ellis, ed.). Academic Press, London and New York.

PATTERSON, K. E. and KAY, J. (1982). Letter-by-letter reading: psychological descriptions of a neurological syndrome. *Quarterly Journal of Experimental Psychology* **34A**, 411-442.

PETRAUSKAS, R. J. and ROURKE, B. P. (1979). Identification of subtypes of retarded readers: a neuropsychological multivariate approach. *Journal of Clinical Neuropsychology* **1**, 17-37.

PETTIT, J. M. and NOLL, J. D. (1979). Cerebral dominance in aphasia recovery. *Brain and Language* **7**, 191-200.

POWELL, G. (1980). *Brain Function Theory*. Gower Press, London.

SAFFRAN, E. M., BOGYO, L. C., SCHWARTZ, M. F. and MARIN, O. S. M. (1980). Does deep dyslexia reflect right-hemisphere reading? In *Deep Dyslexia* (M. Coltheart, K. Patterson and J. C. Marshall, eds). Routledge and Kegan Paul, London.

ST. JAMES-ROBERTS, I. (1981). A reinterpretation of hemispherectomy data without functional plasticity of the brain. *Brain and Language* **13**, 31-53.

SASANUMA, S. (1980). Acquired dyslexia in Japanese: clinical features and underlying mechanisms. In. *Deep Dyslexia* (M. Coltheart, K. Patterson and J. C. Marshall, eds). Routledge and Kegan Paul, London.

SASANUMA, S., ITOH, M., MORI, K. and KOBAYASHI, Y. (1977). Tachistoscopic recognition of kana and kanji words. *Neuropsychologia* **15**, 547-553.

SASANUMA, S., ITOH, M., KOBAYASHI, Y. and MORI, K. (1980). The nature of the task-simulus interaction in the tachistoscopic recognition of kana and kanji words. *Brain and Language* **9**, 298-306.

SHALLICE, T. (1981). Neurological impairment of cognitive processes. *British Medical Bulletin* **37**, 187-192.

SHALLICE, T. and COUGHLIN, A. K. (1980). Modality specific word comprehension deficits in deep dyslexia. *Journal of Neurology, Neurosurgery and Psychiatry* **46**, 866-872.

SHALLICE, T. and WARINGTON, E. K. (1975). Word recognition in a phonemic dyslexic patient. *Quarterly Journal of Experimental Psychology* **27**, 187-199.

SHALLICE, T. and WARRINGTON, E. K. (1977). The possible role of selective attention in acquired dyslexia. *Neuropsychologia* **15**, 31-41.

SHANON, B. L. (1979). Lateralization effects in lexical decision tasks. *Brain and Language* **8**, 380-387.

SHIMUZU, A. and ENDO, M. (1981). Tachistoscopic recognition of kana and hangul words, handedness, and shift of laterality difference. *Neuropsychologia* **19**, 665-673.

SIDTIS, J. J., VOLPE, B. T., HOLTZMAN, J. D., WILSON, D. H. and GAZZANIGA, M. S.

(1981). Cognitive interaction after staged callosal section: evidence for transfer of semantic activation. *Science* **212**, 344-346.

TZENG, O. J. L., HUNG, D. L. and GARRO, L. (1978). Reading the Chinese characters: an information processing view. *Journal of Chinese Linguistics* **6**, 287-305.

TZENG, O. J., HUNG, D. L., COTTON, B. and WANG, S. (1979). Visual lateralisation effects in reading Chinese characters. *Nature, Lond.* **282**, 499-501.

WARRINGTON, E. K. (1981). Concrete word dyslexia. *British Journal of Psychology* **72**, 175-196.

WARRINGTON, E. K. and SHALLICE, T. (1980). Word-form dyslexia. *Brain* **103**, 99-112.

YOUNG, A. W. and ELLIS, A. W. (1981). Asymmetry of cerebral hemispheric function in normal and poor readers. *Psychological Bulletin* **89**, 183-190.

ZAIDEL, E. (1978). Lexical organisation in the right hemisphere. In *Cerebral Correlates of Conscious Experience* (P. Buser and A. Rougeul-Buser, eds). Elsevier, Amsterdam.

ZAIDEL, E. (1982). Reading by the disconnected right hemisphere: an aphasiological perspective. In *Dyslexia: Neuronal, Cognitive and Linguistic Aspects* (Y. Zotterman, ed.). Pergamon Press, Oxford.

ZAIDEL, E. and PETERS, A. M. (1981). Phonological encoding and ideographic reading by the disconnected right hemisphere: two case studies. *Brain and Language* **14**, 205-234.

8

CEREBRAL ASYMMETRY AND THE INTEGRATED FUNCTION OF THE BRAIN

Joseph E. Le Doux

THE INTEGRATED function of the brain is a topic that is often overlooked by those interested in cerebral asymmetry. The emphasis of the field has been on constructing models which partition the human brain and mind into two physical and mental spheres, or more precisely, hemispheres. Such models leave little room for consideration of the integrated function of the brain in other than a trivial or after the (processing) fact sense.

There are good reasons, in my mind, for rejecting the psychological primacy of the hemisphere and for adopting an approach to cerebral asymmetry which favours detailed neurobiological characterisations of the representation of psychological processes in the brain over characterisations at the hemispheric level. In this chapter a model of cerebral asymmetry based on such an approach will be presented. This approach facilitates, if not necessitates, a consideration of the relation between cerebral asymmetry and the integrated function of the brain. First, however, certain misconceptions concerning the nature of cerebral asymmetry must be considered.

Some Misconceptions Concerning Cerebral Asymmetry

A variety of misconceptions have arisen concerning the fact that some processes are represented to a greater or lesser extent in one hemisphere or the other: the

FUNCTIONS OF THE RIGHT CEREBRAL HEMISPHERE
0-12-773250-0
*Copyright © 1983 by Academic Press, London.
All rights of reproduction in any form reserved.*

hemispheres in man function independently; the hemispheres in man function uniquely; the hemispheres in man each represent specialised evolutionary adaptations that mediate different modes of consciousness; human brain organisation is as a result of hemisphere specialisation radically different from non-human brain organisation; hemispheric organisation explains, at least in part, differences in human and non-human mentation. These and a variety of other misconceptions can be traced to the assumption (often treated as fact) that hemisphere asymmetry is synonymous with cerebral asymmetry.

At the level of pure description, there is some truth to the statement that the hemispheres in man are asymmetrically organised. The hemispheres can, after all, be shown to differ. The important question, however, is whether asymmetry at the hemispheric level is a primary or secondary property of hemispheric organisation. As a primary property of hemispheric organisation, asymmetry would be characteristic of the hemisphere itself. As a secondary property, however, asymmetry at the level of the hemisphere would be a by-product of the existence of asymmetric functional representation at a more fundamental level of neural organisation. If our measurement techniques and frame of mind focus on the hemisphere as the proper level of analysis of asymmetry, our results will never uncover anything but hemisphere asymmetry, overshadowing what may be much more basic biological mechanisms involving restricted cell groups within the hemisphere.

In contemporary models, asymmetry is often treated as a primary property of hemispheric organisation. Such models postulate that the two hemispheres are independent and unique information processing units, with each unit having its own unique cognitive style. The cognitive style of the left hemisphere, with its more extensive representation of linguistic processing, has been variably viewed as verbal, analytic, logical, and so forth. The cognitive style of the right hemisphere, in contrast, has been viewed, also variably, as perceptual, synthetic, intuitive, etc., due to the greater representation of non-verbal mechanisms on this side of the brain. There is, however, little agreement as to which adjectives best capture the cognitive style of the hemispheres, with numerous pairs of dichotomous possibilities having been offered (Bogen, 1969).

The notion of the hemispheres as separate cognitive units is derived from studies showing differences in the representation of cognitive processes when the two hemispheres are separately examined. Further consideration of these data, however, reveals that the differences which have been shown to exist are not global, but involve specific cognitive processes and restricted subsets of neurons (see Luria, 1966; Milner, 1975; Moscovitch, 1979; Le Doux, 1982). While the cognitive style of a hemisphere is viewed as a characterisation of hemispheric functions (those functions which are asymmetric), a characterisation of hemispheric functions would obviously have to account for the many processes which are symmetrically organised, as well as the ones which are asymmetrically represented. As Milner (1975) has argued, the parallels between the hemispheres are sometimes overshadowed by the tendency to emphasise the contrasts.

The focus on the hemispheres as asymmetric cognitive units can be traced historically to methodological rather than theoretical considerations. Although asymmetry had been observed much earlier, it was the studies of split-brain patients starting in the 1960s (Gazzaniga *et al.*, 1963, 1965; Levy-Agresti and Sperry, 1968; Levy *et al.*, 1972; Nebes, 1971, 1972, 1973; Zaidel and Sperry, 1973) that led to the current enthusiasm concerning cerebral asymmetry. In split-brain studies, one is methodologically restricted to assessing cerebral asymmetry at the level of hemispheric organisation. The hemisphere is the most detailed level which can be directly evaluated. Studies of patients with focal damage can, however, provide more exacting data. Through an analysis of lesion data it has been and is possible to identify neuronal cell groups which account for differences observed in the psychological capacities of the two hemispheres of split-brain patients (Milner, 1975; Le Doux, 1979).

The heavy reliance of models of cerebral asymmetry on the hemisphere asymmetry focus of split-brain studies has thus led to interpretations of cerebral asymmetry as reflecting overall differences in hemispheric organisation. Even when the data have originated in studies of patients with focal lesions, where more precise intrahemispheric localisation is possible, interpretations have often reverted to the hemispheric level of analysis. The psychology of hemisphere differences has, as a result, flourished, but at an expense. The opportunity to relate specific cognitive processes to specific neural mechanisms in the human brain has often passed by.

The human brain, it should be remembered, is first and foremost a vertebrate brain. And like all other vertebrate brains it does differ from the prototype from which it evolved. The choice at hand, however, is whether we need to postulate that the human brain represents a fundamentally new form of cerebral organisation (Levy, 1977; Bogen, 1969), or whether the human brain should be viewed as a more subtle variation of its evolutionary precursors (Le Doux *et al.*, 1977; Gazzaniga and Le Doux, 1978; Le Doux, 1982). As long as we opt in favour of an approach which assumes, *a priori*, that the hemispheres in man are fundamentally different from each other, as well as from the hemispheres of our evolutionary ancestors, we are not likely to know the answer. It seems we should start with null hypotheses: that the hemispheres of man are not different; that the human brain is not different from the non-human brain. By testing these hypotheses, rather than assuming radical differences, the emphasis is shifted away from the search for elusive cognitive styles in hemispheres which defy their non-human counterparts and towards an effort to: (1) relate specific cognitive processes to specific neural mechanisms in the human brain; (2) identify specific neurobiological differences between the two hemispheres in man; (3) identify specific neurobiological differences between human and non-human brain organisation. This, it seems, is the proper course for neuropsychology.

A Model of Cerebral Asymmetry

The traditional view has been that the major dimensions upon which the hemispheres in man differ are verbal and spatial. Although the list of asymmetries has been extended in a variety of ways, many of which are documented in this volume, some interesting consequences emerge when we attempt to relate the classic psychological distinctions between the hemispheres to specific neural mechanisms. In particular, a model emerges which accounts for many questions concerning the nature and origin of cerebral asymmetry and in addition suggests insights into the relation between human and non-human brain organisation.

Early studies of split-brain humans found the left hemisphere performing poorly on tasks involving spatial processing (Bogen and Gazzaniga, 1965; Gazzaniga *et al.*, 1965; Levy-Agresti and Sperry, 1968; Levy *et al.*, 1972; Nebes, 1971, 1972, 1973). These data were consistent with the well-known clinical observation that right hemisphere damage, particularly right inferior parietal damage, produces disturbances in visuo-spatial perception (see Critchley, 1953; Hécaen and Albert, 1978), suggesting that the intact left hemisphere may be incapable of mediating normal visuo-spatial perception. More recent observations in both split-brain (Le Doux *et al.*, 1977; Gazzaniga and Le Doux, 1978; Le Doux, 1979) and brain-damaged (Le Doux *et al.*, 1980) patients have suggested that the left hemisphere's difficulty with spatial tasks is not so much in visuo-spatial perception, *per se*, but in guiding complex behaviour in space.

For example, many of the tasks used to demonstrate profound differences in spatial ability between the hemispheres of split-brain patients required, in addition to visual perception, the use of the hands in perceiving or constructing spatial stimuli. When these manipulo-spatial demands were relaxed, turning the tasks into pure visuo-spatial tasks, both hemispheres could perform well (Le Doux *et al.*, 1977; Gazzaniga and Le Doux, 1978). The left hemisphere inability is thus not so much in perception as in guiding behavioural interactions with the spatial environment.

A similar conclusion can be drawn concerning the results of studies of patients with focal lesions. We studied a patient with right hemisphere damage and a severe disturbance in visuo-spatial abilities (Le Doux *et al.*, 1980). When asked to draw a clock she placed all the numbers in a vertical array down the right side of a circle. Moreover, she was unable to determine through visual inspection the difference between her clock and the one drawn by the examiner. However, when her clock was presented directly to her left hemisphere through her right visual field, she immediately replied: 'What a funny clock. The numbers are all on the right side.'. Thus, the visuo-spatial disturbance in right hemisphere damaged patients appears not to be due to an inability of the left hemisphere in processing visual patterns. Instead, the problem appears to involve an inability of the left hemisphere to guide behavioural orientation to the spatial world.

It is of particular interest that the lesions of the right hemisphere which result in such disturbances in spatial behaviour are typically in a region which when damaged in the left hemisphere results in extensive deficits in linguistic behaviour (Geschwind, 1965; Luria, 1966). The two processes which are typically viewed as encompassing the essence of cerebral asymmetry are thus dependent in part upon the integrity of homologous areas in opposite hemispheres. The area of concern is the parieto-occipito-temporal junction (POT).

It is interesting to consider the results of studies of POT function in non-human primates. As in man, lesions of POT do not disrupt visual perception as such, but produce disturbances in the regulation of behavioural interactions with the spatial environment: in man and monkey, POT lesions produce disturbances in reaching to specified points in space, optokinetic nystagmus, ocular movements, gaze and fixation control, and environmental orientation (see Le Doux, 1982). The main difference in the representation of these spatial functions in monkey and man is that while the functions are represented in POT in each hemisphere in monkey, only the right POT is involved in man. The left POT in man, as noted, plays a crucial role in language function.

The immediate implication of these observations is that the mechanisms underlying spatial behaviour are bilaterally represented in POT of non-human primates but are represented unilaterally, in the right POT, in man. The less immediate though more tantalizing implication is that the emergence of human language involved a reorganisation of the primate brain such that language development involved adaptations in the spatial mechanisms of the left POT.

Why should language development have involved adaptations in the neural mechanisms underlying spatial behaviour? The answer I would like to propose is that the neural mechanisms underlying spatial behaviour in early humans were preadaptive to language development. Several authors have argued that language development was made possible by multi-modal processing capacities (Geschwind, 1965; Marin et al., 1979). It is thus of interest that the spatial skills characteristic of non-human primates are based on multimodal stimulus integration (Hyvarinen and Poranen, 1974; Mountcastle et al., 1975; Lynch, 1980) made possible by what have been called supramodal cells (Mesulam et al., 1977) in POT. The existence of multimodal processing capacities in POT in ancestral primates in association with spatial functions may have thus set the stage for the later development of language in early man (see Le Doux, 1982).

Although I have used language in the foregoing as if I were referring to the capacities characteristic of contemporary humans, early language was most probably quite different from human speech. In fact, there is considerable evidence that early language may have gone through an initial visuo-gestural phase (Hewes, 1976). It is thus of interest that lesions of the left POT in humans produce disturbances in the production of manual symbolisation (Geschwind, 1965; Kimura, 1979) and the comprehension of visual symbols (Geschwind, 1965; Luria, 1966). POT in early humans may have thus been a primal language zone involved in the production and comprehension of gestural communication (see Le Doux, 1982). The development of speech and the involvement of the anterior speech region (Broca's area) in language processing would have emerged much later. This formulation is non-committal as to why the leftward bias in language lateralisation exists, as well as to why language should be lateralised at all. The focus is instead on the consequences, for human brain evolution and organisation, of the fact that language asymmetry does exist. In telling the story in this way, the evolution of language and cerebral asymmetry is accounted for in a manner which is consistent with what is known about neural organisation in both human and non-human primates. And in specifying the adaptive forces and biological battleground of the evolution of language, we are led to a more general model that accounts for the full range of asymmetries which have been observed.

Specifically, a general model would have to account not only for the representation of language and spatial mechanisms in the two hemispheres, but also for observations of a right hemisphere advantage for perceptual, emotional and mnemonic processing. The asymmetric representation of these processes, as well as of spatial processes, however, can all be viewed as by-products of the representation of language in the left hemisphere, where the neural systems underlying these cognitive processes have undergone adaptations necessary to accommodate linguistic processing. In the right hemisphere, the mechanisms underlying perception, emotion, memory and spatial behaviour follow the prototypical primate organisation pattern. Evolutionary changes in the right hemisphere, which may well be a neurobiological 'missing link', have been of degree rather than kind.

Although the discussion has thus far mainly dealt with left hemisphere language representation, the model is readily adapted to account for other instances by simply shifting the focus away from 'left-right' as the primary feature specified genetically. The alternative is to emphasise the potential for the expression of the language function, with the direction and degree of asymmetry being secondarily determined and even subject to developmental factors. This is certainly suggested by the well known observation, discussed elsewhere in this volume, that following damage to the left hemisphere early in life, the right readily acquires linguistic mechanisms. What is crucial is that language be represented. Where it is represented appears to be less important.

Cerebral asymmetry, in this model, is relegated to a position of secondary importance, being a by-product of the factors which determine where language settles down between and within hemispheres. Viewed in this manner, the right hemisphere advantage on certain tasks is not attributable to evolutionary adaptations in the right hemisphere, but instead reflects the functional adaptations in neural systems required to accommodate linguistic processing.

The focus of this model is thus on specific neural systems as the locus of adaptation. It is not the left hemisphere which is specialised, but specific functions of specific neural systems associated with linguistic processing; and in becoming specialised, these systems have not necessarily sacrificed their prelinguistic function. This is most dramatically illustrated by split-brain patients, whose left hemispheres are, for example, fully capable of visuo-spatial processing, face recognition, and so forth, though perhaps not with the efficiency of right hemisphere visual mechanisms (Gazzaniga and Le Doux, 1978; Le Doux, 1979; Le Doux et al., 1980). As Geschwind (1965) has noted, hemisphere differences on perceptual tasks do not reflect dominance in the sense that the left hemisphere is dominant for speech. This level of efficiency is what was sacrificed in the adaptation of systems for linguistic analysis.

The task at hand, in this view, is one of specifying the specific ways in which the human left hemisphere deviates from the prototypical primate hemisphere, as exemplified by the human right hemisphere. The characterisation, however, should not simply be a psychological profile. Two black boxes are really no better than one. We must attempt to specify in precise terms the nature and extent to which processes are symmetrically as well as differentially represented in the two hemispheres. Through such an approach we will come to understand the evolution and functions of the human brain in terms of adaptations in specific neural systems rather than in terms of global adaptations at the hemispheric level.

Vertebrate brain evolution is as a rule conservative (Hotton, 1976; Welker, 1976). The model put forth here is consistent with this rule. In this model, the human brain follows the prototypical primate pattern of organisation, with deviations from this pattern in contemporary man being directly or indirectly accounted for by the representation of language mechanisms within and between the hemispheres. This contrasts with the widely accepted hemisphere specialisation model, which postulates that with the emergence of the hominids, the phylogenetically ancient pattern of bilaterally symmetric hemispheres was replaced by a pattern involving functionally independent and profoundly asymmetric hemispheres, each undergoing specialisation so that it could function as a complete and unique brain within itself (Levy, 1977; Bogen, 1977). The specialisation hypothesis, however, seems unnecessary in the presence of a simpler, more parsimonious and neurobiologically more detailed model which accounts for cerebral asymmetry without postulating a break with the conservative pattern that characterises brain evolution in vertebrates and which, in fact, views the human brain as lying on a neuroevolutionary continuum with its primary ancestry.

Cerebral Asymmetry and Processing Dynamics

The model put forth in the preceding pages attempts to account in part for the dynamics of brain evolution, but like any model of cerebral asymmetry, it treats brain function in a static, structural, descriptive way. Cerebral asymmetry is, after all, a description of brain organisation, not an explanation of the processing dynamics of the brain in real time cognition and behaviour.

Studies of cerebral asymmetry have told us precious little about the neurological or psychological mechanisms of perception, emotion, memory and so forth, other than that some aspects of these mechanisms are not equally effectively represented on the two sides of the brain. The field has focused on the discovery of asymmetries as an end in and of itself, as if a cognitive taxonomy of hemisphere differences would tell us how the brain works. But cognitive processes in the living brain are not mediated within one hemisphere. As Luria (1966) has argued, 'Complex psychological processes are not "localised" in any one hemisphere but are the result of integration between the two hemispheres.'. And as long as the hemispheres are researched as independent, non-interacting, parallel processors, studies of cerebral asymmetry are not likely to tell us much about the processing dynamics of cognitive mechanisms in the integrated brain.

If, on the other hand, we start with a cognitive system and attempt to understand the underlying neural machinery, in the process of studying the intra- and interhemispheric organisation of that system, we will necessarily have to build into any model which emerges an account of the degree of symmetricity (or asymmetricity, if you choose) of that system. The focus, however, is not on a convenient, arbitrary, dichotomous partition. The focus is, instead, on the neurobiology of cognition in the living, integrated brain.

Cognition and the Integrated Function of the Brain

Vision is useful as a model cognitive system for considering processing dynamics in the integrated brain. In man, as well as all other vertebrates, the visual system is organised such that each hemisphere has a direct representation of the contralateral visual world and an indirect representation, by way of synapse in the opposite hemisphere, of the ipsilateral visual world. How is it, then, that we are aware of only one visual world if there is a double representation of that world in our brains?

This situation is not as bizarre as it may seem. The task of explaining how a unitary sense of awareness of the visual world spans the cerebral midline is no more or less difficult than the task of explaining how unitary percepts emerge from the multiple cortical and subcortical representations of the visual world within a single hemisphere (Le Doux and Gazzaniga, 1981). At the cortical level alone, various retino-topic maps, representing different levels of sensory analysis, exist. The goal of visual physiology is to understand how visual perception is built up from the integration of neural activity in the different regions and a crucial aspect of the problem is the determination of how the various visual representations within the two hemispheres are integrated. Such tasks are more readily approached if we think of vision as a dynamic, integrative process rather than as an activity of a particular part or side of the brain. Particular parts and sides do play a significant and often unique role in cognition, but the neural part in isolation does not explain the neural process. In the final analysis, an understanding of the neurobiology of vision will have to account for the intra- and interhemispheric neural integration which underlies our unified awareness of the visual world. The task is not fundamentally different, though it is admittedly more complicated, when the process is asymmetrically represented.

From Interhemispheric Integration to Intrahemispheric Capacity: A Brief History of Split Brain Studies

The history of experimental studies of the split brain provides an interesting perspective on the issues discussed above. For our purposes, this history begins with Sperry's work on neural specificity (see Sperry, 1948) which by the early 1950s had turned to questions concerning how the visual world is mapped onto the brain. It had been demonstrated that animals trained on a visual discrimination problem with one eye could perform the problem with the other eye, even when the optic chiasm was sectioned (Myers and Sperry, 1953). Since each eye projects solely to the ipsilateral hemisphere following chiasm section, interocular transfer in such animals had to involve interhemispheric integration of visual processing. Subsequent experiments identified the forebrain commissures as the critical pathways of interhemispheric integration and a variety of studies emerged concerning the behavioural (Sperry, 1958; Myers, 1965; Gazzaniga, 1965; Cuenod, 1972; Sullivan and Hamilton, 1973; Doty and Overman, 1976), anatomical (Myers, 1956; Zeki, 1973; Jouandet and Gazzaniga, 1978) and physiological (Berlucchi and Rizzolatti, 1968; Berlucchi et al., 1967) properties of interhemispheric integration, or transfer, as it was called.

This work on the neurobiology of interhemispheric integration was soon overshadowed by the more dramatic demonstration that the unity of experience could also be divided in humans. Gazzaniga, in Sperry's laboratory, had the opportunity to examine epileptics whose forebrain commissures had been sectioned in an effort to relieve intractable epilepsy (Gazzaniga *et al.*, 1963, 1965). These studies confirmed the breakdown of interhemispheric integration observed in animals but also demonstrated, through studies of hemispheric function rather than from the effects of lesions, that the human brain was asymmetrically organised. Though interhemispheric integration has continued to be studied in humans (Mitchell and Blakemore, 1969; Trevarthen, 1974; Le Doux *et al.*, 1977; Le Doux, 1979; Sidtis, 1981), subsequent research on split brain man has shifted from a focus on the mechanisms of interhemispheric integration to a description of the differential capacities of the separated hemispheres (Levy-Agresti and Sperry, 1968; Levy *et al.*, 1972; Nebes, 1971, 1972, 1973; Zaidel and Sperry, 1973, 1975; Franco and Sperry, 1977; Le Doux *et al.*, 1977; Gazzaniga *et al.*, 1977; Greenwood *et al.*, 1980).

Today, it is the split brain contribution to our understanding of the capacities of the separated hemispheres that is the most celebrated. So celebrated is this contribution that models have developed which treat the normal brain as though it were in fact split (Bogen, 1977; Levy, 1977; Galin, 1977; Puccetti, 1981). The split brain, however, shows what a hemisphere in isolation can do, not what the hemisphere in the normally connected brain does. This two brain approach has led to an inappropriate glorification of the role of *the hemisphere* in normal brain function and, somewhat ironically, to a denigration of the role of interhemispheric integration — the phenomenon which gave birth to experimental studies of the split brain.

Beyond the Hemisphere

Cerebral asymmetry has attracted much attention in recent years. Unfortunately, speculation concerning the implications of hemisphere differences has gone well beyond the data. A potpourri of psychological phenomena, from poetic inspiration to jogger's high, from scientific creativity to sexual orgasm and more, have been conveniently explained with the now familiar retort: 'It's a . . . . . . hemisphere function '. The mind is not easily dichotomised in a way that provides much in the way of detailed insight into psychological processes, and it is naïve to think that the brain is any simpler. No one cognitive function is completely dependent on one hemisphere or the other. Complex psychological processes reflect the functioning of both sides of the brain at all levels of the neuraxis, and a theory of how these processes relate to brain mechanisms must account for the integrated functioning of the nervous system. Any model which focuses on cerebral compartmentalisation at the expense of integration would seem to be misdirected.

The model developed in this chapter focuses on neurobiological differences both between human and non-human brain organisation and between the two hemispheres in man. Although we can only begin to specify the nature of these differences, one conclusion of the analysis is that species differences in brain organisation, as well as differences between the hemispheres of man, are best viewed as evolutionary variations of a common vertebrate organisational scheme. This conclusion does not reflect an impoverished view of human nature. It represents the limiting conditions which must be recognised in our efforts to fully understand the origins of, and the neural mechanisms underlying, those adaptations which provide for the unique richness of human behaviour and mentation.

The discovery of differences in the representation of functions in two hemispheres of man has largely been pursued as an end in and of itself. However, the more important questions involve how knowledge that a process is asymmetrically represented contributes to a more general understanding of the relation between brain mechanisms and cognitive processes. In this regard, the challenge facing the field of cerebral asymmetry cannot be viewed as simply documenting hemisphere differences. The challenge is, in short, to move beyond the hemisphere—to elucidate how asymmetry in the representation of psychological processes relates to specific neurobiological mechanisms and to demonstrate how knowledge of these relationships contributes to our understanding of the integrated functioning of the brain in the creation of mind.

References

BERLUCCHI, G., GAZZANIGA, M. S. and RIZZOLATTI, G. (1967). Microelectrode analysis of transfer of visual information by the corpus callosum of cat. *Archives of Italian Biology* **105**, 583-596.

BERLUCCHI, G. and RIZZOLATTI, G. (1968). Binocularly driven neurons in visual cortex of split-chiasm cats. *Science* **159**, 308.

BOGEN, J. E. (1969). The other side of the brain II: an appositional mind. *Bulletin of the Los Angeles Neurological Society* **34**, 135-162.

BOGEN, J. E. (1977). Some educational implications of hemispheric specialization. In *The Human Brain* (N. C. Wittrock, ed.), pp.133-152. Prentice Hall, New Jersey.

BOGEN, J. E. and GAZZANIGA, M. S. (1965). Cerebral commissurotomy in man: minor hemisphere dominance for certain visuo-spatial functions. *Journal of Neurosurgery* **23**, 394-399.

CRITCHLEY, M. (1953). *The Parietal Lobes.* Edward Arnold, London.

CUENOD, M. (1972). Split-brain studies: functional interaction between bilateral central nervous structures. In *Structure and Function of Nervous Tissue*, Vol. 5 (G. Bourne, ed.), Academic Press, New York and London.

DOTY, R. W. and OVERMAN, W. H. (1976). Mnemonic role of forebrain commissures in Macaques. In *Lateralization in the Nervous System* (S. Harnad, ed.), Academic Press, New York and London.

FRANCO, L. and SPERRY, R. W. (1977). Hemisphere lateralization for cognitive processing of geometry. *Neuropsychologia* **15**, 107-113.

GALIN, D. (1977). Hemisphere lateralization and psychiatric issues. In *Evolution and Lateralization of the Brain. Annals of the New York Academy of Science* **229**, 397-411.

GAZZANIGA, M. S. (1965). Some effects of cerebral commissurotomy in monkey and man. *Dissertation Abstracts* **26**, 1.

GAZZANIGA, M. S. and LE DOUX, J. E. (1978). *The Integrated Mind.* Plenum Press, New York.

GAZZANIGA, M. S., BOGEN, J. E. and SPERRY, R. W. (1963). Laterality effects in somesthesis following cerebral commissurotomy in man. *Neuropsychologia* **1**, 209-215.

GAZZANIGA, M. S., BOGEN, J. E. and SPERRY, R. W. (1965). Observations on visual perception after disconnexion of the cerebral hemispheres in man. *Brain* **88**, 221.

GAZZANIGA, M. S., LE DOUX, J. E. and WILSON, D. H. (1977). Language, praxis and the right hemisphere: clues to some mechanisms of consciousness. *Neurology* **27**, 1144-1147.

GESCHWIND, N. (1965). Disconnexion syndromes in animals and man. *Brain* **88**, 237-294, 585-644.

GREENWOOD, P. M., ROTKIN, L. G., WILSON, D. H. and GAZZANIGA, M. S. (1980). Psychophysics with the split-brain subject: on hemispheric differences and numerical mediation in perceptual matching tasks. *Neuropsychologia* **18**, 419-434.

HÉCAEN, H. and ALBERT, M. (1978). *Human Neuropsychology.* Wiley, New York.

HEWES, G. W. (1976). The current status of the gestural theory of language origin. In *Origin and Evolution of Language and Speech. Annals of the New York Academy of Science* **280**, 482-504.

HOTTON, N. (1976). Origin and radiation of the classes of poikilo thermous vertebrates. In *Evolution of Brain and Behaviour in Vertebrates* (B. Masterson, ed.). Wiley, New York.

HYVARINEN, J. and PORANEN, A. (1974). Function of the parietal associative area 7 as revealed from cellular discharges in alert monkeys. *Brain* **97**, 673-692.

JOUANDET, M. and GAZZANIGA, M. S. (1978). Cortical field of origin of the Anterior Commissure in Monkey. *Experimental Neurology* **66**, 381.

KIMURA, D. (1979). Neuromotor mechanisms in the development of human communication. In *Neurobiology of Social Communication in Primates* (H. D. Steklis and M. J. Raleigh, eds). Academic Press, New York and London.

LE DOUX, J. E. (1979). Parietoccipital symptomatology: the split-brain perspective. In *Handbook of Neuropsychology* (M. S. Gazzaniga, ed.). Plenum Press, New York.

LE DOUX, J. E. (1982). Neuroevolutionary mechanisms of cerebral asymmetry in man. *Brain, Behavior and Evolution* **20**, 196-212.

LE DOUX, J. E. and GAZZANIGA, M. S. (1981). The brain and the split brain; a duel with duality as a model of mind. *The Behavioral and Brain Sciences* **4**, 109-110.

LE DOUX, J. E., DEUTSCH, G., WILSON, D. H. and GAZZANIGA, M. S. (1977). Binocular depth perception and the anterior commissure in man. *The Physiologist* **20**, 55.

LE DOUX, J. E., SMYLIE, C. S., RUFF, R. and GAZZANIGA, M. S. (1980). Left hemisphere visual processes in cases of right hemisphere symptomatology. *Archives of Neurology* **37**, 157-159.

LE DOUX, J. E., WILSON, D. H. and GAZZANIGA, M. S. (1977). Manipulo-spatial aspects of cerebral lateralization: clues to the origin of lateralization. *Neuropsychologia* **15**, 743-749.

LEVY, J. (1977). The mammalian brain and the adaptive advantage of cerebral asymmetry.

In *Evolution and Lateralization of the Brain. Annals of the New York Academy of Science* **229**, 264-272.

LEVY, J., TREVARTHEN, C. and SPERRY, R. W. (1972). Perception of bilateral chimeric figures following hemispheric deconnection. *Brain* **95**, 61-78.

LEVY-AGRESTI, J. and SPERRY, R. W. (1968). Differential perceptual capacities in major and minor hemispheres. *Proceedings of the National Academy of Science* **61**, 1151.

LURIA, A. R. (1966). *Higher Cortical Function in Man.* Basic Books, New York.

LYNCH, J. (1980). The functional organization of the posterior parietal association cortex. *The Behavioral and Brain Sciences* **3**, 485-534.

MARIN, O., SCHWARTZ, M. and SAFFRAN, E. (1979). Origins and distribution of language. In *Handbook of Neuropsychology* (M. S. Gazzaniga, ed.). Pleum Press, New York.

MESULAM, M. M., VAN HOESEN, G. W., PANDYA, D. N. and GESCHWIND, N. (1977). Limbic and sensory connections of the inferior parietal lobule in the rhesus monkey. *Brain Research* **136**, 393-414.

MILNER, B. (1975). *Hemisphere Specialization and Interaction.* MIT Press, Cambridge, Massachusetts.

MITCHELL, D. and BLAKEMORE, C. (1969). Binocular depth perception and the corpus callosum. *Vision Research* **10**, 49-54.

MOSCOVITCH, M. (1979). Information processing and the cerebral hemispheres. In *Handbook of Neuropsychology* (M. S. Gazzaniga, ed.). Pleum Press, New York.

MOUNTCASTLE, V. B., LYNCH, J. C., GEORGOPOULOS, A., SAKUTA, H. and ACUNA, C. (1975). Posterior parietal association cortex of the monkey; command functions for operations within extrapersonal space. *Journal of Neurophysiology* **38**, 871-909.

MYERS, R. E. (1956). Localization of function within the corpus callosum. *Anatomical Record* **124**, 339.

MYERS, R. E. (1965). The neocortical commissures and interhemispheric transmission of information. In *Functions of the Corpus Callosum* (G. Ettlinger, ed.), pp.1-17. J. A. Churchill, London.

MYERS, R. E. and SPERRY, R. W. (1953). Interocular transfer of a visual form discrimination habit in cats after section of the optic chiasm and corpus callosum. *Anatomical Record* **175**, 351-352.

NEBES, R. (1971). Superiority of the minor hemisphere in commissurotomized man for the perception of part-whole relations. *Cortex* **7**, 333-349.

NEBES, R. (1972). Dominance of the minor hemisphere in commissurotomized man on a test of figural unification. *Brain* **90**, 633-638.

NEBES, R. (1973). Perception of spatial relationships by the right and left hemispheres of commissurotomized man. *Neuropsychologia* **11**, 285-289.

PUCCETTI, R. (1981). The case for mental duality. *The Behavioral and Brain Sciences* **4** 93-99.

SIDTIS, J. J., VOLPE, B. T., HOLTZMAN, J. D., WILSON, D. H. and GAZZANIGA, M. S. (1981). Cognitive interaction after staged callosal section: evidence for transfer of semantic activation. *Science* **212**, 344-346.

SPERRY, R. W. (1948). Patterning of central synapses in regeneration of optic nerve in teleosts. *Physiological Zoology* **21**, 351-361.

SPERRY, R. W. (1958). The corpus callosum and interhemispheric transfer in the monkey. *Anatomical Record* **131**, 297.

SULLIVAN, M. V. and HAMILTON, C. R. (1973). Interocular transfer of reversed and non-reversed discriminations via the anterior commissure in monkeys. *Physiology of Behavior* **10**, 355-359.

TREVARTHEN, C. (1974). Functional relations of disconnected hemispheres with the brain stem and with each other: monkey and man. In *Hemisphere Disconnexion and Cerebral Function* (W. L. Smith and M. Kinsbourne, eds). Charles Thomas, Springfield, Illinois.

WELKER, W. (1976). Brain evolution in mammals. In *Evolution of Brain and Behavior in Vertebrates* (B. Masterson, ed.). Wiley, New York.

ZAIDEL, E. and SPERRY, R. W. (1973). Performance on Raven's coloured progressive matrices tests by commissurotomy patients. *Cortex* **9**, 34.

ZAIDEL, E. and SPERRY, R. W. (1975). Unilateral auditory language comprehension on the token test following cerebral commissurotomy and hemispherectomy. *Neuropsychologia* **15**, 1-18.

ZEKI, S. M. (1973). Comparison of the cortical degeneration in the visual region of temporal lobe of the monkey following section of the anterior commissure and the splenium. *Journal of Comparative Neurology* **143**, 167-175.

AUTHOR INDEX

Numbers in italics indicate those pages where references are listed in full at the end of the chapter

217

Cioffi, J., 16, *25*, 153, *165*
Clark, R., 152, *168*
Clarkson, D., 74, *86*
Clifford, B. R., 33, *59*
Clyma, E. A., 118, *136*
Code, C., 171, *197*
Cohen, G., 8, *26*, 44, 45, *59*, 101, *106*, 148, *165*, 175, 180, *197*
Cohn, R., 35, *60*
Colbourn, C. J., 123, 133, *136*, 149, *165*
Cole, M., 10, *26*, 35, 39, *60*
Coltheart, M., 97, 101, 160, *165*, 172, 173, 174, 175, 177, 178, 180, 181, 186, 188, 189, 194, 196, *198*, *199*, *200*
Comper, P., *141*
Concannon, M., 129, *144*
Connolly, J., 129, *139*
Cook, M., 33, *58*
Cooper, W., 102, *106*
Corballis, M. C., 117, *136*, 152, *165*
Coren, S., 104, *110*, 127, *143*
Corkin, S., 1, 2, 13, 19, 22, *26*
Costa, L., 40, 41, *60*
Cotton, B., 180, *201*
Coughlin, A. K., 173, *200*
Cox, P. J., 16, *28*
Cranney, J., 124, *136*
Crea, F., 8, *25*
Creutzfeldt, O., *138*, *143*
Critchley, M., 22, *26*, *83*, 97, *106*, *137*, *145*, 206, *213*
Crockett, H. G., 89, 90, *106*
Cuenod, M., 211, *213*
Cullen, J. K. Jr., 122, *136*
Culver, C., 7, *32*
Cunningham, M. R., 126, *137*
Curry, F. K. W., 75, *84*
Czopf, C., 185, *198*
Czopf, J., 96, *106*

d'Élia, G., 118, *137*
Dabbs, J. M., Jr., 129, *142*
Dalby, J. T., 127, *137*, 195, *198*
Damasio, A. R., 122, *137*
Damasio, H., 122, *137*
Daniels, S., 178, *179*, *197*
Dansereau, D. F., 129, *137*
Danta, G., 12, *26*
Darley, F. L., 118, *136*
Das, J. P., 132, *137*

Davidoff, J. B., 1, 2, 8, 9, 12, *26*, 37, *60*
Davidson, R. J., 69, 78, *84*
Davidson, W., 17, *29*
Davies, G. M., 33, 38, 43, 46, *60*, *61*, *63*
Davies-Jones, G. A. B., 10, 11, 19, *30*
Davis, A. E., 154, *165*
Dawson, J. L. M., 104, *107*, 128, *137*
Dawson, M. E., 129, *137*
Dax, M., 114
Day, J., 100, 101, *107*, 180, 181, *198*
De Kosky, S., 54, 55, *60*
De Luca, D., 98, *106*
De Renzi, E., 9, 12, 13, 18, 19, 20, *24*, *26*, 35, 36, 37, *60*, 149, 152, 153, 154, 162, *165*
De Zure, R., 82, *83*, 128, *136*
Demarest, J., 127, *137*
Demarest, L., 127, *137*
Denckla, M. B., 17, *30*, *31*, 153, 155, *167*
Dennis, M., 88, *107*, 152, 155, 162, *165*, *166*
Deręgowski, J. B., 48, *60*
Derouesne, J., 172, *197*, *198*
Desmedt, J. E., 130, *137*
Detre, T., 13, *27*
Deutsch, D., 75, 80, *84*
Deutsch, G., 212, *214*
Di Carlo, D., 126, *144*
Di Stefano, M., 8, *25*
Diamond, R., 37, *62*, 152, 156, 157, 158, 159, *164*, *165*, *166*
Dickerson, J. W. T., *145*, *167*, *168*
Diekhof, G. M., 129, *137*
Dimond, S. J., 13, 16, *24*, *26*, *28*, *62*, *63*, *108*, *109*, 116, 120, 121, 125, *135*, *137*, *139*, *167*
Dixon, M. S., 40, 56, *62*
Dixon, N. F., 8, *28*
Dodds, A. G., 16, *26*
Donchin, E., 130, *137*
Dooling, E. C., 152, *165*
Doty, R. W., 58, *63*, *136*, *137*, *165*, 211, *213*
Doubleday, C., 195, *198*
Ducarne, B., 35, *62*
Dumas, R., 82, *84*
Dunne, J. J., 36, *62*
Durnford, M., 11, 12, *26*, *28*, 37, *62*
Dyer, F. N., 13, *26*

Earle, J., 78, *84*
Edwards, B., 82, *84*

SUBJECT INDEX